T0231244

Emerging Trends
in Psychological Practice
in Long-Term Care

Emerging Trends in Psychological Practice in Long-Term Care has been co-published simultaneously as *Clinical Gerontologist*, Volume 25, Numbers 1/2/3/4 2002.

Emerging Trends in Psychological Practice in Long-Term Care

Margaret P. Norris, PhD
Victor Molinari, PhD
Suzann Ogland-Hand, PhD
Editors

Emerging Trends in Psychological Practice in Long-Term Care has been co-published simultaneously as *Clinical Gerontologist*, Volume 25, Numbers 1/2/3/4 2002.

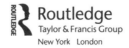

Routledge
Taylor & Francis Group
New York   London

Emerging Trends in Psychological Practice in Long-Term Care has been co-published simultaneously as *Clinical Gerontologist*™, Volume 25, Numbers 1/2/3/4 2002.

The development, preparation, and publication of this work has been undertaken with great care. However, the publisher, employees, editors, and agents of The Haworth Press and all imprints of The Haworth Press, Inc., including The Haworth Medical Press® and Pharmaceutical Products Press®, are not responsible for any errors contained herein or for consequences that may ensue from use of materials or information contained in this work. Opinions expressed by the author(s) are not necessarily those of The Haworth Press, Inc. With regard to case studies, identities and circumstances of individuals discussed herein have been changed to protect confidentiality. Any resemblance to actual persons, living or dead, is entirely coincidental.

First published by

The Haworth Press, Inc., 10 Alice Street, Binghamton, NY 13904-1580 USA

This edition published 2012 by Routledge

Routledge
Taylor & Francis Group
711 Third Avenue
New York, NY 10017

Routledge
Taylor & Francis Group
27 Church Road, Hove
East Sussex BN3 2FA

Cover design by Lora Wiggins

Library of Congress Cataloging-in-Publication Data

Emerging trends in psychological practice in long-term care / Margaret P. Norris, Victor Molinari, Suzann M. Ogland-Hand.
        p.cm.
Includes bibliographical references and index.
    ISBN 0-7890-2004-1 (alk.paper)–ISBN 0-7890-2005-X (pbk.: alk.paper)
    1. Aged–Mental health. 2. Aged–Long-term care. 3. Geriatric psychiatry. I. Norris, Margaret, 1952- II. Molinari, Victor, 1952- III. Ogland-Hand, Suzann.
        RC451.4.A5 E445 2002
        362.2´ 084´ 6–dc21
                                                                    2002152088

Emerging Trends in Psychological Practice in Long-Term Care

CONTENTS

ABOUT THE EDITORS

Margaret P. Norris, PhD, is Associate Professor and psychologist in private practice with more than 20 years experience in geropsychology. Dr. Norris consults in numerous long-term care facilities, providing direct clinical services to patients and their families, as well as consultation to staff. She has national prominence in the area of clinical geropsychology. Dr. Norris is currently President of Psychologists in Long-Term Care, the premier organization devoted to establishing excellence in psychological services, research, and training in long-term care settings. In addition, she serves on the American Psychological Association's Medicare Task Force. Dr. Norris is also Treasurer and Chair of the Public Policy Committee for the Clinical Geropsychology Section of the American Psychological Association and has served in leadership roles in the Mental Health Practice and Aging section of the Gerontological Society of America. As Associate Professor, Dr. Norris has published extensively in the area of the mental health of older adults and trains future geropsychologists.

Victor Molinari, PhD, is Professor in the Department of Aging and Mental Health at the Louis de la Parte Florida Mental Health Institute of the University of South Florida. He was previously the Director of Psychology Training at the Houston Veterans Affairs Medical Center and Clinical Associate Professor of Psychiatry and Behavioral Sciences at Baylor College of Medicine. Dr. Molinari is the former coordinator for Psychologists in Long-Term Care, and President-elect of the American Psychological Association's section on clinical geropsychology. In 1997, he received the Houston chapter of the Alzheimer Association's Harry E. Walker Award for Professional Excellence. He is editor of *Professional Psychology in Long Term Care* and has published over 75 articles in geriatric mental health journals.

Suzann Ogland-Hand, PhD, is a geriatric consultant and Supervising Geropsychologist with Pine Rest Christian Mental Health Services in Grand Rapids, Michigan, and Adjunct Assistant Professor in the Department of Psychiatry at Michigan State University. She has been working in the field of geropsychology for ten years, working across the continuum of care from long-term to acute care settings. She served as Secretary for Psychologists in Long-Term Care (PLTC) for six years and has presented nationally on caregiver and mental health issues. In 2002, she published *Assessing and Treating Late-Life Depression: A Casebook and Resource Guide.*

Introduction:
Emerging Practices for Psychologists
in Long-Term Care

Margaret P. Norris, PhD

This volume on long-term care is intended to bring geropsychologists up to date on the ever-evolving field of geriatric mental health in long-term care settings. The articles are a product of our highly valued scientist-practitioner model, as they are authored by experts who practice in geriatric settings where clinical service cultivates empirical and scholarly advances in geropsychology. An underlying theme emerges throughout these articles; that is, the field of geropsychology is in a continuous process of evolution in the midst of multiple complex systems. The patient population is perpetually redefined by changing demographics, advances in medical technology, and sociopolitical transitions. In addition, the settings where services to older adults are provided are in flux, blurring existing definitions of long-term care. Finally, we face a new era of mental health care that is challenged by persistent reminders of accountability from the systems that finance health care.

In all the articles of this publication, the uniqueness of geropsychology practice is demonstrated. In particular, the authors highlight multifaceted ways in which direct clinical services must be modified from traditional outpatient services for this population, and how these services differ in the context of settings that inherently entail collaborative efforts within multidisciplinary environments. All authors recapitulate

---

Margaret P. Norris is affiliated with the Department of Psychology, Texas A&M University.

[Haworth co-indexing entry note]: "Introduction: Emerging Practices for Psychologists in Long-Term Care." Norris, Margaret P. Co-published simultaneously in *Clinical Gerontologist* (The Haworth Press, Inc.) Vol. 25, No. 1/2, 2002, pp. 1-11; and: *Emerging Trends in Psychological Practice in Long-Term Care* (ed: Margaret P. Norris, Victor Molinari, and Suzann Ogland-Hand) The Haworth Press, Inc., 2002, pp. 1-11. Single or multiple copies of this article are available for a fee from The Haworth Document Delivery Service [1-800-HAWORTH, 9:00 a.m. - 5:00 p.m. (EST). E-mail address: getinfo@haworthpressinc.com].

1

how the practices that govern geropsychology mental health care are different from and similar to those that prevail in traditional private practice, outpatient delivery systems.

One important difference concerns the epidemiology of mental illness in older adults. Rates of mental disorders among older adults are estimated to be approximately 18%-28% (Gatz, 1995). Other than organic brain disorders, rates of almost all categories of mental disorders are lower in older adults than in younger adults. However, these rates of mental illness in today's elderly generation pale in comparison to the rates observed among long-term care residents. Approximately 65% of residents in long-term care suffer from mental health problems (Burns et al., 1993).

Why are so many residents in long-term care in need of mental health services? In great part, the need reflects the high co-morbidity of physical and mental illnesses. Pain, progressive dementias, and disabling illnesses such as diabetes, strokes, and hip fractures all dramatically increase the risk of depression, anxiety, and behavioral disturbances. By and large, these illnesses and their sequelae cause serious declines in daily functioning and independence, which subsequently may trigger emotional problems. It is interesting to note that the rate of physical disability in older adults is currently declining. In 1992, more than one-quarter of older adults were chronically disabled; in contrast, in 1999 only 19% were chronically disabled (Nyberg, 2001). This is clearly a positive trend; however, the impact of this decline on the rate of mental illness remains unknown. Clearly, this decline is not mirrored in long-term care residents. Indeed, the proportion of nursing home residents with impairments in three or more activities of daily living increased from 72% to 83% between 1989 and 1996 (Institute of Medicine, 2001), and this trend is expected to continue.

While advances in medical technology are affording longer years of health and independence, there are parallel converse effects. The demand for long-term care will increase as medical advances help more people survive previously life-threatening conditions (e.g., AIDS, spinal cord injuries). The most frail and disabled are the old-old (age 85 and older), and this population's rapid growth will have a major effect on the supply and demand of long-term care services. This demand for long-term care services will be further magnified as the baby boomers reach old age. According to the 1990 and 2000 census data, the most rapid increase in any age group in the last 10 years was roughly a *50%* jump in the 45-54-year-old population (Nyberg, 2001). The media frequently warns us that the tidal wave of aging baby boomers will soon overload the Medicare health insurance system. Projections estimate that the number of disabled older adults who will need care will be 2-4 times the current numbers (General Accounting Office, 2001). Moreover, the baby boomers' relatively higher rates of depression, anxiety, and substance abuse predict an increase in the prevalence of mental disorders as this cohort reaches old age.

The articles of this volume also highlight the impact of the settings in which older adults often receive mental health care. Long-term care is commonly equated with skilled nursing home; in fact, these settings are not synonymous. Skilled nursing care represents one type of long-term care setting, although it is certainly not the most common. In fact, only 20% of older adults who require assistance with daily care receive that care in skilled nursing homes; the remaining 80% receive care in community-based settings or at home (General Accounting Office, 2001). And while institutional care is the exception rather than the rule, institutionalized care remains the biggest financial burden (Burwell, 2000). Institutional care represented 73% of Medicaid long-term care spending, compared to the more common but less expensive home- and community-based care, which was only 27% of the long-term care expenditures. However, in 2000, Medicaid expenditures for home- and community-based services increased 14.6%, making it the most rapidly growing Medicaid long-term care service. This emphasis on non-institutionalized care will become even stronger in view of the Supreme Court's 1999 decision, known as Olmstead. This decision ruled that states are violating the Americans with Disabilities Act if people with disabilities in institutional settings can be appropriately cared for at home or in the community (General Accounting Office, 2001). The article by Drs. Ogland-Hand and Florsheim, which highlights the critical role of family caregivers in long-term care, is especially applicable to home- and community-based care.

The interplay of long-term care and mental health care is especially realized in skilled nursing homes. In many ways, skilled nursing homes are becoming inpatient psychiatric care units for older adults. By 1977, the number of older adults with mental disorders in nursing homes had surpassed the number in state mental health facilities (Gatz & Smyer, 1992). Perhaps one reason nursing homes are becoming psychiatric facilities is because outpatient services dramatically underserve older adults in need of mental health services. The proportion of elderly clients served in community mental health services is fewer than 6% and also among private mental health professionals it is only 5% (Colenda & van Dooren, 1993). Therefore, it is not surprising that large percentages of residents in long-term care settings have significant psychiatric needs.

In reaction to the prevalence of behavioral and emotional disturbances in long-term care residents, the Omnibus Budget Reconciliation Act of 1987 mandated restricted use of physical and chemical restraints in nursing homes, opting instead for psychological and behavioral interventions, which have far fewer iatrogenic effects. All the articles in this volume depict the important role psychologists are playing in long-term care settings where more ethical and effective psychosocial interventions may rectify the unsanctioned reliance on chemical and physical restraints.

The articles in this collection are divided into three sections. The first section reviews modifications of traditional psychotherapy techniques for elderly clients. The second section addresses issues unique to multidisciplinary settings and presents systemic therapy approaches that often define long-term care mental health services. Finally, the third section addresses the ethical and confidentiality quandaries that are inherently more complex in long-term care settings.

Dr. Victor Molinari provides an integrated and comprehensive examination of group treatment in long-term care covering four germane topics. He first delineates the types of group treatment that are well suited for long-term care residents including remotivation, reality orientation, medication maintenance, nursing home adjustment socialization, reminiscence, traditional treatment, and family support groups. He insightfully applies Yalom's "common curative factors" to group work with older adults. In doing so, the reader is reminded of powerful achievements that can be attained in group treatment with long-term care residents. These gains may include helping residents cope with and accept natural age-related physical changes, find meaning in their late-life experiences, and especially salient, accept the nursing home as their new home with the potential for intimate personal relationships and care. Next, Molinari outlines important modifications for using group therapy with this population. Practical suggestions may greatly enhance therapy effectiveness such as scheduling therapy during times that will maximize functioning and alertness, assuring privacy and avoiding extraneous distractions, providing more structure, modeling of open discussion, and setting individually appropriate treatment goals. Finally, Molinari provides a candid review of the empirical literature on group treatment with older adults. He calls for improved methodology, i.e., larger sample sizes, controlled comparisons across therapies, and follow-up studies. Only by these investigative techniques will we learn what types of group therapy are best, for whom, in what types of long-term care settings (e.g., rehabilitation versus chronic care facilities), and what patient characteristics (e.g., cognitive functioning level, diagnostic mix) portend effective group therapy outcomes.

Dr. Brian Carpenter and his colleagues provide a stellar example of the process for developing an empirically-based treatment specifically designed for this unique population. Developed at the Philadelphia Geriatric Center, they present the Restore-Empower-Mobilize (R-E-M) brief psychotherapy treatment of depression for long-term care residents who have mild to moderate dementia. They adopted a procedure for developing this new integrated model of therapy, which serves as an example for other geropsychology scientist-practitioners to follow. After consulting with numerous colleagues, they drafted a treatment manual, conducted a preliminary clinical trial, gathered feedback from participating clinicians, collected further commentary from national geropsychology experts, revised their treatment manual, and finally conducted a larger pilot study using this carefully modified and standardized treatment. The results are presented in their manuscript. The process was meticulous and deserves special recognition. Their R-E-M therapy integrates theory and technique from multiple perspectives including cognitive, behavioral, humanistic, psychodynamic, as well as critical "nonspecific" or "common" factors. The R-E-M therapy incorporates three goals: restore self-esteem; empower residents to activate their abilities, strengths, and control; and mobilize both residents and staff to take actions that will make their environment more rewarding and therapeutic. Finally, Carpenter and his colleagues present empirical findings from their pilot study which documents reduced depression and increased participation in activities. Interestingly, the authors' data further corroborate the need for follow-up treatment (i.e., booster sessions) that may be necessary to maintain gains and prevent relapse in this vulnerable population.

Dr. Lee Hyer and his colleagues present a treatment for long-term care residents which utilizes salient positive memories from the individuals' early life to structure psychotherapy's goal of enhanced self-esteem. The authors first provide a broad overview of memory processes in late life. They then review, in detail, the theoretical underpinnings of major autobiographical memory techniques that have been used in the context of psychotherapy including reminiscence, life review, narrative therapy, and life story. The common ingredients of these strategies are apparent; Hyer and his colleagues delineate their distinguishing and subtle differences both in approach and goals. They have developed an autobiographical memory technique, positive core memories (PCM), applied to a cognitive-behavioral treatment model, in which patients elicit a salient positive memory that represents a critical aspect of their identity. Used in group therapy, the long-term care residents are encouraged to be reflective, to use their memories to validate a stable and positive self-image, and apply this to their current and future sense of self. Results of their pilot study are encouraging. Depressive symptoms were significantly reduced in the treatment group but not in the control group. The authors' examination of this type of treatment highlights the value of autobiographical memories in long-term care residents who have long lives of rich memories that can integrate meaning and purpose, and they de-emphasize a focus on disability and loss.

In the final article in this section, Dr. Michael Duffy addresses the common problem of disruptive behaviors among long-term care residents. He argues for strategic, counterintuitive solutions to problems such as depression, demanding behavior, dependency, hypochondriacal behavior, narcissistic behavior, and aggression. Recognizing the complex forces that drive these behaviors is necessary to identify tactics that will reduce these behavior problems, rather than intensify them. For example, the caregiver who avoids interacting with a particularly demanding patient may inadvertently sustain persistent requests from the patient, resulting in a vicious cycle of reciprocal discontentment felt by both patient and caregiver. A counterintuitive response of approaching and connecting with the patient may be far more effective in accommodating the patient's emotional needs, and thus, reduce the intensity of the patient's demands. Similar recommendations are made in therapeutically responding to hypochondriacal patients whose anxiety will not be reduced by ignoring their physical complaints, aggressive patients who should not be approached in an authoritative manner, narcissistic patients who need empathy to fill the void of emotional deprivation, and so forth. These emotional problems within nursing home residents are quite complex, and nursing home staff often rely on the expertise of a psychologist to help them understand the therapeutic (and non-therapeutic) effects of their responses to these patients.

The second series of articles address systemic interventions, which are so critical in long-term care settings. Drs. Suzann Ogland-Hand and Margaret Florsheim review family therapy. They emphasize the important role that family members continue to have in caring for their loved one after placement in long-term care facilities. The authors describe a number of family concerns that may come to the attention of the psychologist. For example, geropsychologists may work with family members who are experiencing guilt or depression following placement, struggling to adopt new identities as caregivers, re-experiencing long-standing family conflicts and pathology, or accepting their role as active agents of the residents' treatments (e.g., complying with dietary restrictions, assisting with end-of-life care decisions). These family issues are cogently illustrated with rich examples. Finally, Ogland-Hand and Florsheim articulate some of the challenges that geropsychologists confront when working with families in long-term care settings. For example, psychologists consulting in long-term care settings may have limited time and reimbursement sources for working with staff who have the most contact with family members. Psychologists are also reminded of the importance of attending to multiple perspectives including those of staff, patients, and families, as well as the impact of diverse cultural and ethnic backgrounds of residents and staff. The authors end with a compelling case example that illustrates an "interactional model of systematic communication." They remind the reader that many problems brought to the attention of a psychologist are not simply problems of an individual resident, but are strained interactions between parties. Resident and staff experience each other differently (as examined in detail by Drs. Parr and Green), contribute simultaneously to dysfunctional and functional interactions, and thus, provide the psychologist with multiple points of intervention.

Drs. Suzanne Meeks and Colin Depp present the theoretical and empirical foundation of a pleasant event-based behavioral treatment for depression that emphasizes systemic rather than individual interventions. Their therapeutic approach has its foundations in the seminal works of Linda Teri and Peter Lewinsohn, which are reviewed in detail in this article. Based on their empirically supported treatment of depression in patients with dementia, which trains family caregivers to increase pleasant events in the lives of elders with dementia, these authors present a translation of this therapy to long-term care patients whose caregivers are primarily professional staff. The application of this behavioral intervention for depression in long-term settings is potentially rich because these environments have institutional obstacles that inadvertently foster inactivity, social isolation, and dependency. Treatment goals are formed to change institutions to health-promoting environments. Thus, interventions are taught to and implemented by staff, especially social service and activity therapy staff. They are taught to understand depression and dementia, and their associated behavior problems, understand the important connection between pleasant events and positive mood states, and implement activities tailored to the patient's abilities, limitations, and preferences. Finally, outcome is assessed at the institutional level to evaluate the success of the interventions.

Drs. Joyce Parr and Sara Green approach the systemic characteristics of long-term care settings by comparing the perceptions of residents and staff. They asked residents and staff what characteristics of the setting contributed to quality of the facility. Factor analysis revealed five factors: relationships with staff, relationships among residents, personal services (food quality, food service, and maintenance services), physical and programmatic environment, and resident involvement and influence in the facility. Interestingly, both residents and staff rated resident satisfaction, on average, between good and very good. However, staff underestimated the degree of control that residents feel they have in their lives. Surprisingly, the best predictor of overall satisfaction with the facility for residents was the quality of the food, food service, and maintenance service. In contrast, staff perceived multiple variables as contributing to resident satisfaction. Interestingly, residents and staff also may perceive the sources for resident control differently. Residents related their feelings of control in their life to their relationships with staff, whereas staff believed residents acquire their sense of control primarily from facility variables. In discussing their findings, the authors suggest differences in staff and resident perceptions, while perhaps inevitable, may contribute to poor quality of care. Recommended remediations include an interdisciplinary team approach to care and training opportunities that include both staff and residents.

[The following articles will appear in Part II, volume 25, numbers 3/4.]

In keeping with the emphasis on systemic interventions, Dr. Donald Slone details a team approach when working with patients with dementia. He presents fundamental principles and practical guidelines for implementing a treatment team. The critical reasons for a team approach are delineated, i.e., to elicit complex, multifaceted, and creative solutions from numerous caregivers. Readers are reminded that the composition of the team is critical and must especially include nursing assistants who provide the most direct care, have ample opportunity to observe residents, and are the most vital staff in implementing intervention strategies. The team remains active not only during treatment planning but also during implementation in order to monitor intervention effectiveness. He further recommends that the mechanism for teamwork coordination be better conceptualized as "behavior rounds" rather than the traditional treatment planning meetings that may succumb to merely satisfying documentation requirements. The strength of Slone's message comes especially from fostering an attitude toward acceptance of a team approach. He promotes a "specialist mentality," that is, recognizing that treating patients with dementia requires specialized knowledge of dementia, an atmosphere of creative experimentation, and a receptive openness to other staff members' perspectives.

This section ends with the article by Drs. Lee Hyer and Amie Ragan, who offer a unique philosophical essay about the scant methods available for training long-term caregivers in behavioral techniques. Embedded in their contemplative exploration of this problem facing caregivers are sobering facts. For example, among directors of nurses surveyed, only 15% felt satisfied with their current level of expertise in handling disruptive behaviors. They review training models, which seemingly offer more overlap than solutions. Advances in long-term care, particularly those arising from OBRA regulations, are acknowledged. Hyer and Ragan underscore the limited outcomes measured by such regulations (e.g., cleanliness, safety) and call attention to the neglected psychosocial aspects of care that ultimately contribute to quality of care. Unfortunately, regulation of skilled nursing homes may have little effect on quality of care for the patients who are struggling to maintain some semblance of dignity, self-control, and independence. As they point out, psychologists spend as much time with the staff in long-term care settings as with the patients; thus, it behooves the profession to be innovative in developing behavioral techniques that capitalize on patients' spared abilities.

The final section on professional ethics is a provocative reminder to psychologists that the ethical dilemmas faced in long-term care settings are entangled in subtle complexities produced by the unique characteristics of the patient population and the multidisciplinary care setting. As a psychologist and attorney, Dr. Martin Zehr begins this discussion with an expert perspective on the legal definitions and requirements of informed consent. Zehr reviews the legal underpinnings of informed consent, instructing the reader that informed consent requires three components: disclosure of information regarding the proposed treatment, voluntary choice of treatment alternatives, and sufficient competence of the patient to comprehend the nature and consequences of the proposed treatment alternatives. He further suggests critical elements that should be discussed with patients in order to assure that informed consent has been fully achieved. The reader will find these practical guidelines highly germane to the unique challenges of treating cognitively impaired patients in settings where it is not appropriate to assume that all patients desire psychological interventions.

Dr. Margaret Norris's article details the confidentiality dilemmas that characterize long-term care practice. In multidisciplinary settings, the psychologist must balance the multiple roles of providing direct clinical services to patients, while simultaneously coordinating treatment efforts with other health care providers and family members. Psychologists must recognize that obtaining release of confidential information may need modifications for this special population. For example, they must be cognizant that in inpatient settings, patient information is revealed to the psychologist, typically without the patient's explicit consent to release this information to the psychologist. Norris reviews a number of professional and legal standards that address confidentiality regulations, pointing out that professional standards may be at odds with state law. She concludes with a series of cases that illustrate recommended practices, emphasizing that all patient information should not be treated uniformly. Patients and the psychologist should agree what information will and will not be communicated to staff and family, and the psychologist should exercise caution by communicating general information in charts and to staff, rather than specific and deeply personal information.

This final section on ethics concludes with Dr. Michael Duffy's cogent article, which makes the reader acutely aware of the controversial nature of topics such as informed consent and confidentiality in long-term care settings. Beginning with the position that these standards are more easily maintained in the orderly world of the outpatient psychotherapy office than in the "hurly burly world" of a typical nursing home, Duffy asks whether the ethical geropsychologist can *not* communicate and collaborate with staff. While at first glance, it may appear that Dr. Duffy's position is at odds with those articulated by Drs. Zehr and Norris, such a conclusion would be simplistic. Duffy emphasizes the difference between ethical principles and ethical regulations, cautioning geropsychologists to always keep in mind the principles that ultimately become defined and shaped into regulations. He uses example scenarios to point out that a legalistic application of ethical regulations may be at odds with client well-being. By striving to deliver altruistic services, geropsychologists tackle the complicated ethical dilemmas that our regulations do not always address.

In conclusion, these thought-provoking articles underscore major themes in mental health and long-term care. Geropsychology continues to evolve into newly defined practices and standards. In addition, complex service delivery is the rule rather than the exception in working with this frail elderly population, creating a necessity for coordinated, collaborative team efforts. Psychologists in long-term care are rewarded with creative challenges for which training and skilled preparation can prepare them to boldly and successfully meet.

REFERENCES

Burns, B., Wagner, H. R., Taube, J. E., Magaziner, J., Permutt, T., & Landerman, L. R. (1993). Mental health service use by the elderly in nursing homes. *American Journal of Public Health, 83,* 331-337.

Burwell, B. (2001). Medicaid long term care expenditures in fiscal year 2000. *The Gerontologist, 41,* 687-691.

Colenda, C. & van Dooren, H. (1993). Opportunities for improving community mental health services for elderly persons. *Hospital and Community Psychiatry, 44,* 531-533.

Gatz, M. (1995). Introduction. In M. Gatz (Ed.), *Emerging Issues in Mental Health and Aging.* (pp. xv-xx). Washington, DC: American Psychological Association.

Gatz, M. & Smyer, M. (1992). The mental health system and older adults in the 1990s. *American Psychologist, 47,* 741-751.

General Accounting Office (2001). *Long Term Care: Implications of Supreme Court's Olmstead Decision Are Still Unfolding.* Testimony before the Special Committee on Aging, U. S. Senate. (GAO-01-1167T).

Institute of Medicine (2001). *Improving the quality of long term care.* Washington, DC: National Academy Press.

Nyberg, J. (2001). Longevity news and trends in the United States and abroad. *The Gerontologist, 41,* 692-694.

SECTION ONE:
MODIFICATIONS OF TRADITIONAL PSYCHOTHERAPY TECHNIQUES

Group Therapy in Long Term Care Sites

Victor Molinari, PhD

SUMMARY. Group therapy is an intervention that is particularly suited for residents in long term care settings, because it can reduce social isolation and efficiently address the common issue of adjustment to institutional living. This article first specifies the types of groups that should be offered in long term care settings as a function of therapeutic aims and resident composition. It then enumerates Yalom's common curative factors and how they are reflected in the group process with frail nursing home residents. The unique elements in doing group therapy within long term care sites are then discussed. Next, the meager research on group psychotherapy in long term care sites is summarized, and a plea is made for more empirical studies to be conducted in this exciting but neglected

Victor Molinari is Professor in the Department of Aging and Mental Health, Louis de la Parte Florida Mental Health Institute, University of South Florida. This paper was presented as part of a symposium on "Psychology in nursing homes: New techniques in assessment and treatment" (Chairs, L. Hyer & S. Sohnle) at the American Psychological Association Meeting, Washington DC, August 2000.

[Haworth co-indexing entry note]: "Group Therapy in Long Term Care Sites." Molinari, Victor. Co-published simultaneously in *Clinical Gerontologist* (The Haworth Press, Inc.) Vol. 25, No. 1/2, 2002, pp. 13-24; and: *Emerging Trends in Psychological Practice in Long-Term Care* (ed: Margaret P. Norris, Victor Molinari, and Suzann Ogland-Hand) The Haworth Press, Inc., 2002, pp. 13-24. Single or multiple copies of this article are available for a fee from The Haworth Document Delivery Service [1-800-HAWORTH, 9:00 a.m. - 5:00 p.m. (EST). E-mail address: getinfo@haworthpressinc.com].

13

area. Finally, reimbursement issues for group therapy in nursing homes are briefly considered. *[Article copies available for a fee from The Haworth Document Delivery Service: 1-800-HAWORTH. E-mail address: <getinfo@haworthpressinc.com> Website: <http://www.HaworthPress.com> © 2002 by The Haworth Press, Inc. All rights reserved.]*

KEYWORDS. Group therapy, nursing homes, long term care, frail older adults

The Omnibus Budget Reconciliation Act (OBRA) legislated that long term care (LTC) facilities must address the psychological needs of their residents. This inspired many geriatric mental health professionals to consult with nursing homes who were faithfully seeking to fulfill this mandate. Available treatments run the gamut from psychosocial to psychopharmacological, but group therapy is well-suited for LTC residents for three basic reasons. One, social isolation is surprisingly prevalent in nursing homes. Groups are obvious interpersonal situations in and of themselves, enhance a sense of belonging, and provide a benign forum for constructive feedback concerning social behavior and reality testing. Two, given the frequent lack of trained mental health personnel in nursing homes, group therapy allows a lone geriatric specialist to treat a number of residents at the same time. And three, the common issue of adjustment to institutional living lends itself to processing in a supportive group therapy format.

It is important to note that the conduct of group therapy is a unique treatment practice, and should not be construed as individual therapy in a communal context where other members merely observe and vicariously benefit. Rather, a special aspect of group work is reflected in the ongoing interpersonal processes that are emphasized in the "here and now." However, given that approximately half of LTC residents have dementia (Magaziner et al., 2000), the traditional group approach must be modified to take account of age-related cognitive impairment and sensory changes. Nonetheless, it should always be kept in mind that empathizing and validating a person's worth, especially when the person is cognitively impaired (Feil, 1989), is the foundation for all good therapy.

TYPES OF GROUPS

The positive response of residents, family members, and staff to the more stimulating atmosphere engendered by group activities has provided incentives for many LTC facilities to incorporate formal group programs into their routine. The support of both the LTC administration and nursing staff are absolutely necessary for an effective program to be developed (Abramson & Mendis, 1990; Ruckdeschel, 2000). It therefore behooves mental health consultants to expend a good portion of time during their initial visits to an LTC institution in meetings with administrators to determine their commitment to a group modality of care.

The types of groups offered in a particular LTC site should depend on the purpose of the facility, primary reasons for referral, resident composition (e.g., psychiatric/medical diagnoses, extent of cognitive impairment), and staff expertise in mental health interventions. For example, with hospitals now discharging patients from acute beds after brief inpatient stays, some LTC facilities have begun to specialize in physical and neurological rehabilitation and pay heightened attention to motivational factors that can affect intermediate care outcome. The ultimate goal of discharge back to the community (which can still take months to accomplish) is different from the chronic care of the traditional nursing home where residents are expected to remain for the rest of their lives. The group therapy program should, of course, reflect such differences in aims, with perhaps greater prominence given to addressing current dynamics affecting treatment compliance, earmarking patients with specific disabilities for particular groups, and hiring staff with expertise in designated areas (e.g., stroke support groups).

Due to the aforementioned factors, there are a wide variety of different kinds of LTC groups (Burnside, 1978), and only the most common ones that focus on mental health will be detailed here. (See Table 1). Remotivation groups can help rekindle interest in the outside world for residents and reduce the "institutionalization syndrome." Reality orientation groups (Taulbee & Folsom, 1966) attempt to keep residents current with basic facts of daily life, and should be planned as part of an overall milieu that promotes the cognitive strengths of residents. Medication maintenance groups may be helpful in managing physical symptoms, explaining medical diagnoses and the necessity of LTC, and encouraging compliance with medication regimens. By offering sessions immediately upon admission to new residents and their families, nursing home adjustment groups may ease the transition from community to institutional living. Socialization groups can have both content dimensions (i.e., teaching residents new social skills) and process dimensions (i.e., utilizing the interaction displayed in the group for members to provide constructive feedback to each other concerning interpersonal styles).

Reminiscence groups offer predetermined topics to be discussed that are relevant to the members' past and allow them to relive glory days in a conversational, informal format. Such groups are popular but should

TABLE 1. Types and Goals of Groups in LTC Settings

Types	Targeted Population	Goals
Remotivation	Chronic schizophrenics	Rekindle interest
Reality orientation	Demented residents	Stabilize mental status
Medication maintenance	Medically ill	Encourage compliance
Nursing home adjustment	Newly admitted	Expedite adjustment
Socialization	All patients	Improve sense of community
Reminiscence	Cognitively intact	Relive "good" times of past
Psychotherapy	Repressed/anxious patients	Address losses
Family support	Stressed family caregivers	Aid transition to care manager

be distinguished from life review groups that are professionally led and encourage comprehensive evaluation of members' past experiences. The ultimate aim of life review groups is to reduce group members' recriminations, affirm their histories, gain continuity with the past, and achieve personal integration. To achieve such lofty goals, group members must therefore be selected carefully for motivation to participate, ego strength, and positive personality variables (e.g., openness to experience), or there may be a danger of a negative therapeutic reaction (Hewett, Asamen, Hedgespeth, & Dietch, 1991; Molinari, 1999). Psychotherapy groups are also professionally led and typically address the losses in members' lives (e.g., home, health, work status, regular contact with family, etc.). Strategies to avoid boredom, deal with abandonment fears, and replace losses become preeminent. Finally, family support groups engage the feelings of family members concerning nursing home placement, particularly guilt over this decision, but also emotional reactions about seeing their loved ones physically and psychologically deteriorate. The critical importance of the family's new role as care managers may need to be processed, in particular their functioning as a liaison to nursing home staff to help them to understand the individual person behind the dementia and the necessity of personalized care.

YALOM'S COMMON CURATIVE FACTORS

Yalom (1975) has proposed a number of "common curative factors" for group therapy that have applicability to group work with older adults. (See Table 2). Imparting information can be helpful in assisting residents to understand why they are in nursing homes, that their families have not abandoned them, and that age-related physical changes are natural. Instillation of hope allows residents to recognize that positive meaning can be distilled from any human experience and that nursing homes are not just places to die. The universality factor provides a broader context to view LTC experiences. Residents can understand that they are in a new stage of life which proffers different challenges. Their problems are not unique since common aging losses necessitate LTC. Group therapy allows modeling by the therapist and by more psychologically-minded residents to demonstrate to other group members that it is okay to express emotions. The leader's competence in negotiating interpersonal encounters may "rub off" on some introverted residents with avoidant or schizoid tendencies who reluctantly find themselves confined in a stressful social environment. The development of socialization skills is thus another healing factor, with informal interaction outside of the group thereby encouraged.

Sometimes, even at this late stage of life, unresolved family conflicts can be addressed. In LTC sites, it is usually long-standing marital difficulties or the relationship between the resident and adult children that needs attention. Sporadic visiting schedules may more properly be framed as family members having competing demands rather than being unconcerned about residents. Given the frequency of dementia in

TABLE 2. Yalom's (1975) Common Curative Factors for Group Therapy

1. Imparting information
2. Instillation of hope
3. Universality
4. Altruism
5. Modeling
6. Development of socialization skills
7. Correction of unresolved family conflicts
8. Catharsis
9. Existential factors
10. Interpersonal living
11. Group cohesion

LTC sites, catharsis must be used judiciously to keep residents from being flooded with negative emotions without adequate coping mechanisms. Intense emotional or spontaneous expression can be healing in certain contexts (Serok, 1986), but must be linked with cognitive understanding. A resident's acceptance of limitations and dependency, the inevitability of death, and the desire to leave a legacy are existential curative factors that may be poignantly addressed in higher-level groups.

But the final factors, interpersonal living and group cohesion, are probably the most salient ones that can aid residents in accepting the nursing home as their new home. Interpersonal living offers the opportunity to receive feedback concerning a member's relational behavior that is so essential in a communal living situation. Group cohesion is the strength of the emotional bond to the group that should always be fostered in LTC sites. To promote social ties, Ruckdeschel (2000) recommends that LTC groups have memberships that are closed, with participants manifesting similar cognitive capacity and attending group at the same time in the same place. Periodically restating group goals and rules of respect for each other go a long way to assure that all members will feel valued and comfortable in risking expressing their true selves to the other residents.

UNIQUE ELEMENTS OF GROUP THERAPY IN LTC SITES

In order for group therapy to be effective in LTC sites, therapeutic technique must be modulated to take account of the unique characteristics of this population such as cognitive and physical limitations. (See Table 3). Group schedules should be organized around the maximum functioning portion of the day. It is probably not wise to run a group just after meals or at later "sundowning" times. There must be a more leisurely therapeutic pace, because older adults learn, albeit, more slowly. The environment should be carefully planned to achieve privacy with as few extraneous noises as possible. Seating members in a tight circle promoting face to face viewing has been recommended (Speer & O'Sullivan, 1994). Common sensory and physical ailments can affect the rhythm of a group. Obviously, absenteeism should not be automatically attributed to resistance.

Most of the time the leader will need to be active and provide more structure, because older adults are in general less knowledgeable about therapy and often uncomfortable revealing private matters (particularly to non-professional acquaintances who may also be group members).

TABLE 3. General Differences in Group Work with LTC Residents

Conducted at maximum functioning of day
Environment needs to be carefully planned
Slower pace
Sensory deficits and physical ailments common
Ego enhancement rather than confrontation
Outside the group socializing more acceptable
More limited goals
Losses and boredom are constant themes
Leader: more directive, flexible, disclosing, supportive

Indeed, modules have been developed over the years that teach older adults what to do in therapy for the purpose of reducing their anxiety in this novel situation (Orne & Wender, 1968). Providing food and drink can create a convivial atmosphere that allows the group leader to offer residents sustenance before soliciting their personal contributions. Leaders may be expected to share more of themselves and their feelings concerning how the subject matter affects them. This could help participants focus on their own personal responses, and improve rapport by "bridging the generation gap" between younger therapists and older residents. Long silences with expectations that this will provide "grist for the therapeutic mill" are rarely productive with LTC residents. Chit-chat in the first few minutes of the group is more tolerated, and outside the group socializing is promoted, because increased interaction is often a therapeutic aim.

It is important to note that objectives should always be clearly stated when the group is being promoted so that residents can make informed choices about participation (Ruckdeschel, 2000; Zarit, 1978). In general, the LTC group therapist should countenance more limited treatment goals. Short-term and supportive approaches are preferred. For most residents, major personality change is not a realistic option, so ego enhancement strategies that promote building up defenses rather than tearing them down are desired therapeutic modes. Confrontation should be infrequent and gentle. Perhaps self-actualization is unrealistic, but adjustment to nursing home living may be a pragmatic and achievable goal. To summarize, group therapists in LTC sites must be more flexible, supportive, directive, disclosing, and less confrontative with frail and disabled nursing home residents.

RESEARCH

Reviews of the geriatric literature have consistently found psychotherapy with older adults to be just as effective as with younger adults (Gatz et al., 1998; Niederehe & Schneider, 1998). Empirical studies have also specifically demonstrated the efficacy of group treatment for community dwelling older adults (Ingersoll & Silverman, 1978). Unfortunately, most research on group therapy with LTC residents is qualitative and anecdotal. However, some research does suggest that group therapy practice with LTC residents may be viewed as evidence-based, and a few of these studies will be briefly described below (n.b., this is not an exhaustive review of the literature).

Moran and Gatz (1987) conducted a study comparing the effects of task-oriented, insight-oriented, and waiting list control groups on the psychological functioning of 59 nursing home residents. Although there was no improvement in the behavioral attributes of psychosocial competence, participants in the task condition enhanced their sense of internal control and life satisfaction; those in the insight condition increased in internal locus of control and trust, while those in the waiting list control decreased in trust. Although the results are marred by a small sample size and lack of follow-up data, it should be noted that in addition to the quantitative gains, the residents appeared to enjoy the group experience and exhibited a low attrition rate.

Reminiscence groups have also undergone some empirical scrutiny. Cook (1991) offered a reminiscence group in a nursing home setting and found a trend towards increased ego integrity for the 56 resident/participants. In a series of studies, Haight and her colleagues (Haight, 1992; Haight, Michel, & Hendrix, 1998; Haight, Michel, & Hendrix, 2000) measured the short- and long-term effects of a life review intervention, and documented the continued positive effects on depression, hopelessness, and long life satisfaction three years after implementation. However, it should be noted that due to high mortality rates in nursing homes, follow-up analyses were conducted on only a small percentage of the original cohort. Unfortunately, other authors have been unable to detect significant positive changes with reminiscence groups (Hedgepeth & Hale, 1983; Youssef, 1990). Perhaps a clearer delineation of the specific interventions and suitable membership (e.g., whether it is truly reminiscence or life review; which nursing home candidates are appropriate for an intensive life review intervention) may pave the way for a synthesis of the contradictory findings in this literature.

As has been well-known for years, research has strongly indicated that 24-hour-a-day orientation groups (Hahn, 1980) are helpful in improving cognition and behavior for patients with dementia, but its effects are not lasting when the program is withdrawn (Gilewski, 1986; Spector, Davies, Woods, & Orrell, 2000). Interestingly, some authors have attempted to go beyond simple reality orientation and to extend some types of group work typically reserved for higher functioning residents to those with significant cognitive impairment. Lantz, Buchalter, and McBee (1997) offered a one-session well-being group to demented nursing home residents. The intervention was designed to enhance self-awareness, self-esteem, and body awareness via meditation, relaxation, sensory awareness, and guided imagery techniques. Compared to a control group, the intervention group manifested a significant reduction in total agitation scores. Unfortunately, the latter analysis was done on only a few of the residents and the results must therefore be deemed preliminary. Goldwasser, Auerbach, and Harkins (1987) developed a group intervention that integrated "training group" and "therapy group" elements via utilizing exercises to stimulate reminiscence activity in significantly demented nursing home residents. Participants' depression levels were reduced at post-test, but these effects were less detectable at follow-up. Finally, Hepburn et al. (1997) developed a "Family Stories Workshop" to encourage family members of residents with dementia to use narrative materials to convey information to nursing care providers about the uniqueness of their family member. It was reasoned that nursing staff's knowledge of the history of the residents they are caring for will result in more personalized care. The authors conclude that the program eased residents' integration into the institution by allowing family members to regain a sense of the meaning of the resident's life which was thereby conveyed to staff members who learned to appreciate the resident as an individual. Unfortunately, the materials used for program evaluation were largely qualitative rather than quantitative in nature, preventing easy replication of the results.

REIMBURSEMENT ISSUES

Medicare reimbursement for group therapy in nursing homes is per each person in the group, with a minimum of three and a maximum of eight members. Payment is at 50% of the Medicare allowable. Reimbursement is routine for group psychotherapy if the patient is appropriate for, can benefit from, and has the capacity to participate in psychotherapy on a group level. That is, the procedure must meet criteria for medical necessity (i.e., there is a psychiatric reason/diagnosis, there is a professional therapeutic intervention, and there is a desired outcome or progress expected from the procedure). Each patient must have a progress note for the session, substantiating the medical necessity for the group on that particular date (J. Casciani, personal communication, May 14, 2001).

To underscore the above, it should be noted that a 1996 report by the Office of Inspector General (Dunn, 2000) singled out inappropriate billing for group psychotherapy with demented patients as one of the two major causes for concern (just behind psychological testing with demented nursing home residents). Those conducting group therapy with LTC patients should be ever-mindful of the need to assure that the therapy being offered is well-reasoned and of likely benefit to all the group members. By keeping in mind that different types of groups are earmarked for different problems in nursing home settings, therapists may be better able to justify their practice by adjusting their interventions to the unique needs of this frail population.

CONCLUSION

Although many clinicians have been creatively attempting to address the myriad mental health problems of LTC residents with cutting-edge interventions, the empirical foundation of group therapy with nursing home residents remains weak. Rigorous quantitative assessment must be integrated with qualitative analysis in order to assure reimbursement rates commensurate with professional expertise. Future studies must use larger sample sizes, identify the theoretical rationale for utilization of particular interventions (e.g., reminiscence versus life review) with the targeted nursing home population, and incorporate adequate follow-up. There are too few controlled studies on the effectiveness of group therapy in LTC settings, and many basic questions remain unanswered. We still do not know whether group formation proceeds in similar fashion and rate as among younger persons or as among community dwelling older individuals. There is sparse literature on religious issues groups in LTC sites, which is surprising as older adults in this cohort are more traditionally religious and are in a stage of life that may prompt spiritual yearnings (Erikson, Erikson, & Kivnick, 1986). There is also little research on contraindications for group therapy in LTC settings. Zarit (1978) has suggested that assertiveness groups may not be appropriate for some institutional settings where residents may be "punished" for such behavior. What other types of groups should generally be avoided? What types of group are most and least appropriate for frail older adults in rehabilitation versus chronic care facilities? What is the best diagnostic mix for membership in LTC groups? At what cognitive level should an individual be triaged to a low versus high functioning group? What types of group therapy training renders the most positive results? The answers to these questions will guide clinicians in this relatively uncharted professional territory, buttress mental health public policy advocacy efforts, and dramatically affect the quality of life for LTC residents.

REFERENCES

Abramson, T. A., & Mendis, K. P. (1990). The organizational logistics of running a dementia group in a skilled nursing facility. In T.L. Brink (Ed.), *Mental health in the nursing home* (pp. 111-122). New York: Haworth Press.

Burnside, I. (1978). *Working with the elderly: Group process and technique.* Massachusetts: Roxbury Press.

Cook, E. (1991). The effects of reminiscence on psychological measures of ego integrity in elderly nursing home residents. *Archives of Psychiatric Nursing, 5,* 292-298.

Dunn, R. (2000, June). Mental health services in nursing homes. Presented as part of a symposium on "Policy implications from the payment systems perspective" (Chair, J. Streim) at the *Providing optimal mental health services in long term care consensus conference,* Washington, DC.

Erikson, E., Erikson, J., & Kivnick, H.Q. (1986). *Vital involvement in old age.* New York: Norton.

Feil, N. (1989). Validation: An empathetic approach to the care of dementia. *Clinical Gerontologist, 8,* 89-94.

Gatz, M., Fiske, A., Foz, L.S., Kaskie, B., Kasl-Godley, J.E., McCallum, T.J., & Wetherell, J.L. (1998). Empirically validated psychological treatments for older adults. *Journal of Mental Health and Aging, 4,* 9-46.

Gilewski, M. (1986). Group therapy with cognitively impaired older adults. In T.L. Brink (Ed.), *Clinical gerontology: A guide to assessment and intervention* (pp. 281-296). New York: Hatherleigh Press.

Goldwasser, A.N., Auerbach, S. M., & Harkins, S.W. (1987). Cognitive, affective, and behavioral effects of reminiscence group therapy on demented elderly. *International Journal of Aging and Human Development, 25,* 209-222.

Hahn, K. (1980). 24-hour reality orientation. *Journal of Gerontological Nursing, 6*(3), 130-135.

Haight, B.K. (1992). Long-term effects of a structured life review process. *Journal of Gerontology: Psychological Sciences, 47,* P312-P315.

Haight, B.K., Michel, Y., & Hendrix, B.K. (1998). Life review: Preventing despair in newly relocated nursing home residents. *International Journal of Aging and Human Development, 47,* 119-142.

Haight, B.K., Michel, Y., & Hendrix, B.K. (2000). The extended effects of the life review in nursing home residents. *International Journal of Aging & Human Development, 50*(2), 151-168.

Hedgepeth, B.E., & Hale, D. (1983). Effects of a positive reminiscing intervention on affect, expectancy, and performance. *Psychological Reports, 53*, 867-870.

Hewett, L., Asamen, J. K., Hedgespeth, J., & Dietch, J.T. (1991). Group reminiscence with nursing home residents. *Clinical Gerontologist, 10*, 69-72.

Ingersoll, B., & Silverman, A. (1978). Comparative group psychotherapy for the aged. *The Gerontologist, 18*, 201-206.

Lantz, M.S. Buchalter, E.N., & McBee, L. (1997). The wellness group: A novel intervention for coping with disruptive behavior in elderly nursing home residents. *The Gerontologist, 37*, 551-556.

Magaziner, J., German, P., Zimmerman, S. I., Hebel, J. R., Burton, L., Gruber-Baldini, A.L., May, C., & Kittner, S. (2000). The prevalence of dementia in a statewide sample of new nursing home admissions aged 65 and older: Diagnosis by expert panel. *The Gerontologist, 40*, 663-672.

Molinari, V. (1999). Using reminiscence and life review as natural therapeutic strategies in group therapy. In M. Duffy (Ed.), *Handbook of counseling and psychotherapy with older adults*. New York: John Wiley & Sons Inc.

Moran, J.A., & Gatz, M. (1987). Group therapies for nursing home adults: An evaluation of two treatment approaches. *The Gerontologist, 27*, 588-591.

Niederehe, G., & Schneider, L.S. (1998). Treatments for anxiety and depression in the aged. In P. Nathan & J.M. Gorman (Eds.), *A guide to treatments that work*. New York: Oxford University Press, pp. 270-287.

Orne, M. T., & Wender, P. H., (1968). Anticipatory socialization for psychotherapy: Method and rationale. *American Journal of Psychiatry, 124*, 1202-1212.

Ruckdeschel, H. (2000). Group psychotherapy in the nursing home. In V. Molinari (Ed.), *Professional psychology in long term care: A comprehensive guide* (pp. 113-131). New York: Hatherleigh Press.

Serok, S. (1986). Application of gestalt therapy to group work with the aged. In T.L. Brink (Ed.), *Clinical gerontology: A guide to assessment and intervention* (pp. 231-243). New York: Hatherleigh Press.

Spector, A., Davies, S., Woods, B., & Orrell, M. (2000). Reality orientation for dementia: A systematic review of the evidence of effectiveness from randomized control trials. *The Gerontologist, 40*, 206-212.

Speer, D.C., & O'Sullivan, M. (1994). Group therapy in nursing homes and hearing deficit. *Clinical Gerontologist, 14*(4), 68-70.

Taulbee, L.R., & Folsom, J.C. (1966). Reality orientation for geriatric patients. *Hospital and Community Psychiatry, 17*, 133-135.

Yalom, I. (1975). *Theory and practice of group psychotherapy*. New York: Basic Books.

Youssef, F. (1990). The impact of group reminiscence counseling on a depressed elderly population. *Nurse Practitioner, 15*, 32-38.

Zarit, S. (1978). *Aging and mental disorders: Psychological approaches to assessment and treatment*. New York: Free Press, p. 335.

R-E-M Psychotherapy:
A Manualized Approach
for Long-Term Care Residents
with Depression and Dementia

Brian Carpenter, PhD
Katy Ruckdeschel, PhD
Holly Ruckdeschel, PhD
Kimberly Van Haitsma, PhD

SUMMARY. Although depression and dementia are common comorbid illnesses among long-term care residents, psychotherapeutic services for these individuals have not been tailored for their particular needs and circumstances. In this article we present a new model for brief individual psychotherapy–Restore, Empower, Mobilize, or R-E-M–to treat depression in long-term care residents who have mild to moderate dementia.

Brian Carpenter is affiliated with the Department of Psychology, Washington University in St. Louis. Katy Ruckdeschel is affiliated with the Department of Psychiatry at the University of Pennsylvania. Holly Ruckdeschel is affiliated with Transitional Care and Rehabilitation, Coatesville Veterans Affairs Medical Center. Kimberly Van Haitsma is affiliated with the Polisher Research Institute of the Madlyn and Leonard Abramson Center for Jewish Life.

The authors would like to thank Drs. Loren Connelly, Michelle Gagnon, and David Payne for their extensive contributions to the treatment model and empirical trial. For their support of this project the authors also are grateful to Dr. Ira Katz at the University of Pennsylvania (NIMH grant 5-P30-MH52129) and The Harry Stern Family Center for Innovations in Alzheimer's Care at the Philadelphia Geriatric Center.

[Haworth co-indexing entry note]: "R-E-M Psychotherapy: A Manualized Approach for Long-Term Care Residents with Depression and Dementia." Carpenter, Brian et al. Co-published simultaneously in *Clinical Gerontologist* (The Haworth Press, Inc.) Vol. 25, No. 1/2, 2002, pp. 25-49; and: *Emerging Trends in Psychological Practice in Long-Term Care* (ed: Margaret P. Norris, Victor Molinari, and Suzann Ogland-Hand) The Haworth Press, Inc., 2002, pp. 25-49. Single or multiple copies of this article are available for a fee from The Haworth Document Delivery Service [1-800-HAWORTH, 9:00 a.m. - 5:00 p.m. (EST). E-mail address: getinfo@haworthpressinc.com].

25

R-E-M treatment has three goals: (1) restore self-esteem and support a positive self-concept, (2) empower residents to make use of their existing abilities, and (3) mobilize residents and the environment to achieve and maintain long-term mental health. We describe the interventions of R-E-M treatment, the construction of a treatment manual, and a pilot evaluation of the treatment with three nursing home residents. Positive outcomes in the pilot have encouraged us to pursue additional treatment development and evaluation. Standardized treatments, such as R-E-M, that yield measurable gains are needed to ensure that long-term care residents with depression and dementia receive the mental health services they require and deserve. *[Article copies available for a fee from The Haworth Document Delivery Service: 1-800-HAWORTH. E-mail address: <getinfo@haworthpressinc.com> Website: <http://www.HaworthPress.com> © 2002 by The Haworth Press, Inc. All rights reserved.]*

KEYWORDS. Individual psychotherapy, depression, dementia, long-term care

Dementia and depression are common psychiatric syndromes in older adults living in institutional settings. Among nursing home residents, for instance, the prevalence of dementia is estimated to range from 50% to 75% (Mega & Cummings, 1996; Parmelee, Katz, & Lawton, 1989), while the prevalence of major and minor depression is estimated to range from 5-50% (Borson & Fletcher, 1996). Not surprisingly, dementia and depression are common comorbid illnesses. Up to 87% of older individuals with Alzheimer's disease (AD) also experience depression, with modal estimates near 30% (Parmelee, Katz, & Lawton, 1992; Teri & Wagner, 1992; Wragg & Jeste, 1989). The subjective distress of depression is compounded by the disorder's contribution to excess disability–secondary effects that exacerbate problems such as poor physical health (Schleifer, Keller, Bond, Cohen, & Stein, 1989), pain (Parmelee, Katz, & Lawton, 1991), and impaired cognitive functioning (Borson & Fletcher, 1996). In this article we briefly review the literature on psychosocial treatments for depression with individuals who have dementia, and we introduce a new treatment model designed specifically for these clients. Further, we discuss the process of treatment development and results from a recent pilot evaluation.

In a recent consensus statement an NIH panel identified as a priority the "development of psychotherapeutic treatments tailored to the physical illness and disability status of depressed older patients" (Lebowitz et al., 1997, p. 1189). Presumably this includes persons with cognitive impairment. One important approach in the treatment of depression in long-term care residents is pharmacologic intervention. A variety of medications are effective in treating depression in older adults (Katz, Simpson, Curlik, Parmelee, & Muhly, 1990; Majeroni & Hess, 1998; Reynolds, 1997), including persons with dementia (Katona, Hunter, & Bray, 1998; Taragano, Lyketsos, Mangone, Allegri, & Comesana-Diaz, 1997). Unfortunately, pharmacokinetics in older adults may increase susceptibility to side effects and medication interactions (Streim & Katz, 1996). A treatment strategy that avoids the risk of side effects and that may complement pharmacological treatment is psychotherapy.

PSYCHOTHERAPY FOR OLDER ADULTS WITH DEMENTIA AND DEPRESSION

Despite the common belief that cognitive impairment is a barrier, dementia is not necessarily a contraindication for psychotherapy with older persons (Fisher & Carstensen, 1990). Individuals with mild to moderate dementia can benefit from psychotherapy to improve emotional control, maintain self-esteem, foster positive adjustment to increased dependence, and reestablish a sense of identity (for reviews see Kasl-Godley & Gatz, 2000; Teri & McCurry, 1994; and Zweig & Hinrichsen, 1996). For treatment to be successful, however, clinicians must be mindful of the impact of dementia on memory, attention, expressive and receptive language, and executive functions such as planning and judgment. Furthermore, they must consider how the goals, strategies, and scope of treatment of persons with dementia need to be modified. Goals may be pragmatic as well as psychologically enriching, strategies more active and direct, and the scope broader to incorporate the larger long-term care system.

A variety of psychotherapeutic approaches for treating depression have been used with older adults, both with and without dementia. Thompson and Gallagher-Thompson have demonstrated positive outcomes with cognitive-behavioral interventions with non-demented, depressed older adults (e.g., Gallagher & Thompson, 1983; Thompson, Gallagher, & Breckenridge, 1987). Meanwhile, Teri and colleagues have developed an extensive research program affirming the efficacy of behavioral interventions in depressed older adults with dementia (e.g., Teri & Gallagher-Thompson, 1991; Teri, Logsdon, Uomoto, & McCurry,

1997). Interpersonal therapy has been found to enhance pharmacological treatment response in non-demented, depressed older adults (Reynolds et al., 1992). Reminiscence and life review are two other approaches commonly used with older adults, including nursing home residents (Fielden, 1990; Lappe, 1987; Rattenbury & Stones, 1989). Brief insight-oriented psychotherapy appears to reduce symptoms of mild depression in older adults (Lazarus et al., 1987), while brief counseling has been shown to bolster self-esteem and continuity of self in nursing home patients (Frey, Kelbley, Durham, & James, 1992; Marson, 1995). A number of theorists have suggested that psychodynamic interventions, including a focus on object relations and self psychology, may be helpful with depressed and demented individuals, who may suffer a decline in self-concept (Jones, 1995; Sadavoy & Robinson, 1989; Unterbach, 1994). Hausman (1992) has written explicitly on dynamic psychotherapy for depression in the context of Alzheimer's disease. Feil's validation therapy is another dynamically-oriented treatment for depression in older adults (Feil, 1989, 1992).

These approaches make important contributions to the treatment of depression in general and comorbid depression and dementia in particular. However, in their adherence to specific models they may not take full advantage of the range of available interventions (Dobson & Shaw, 1988). For example, behavioral approaches acknowledge the value of a positive relationship between the patient and care provider but do not view the relationship as an agent of change and so fail to capitalize on its potential value. Other approaches minimize the contribution that persons with dementia may make to establishing goals and carrying out the plan of treatment, thereby missing an opportunity for enhancing control, mastery, and self-worth. Approaches that depend on interventions directed by caregivers may be limited in their applicability by excluding the large number of persons who lack family or informal support. Moreover, these interventions primarily focus on persons served in outpatient or community settings, overlooking residents of long-term care facilities for whom formal providers assume the majority of care responsibilities. In sum, a psychotherapeutic approach that is broad and integrative may be able to take full advantage of the features of many theoretical perspectives. Integration may be particularly important when treating long-term care residents, who represent a neglected population in psychotherapy research.

Previous theory and research have not addressed in much detail contributions to the etiology and challenges to the treatment of depression presented by institutional life. Moving to and living in a long-term care facility may pose unique risks for depression. For instance, numerous losses precipitate and accompany entry into a long-term care facility. Residents are faced with a new and unfamiliar physical and human environment and may be required to share intimate living space with a stranger. Social interaction, in general, is with individuals one might not have chosen as friends, but with whom one shares proximity. Residents' daily schedules often are determined by institutional demands, ignoring the residents' wishes for particular routines or specific activities. Each institutional decision that imposes structure or limitations on residents strips them further of autonomy and a sense of control over their world. Although some limits are essential to maintain residents' safety, many restrictions represent overreaching attempts to achieve organizational efficiency.

Another loss often related to nursing home entry, that of physical disability, can color one's every experience. A decline in physical health may trigger depression through its impact on everyday activities (e.g., the need for assistance in using a bathroom, restrictions on social contact) or by precipitating existential crises (e.g., a heightened awareness of approaching death). Parallel to its influence on the etiology of depression, physical illness influences the treatment of depression in long-term care facilities at levels from the mundane (e.g., holding therapy sessions at bedside) to the profound (e.g., revising personal definitions of "productivity" in light of new physical limitations).

When intervening in the long-term care setting it is essential to consider the larger system in which the resident is embedded, as the system influences both the need for and the process of treatment. This requires collaborating with direct care nursing staff, social workers and activity therapists, resident councils, volunteer services, and families, and paying attention to the physical environment (see Molinari, 2000, for several useful chapters). In planning treatment, input should be solicited from the entire interdisciplinary care team and interventions may target adaptation in multiple areas of functioning. Resident outcomes also need to be assessed across disciplines. As residents' physical and psychosocial worlds are likely to be somewhat constricted, care providers may need to look for subtle signs of improvement within a narrowed range of behaviors. The issues noted above are but an outline of some of the influences that converge when an older adult has depression and dementia and finds himself living in a long-term care setting. It is those issues we have tried to address in our treatment.

A NEW TREATMENT MODEL

Drawing upon our experience in the nursing home at the Philadelphia Geriatric Center, we have developed and begun testing a new model of psychotherapeutic intervention that addresses depression in demented residents by taking into account the multiplicative factors associated with aging, dementia, and institutional life. The treatment is based on a theory of depression that acknowledges that, in the presence of a variety of risk factors, multiple losses can trigger depression among long-term care residents. A depressive syndrome can result when cognitive and affective mechanisms (e.g., negative cognitions, loneliness due to decreased social support) interact with a diminished capacity to cope with loss because of cognitive impairment. Consider the following example.

> *Mr. Clarke had an episode of major depression two years ago, and staff are now concerned that his depression is recurring. Arthritis causes him great discomfort and limits his ambulation and ability to attend social activities in the nursing home. He also has difficulty leaving the nursing home when his family wants to take him out. Simultaneously, Mr. Clarke has been told by other frustrated residents that he repeats stories often, and he has begun to doubt his ability to conduct a normal conversation without embarrassing himself. Consequently, Mr. Clarke has been spending more and more time in his room, discouraged by the "betrayal" of his body and mind. Frustrated about not being able to keep up his social contacts, he is increasingly pessimistic and despondent. Although previously Mr. Clarke was able to cheer himself up and motivate himself to stay active, he seems less able to do so now that mild cognitive impairment has emerged.*

Figure 1 depicts our theory of depression as illustrated in Mr. Clarke's circumstances. He has experienced a number of losses (mobility, social connectedness) that interact with risk factors (pain, a history of depression) to evoke depressogenic mechanisms (negative cognitions, decreased self-esteem), which lead to a depressive syndrome. In addition, Mr. Clarke's cognitive impairment limits his ability to use adaptive coping strategies that have been helpful to him in the past. This is an oversimplified example, but it demonstrates the cascade of factors that can contribute to the development of depression in the context of dementia.

Our model for the treatment of depression in dementia consists of three phases of intervention–Restore, Empower, and Mobilize–and is

FIGURE 1. An Example of the Etiology of Depression

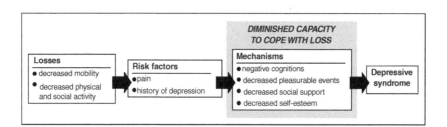

known by the acronym R-E-M. This treatment model is not a novel approach to psychotherapy with demented elders; rather, it integrates theory and technique from multiple perspectives. R-E-M incorporates aspects of cognitive, behavioral, humanistic, and psychodynamic treatments and also acknowledges the importance of a systems perspective when working in residential settings with clients who depend on others for assistance in meeting their daily needs. The treatment is sensitive to the challenges posed by normal aging, including potential sensory deficits, medical illness, medications and their side effects, and other physical needs or impairments that may influence the process of therapy (the reader is referred to Knight [1996] for a more detailed discussion of these issues). It also reflects the belief that individuals with cognitive impairment retain an ability to participate in their psychotherapeutic treatment. Furthermore, R-E-M formally incorporates some of the "nonspecific" or "common" factors that may be beneficial in psychotherapy (Floyd & Scogin, 1998; Omer & London, 1989).

In brief, nonspecific factors may be conceptualized in terms of three categories: support factors (e.g., aspects of the therapeutic alliance), learning factors (e.g., changing expectations for personal effectiveness), and action factors (e.g., practicing and achieving mastery) (Lambert & Bergin, 1994). Nonspecific factors are anticipated to have the same influence on older, depressed, and demented clients as they would on younger individuals. Which common factors are most salient, however, might be different for older clients. For example, the therapeutic relationship might be more important for older adults, who have less experience with psychotherapy and who are socially isolated because of their depression and their living situation. Expectancy effects, on the other hand, might be variable because of cognitive impairment that compromises beliefs (of both the client and the therapist) about therapy's potential effectiveness. R-E-M therapy attempts to capitalize on nonspecific factors by explicitly incorporating them into both the theoretical structure and the therapeutic activities of treatment. By doing so, R-E-M treatment highlights the healing value of the therapeutic relationship, the mediating role of the sense of self in depression, the importance of providing opportunities to gain a sense of mastery and control, and the unique challenges–both intra- and extrapersonal–of institutional life.

WHO SHOULD RECEIVE R-E-M TREATMENT?

R-E-M therapy is designed for older adults who are depressed, have mild to moderate cognitive impairment, and live in a nursing home or other institutional setting. This treatment can be used for a range of disorders in the depression spectrum, including major depression, adjustment disorder with depressed mood, and dysthymia. R-E-M is likely to be less effective with residents who have depression with psychotic features or other psychiatric symptoms more primary than depression. For instance, substance dependence might require attention before depression can be addressed effectively. Personality disorders, on the other hand, would not necessarily prevent a resident from benefiting from R-E-M treatment. The therapist would have to monitor a more complex set of factors in these cases.

R-E-M treatment recognizes the role that cognitive impairment can play in the development and exacerbation of depression. R-E-M also acknowledges that cognitive impairment poses a challenge to traditional "talk" psychotherapies. Necessary modifications might include conducting shorter and more frequent sessions, reviewing material frequently, using written materials to enhance recall, and slowing and simplifying the presentation of information (see Hausman, 1992, for additional suggestions). Individuals with mild to moderate cognitive impairment can reasonably participate in this treatment. The specific range of scores on the Mini-Mental State Examination (MMSE; Folstein, Folstein, & McHugh, 1975) for which R-E-M is appropriate remains an unanswered question. As shown in the data presented at the end of this article, we achieved some therapeutic success with a resident scoring 11 on the MMSE. More important than the MMSE score, however, is patients' minimally preserved ability to engage with the therapist and to learn and remember. Regardless of cognitive level, therapeutic interventions can be adapted to match the cognitive skills of the resident, and the phases of treatment may be emphasized differently given a resident's needs and preserved abilities.

Although some aspects of R-E-M treatment are applicable to older adults regardless of where they live, the treatment is designed for older adults in nursing homes or assisted living facilities. The treatment helps older adults cope with the challenges of living in institutional settings that may compromise their autonomy but that also provide the assistance and care required by their current life circumstances.

OVERVIEW OF R-E-M TREATMENT

R-E-M involves three overlapping phases, each of which includes a different focus of treatment. The phases are conceptualized to occur in a certain order–Restore, Empower, then Mobilize–although in practice the therapeutic work in early phases is likely to continue in subsequent phases. Likewise, the duration of each phase and the specific therapeutic activities within each will vary across residents depending on their particular needs. In this section we provide a brief introduction to the theory and practice of R-E-M in each of its phases.

Phase I: Restore

People with dementia who live in institutions are faced with a host of losses that undermine their sense of self and may lead to depression depending on their resources and stress threshold. Losses exert an influence in at least two ways. First, losses change everyday life. Having fewer social contacts, being confined to a particular room or floor, needing to be reminded how to get to the dining room, depending on others for assistance with daily needs, living with continuous pain–these everyday challenges can contribute to depression. Second, when individuals reflect on their losses they may feel inept or worthless. Even residents with cognitive impairment may be aware that they are not the same person they used to be (Kitwood, 1998). This awareness may prompt a decline in self-confidence and feelings of self-worth. In light of losses, the goals of the Restore phase are to develop a strong therapeutic relationship and instill hopefulness, to provide empathic acknowledgment of the resident's experience, and to restore a coherent sense of personal identity and self-esteem.

All theoretical traditions emphasize the importance of the therapeutic alliance, and it is no less important with individuals who have cognitive impairment. In fact, establishing an empathic relationship with the resident is one way to take advantage of preserved social and emotional capabilities (Hausman, 1992). Naturally the therapeutic relationship develops throughout one's work with a resident, but efforts to strengthen the relationship are particularly important during the initial sessions of therapy. The therapist should be warm and sincere, arrive on time for appointments, and attend to nonverbal communication (e.g., use empathic touch). The therapist can encourage positive associations with psychotherapy by meeting at the same place and time for each appointment, following a similar routine during each session, and engaging in social pleasantries. While these recommendations may seem simple, they can have a powerful impact on individuals with dementia by countering the depersonalizing effects of institutional living. Given the significance of losses, the therapist might begin therapy by taking a formal or informal inventory of them. Affirming losses communicates to the resident that they are real, that the losses are difficult to cope with, and that it is understandable that they can make a person feel depressed. During the first sessions the therapist can promote feelings of hopefulness and optimism that enhance the resident's motivation by reiterating a belief in the usefulness of therapy and the ways in which the process can be helpful to the resident.

Another goal of the Restore phase is to help residents rejuvenate their self-esteem. People tend to be happier and more resilient to stressors if they have an internalized sense of themselves as being competent, worthwhile, and valued (Tobin, 1999; Vittoria, 1998). Losses can bring about a decline in self-esteem and, more generally, a deterioration of one's sense of self (McAdams, 1993). Interventions during the Restore phase focus on establishing a sense that residents remain connected to their past and continue to have a valuable present. Strategies for bolstering self-esteem and preserving continuity of self include: encouraging reminiscence to identify significant accomplishments and capabilities, encouraging awareness and expression of emotions, and facilitating the resident's search for meaning in life.

In summary, the relationship between therapist and client is a major focus in the Restore phase. At a time when a resident may have few close confidantes, the therapist can become someone who, through word and behavior, communicates to the resident that her problems are real, that she remains a worthwhile person, and that she deserves to overcome her current psychological distress. Note that these strategies combine elements of a variety of theoretical traditions such as life review, psychoeducational and supportive counseling approaches, and existential theories. Again, R-E-M is not a novel theoretical approach but instead simply codifies beneficial aspects of other approaches and makes explicit the strategies clinicians may already use with older adults.

Phase II: Empower

The second phase of treatment builds upon the therapeutic gains from the Restore phase. As the resident's sense of self is enhanced, therapeutic attention shifts to helping the resident become an active, positive agent in her own well-being. Life in an institution can threaten feelings of efficacy and reinforce dependency (Baltes, 1988), both of which can contribute to the development and maintenance of depression. A key aspect of the Empower phase is encouraging residents to see themselves as effective, powerful people who have the skills to make their lives more satisfying. Residents should begin to feel that they have control over their lives and that they can face problems and challenges confidently. Perceptions of personal control are important for older adults' quality of life (Haley, 1983; Perlmuter & Eads, 1998), even when control revolves around the simplest of daily choices and routines. Beliefs by themselves, though, are not enough. The Empower phase also begins to put beliefs into action. Interventions in the Empower phase focus on enhancing the resident's personal control by reviewing past successes, emphasizing current strengths, investigating personal preferences, identifying current circumstances where control is possible, and encouraging the resident to state her concerns.

For example, being told by staff that he or she must take a bath may upset a resident who prefers showers and has not taken a bath since childhood. Being "pressured" to take a bath may feel like an affront to autonomy and dignity. While a bathing routine may seem like a small concern, it is important enough to some residents to cause significant emotional distress. Empower interventions in this case might involve identifying the resident's specific preferences, exploring fears about raising the issue with staff, and engaging in role-play exercises of how to approach staff and communicate requests.

When residents feel competent and in control, they are more prepared to make changes in their lives. However, being ready does not mean one knows the best way to make changes. Therefore, a second goal of the Empower phase is to assist the resident in determining how to create changes that will enhance well-being. Therapy focuses on facilitating the development of effective coping strategies to bring about the desired changes. Problem identification, brainstorming, and assertiveness and social skills training are some of the techniques that may be utilized in this phase. As another example, a resident may need assistance being assertive with family members about the frequency, timing, duration, and content of their visits to the facility. Empower strategies may involve coming to an understanding of past family dynamics as well as skills training to help the resident express concerns in an adaptive manner. Naturally, some of these strategies may be more appropriate for residents with mild cognitive impairment, while other strategies which are less cognitively demanding (e.g., relaxation training with prompts provided) may be appropriate for individuals with more severe decline.

Phase III: Mobilize

By this phase of treatment the resident should be experiencing an improvement in mood and related functioning. This final phase takes advantage of those gains by bringing in the institutional environment to support the resident's progress. This phase borrows from systems theories of psychology in recognizing the significance of the broad social (and physical) context in which the residents live. In order to be realistic and effective in implementing Mobilize interventions, it is essential that the therapist perform an assessment of the resident's environment early in the treatment process. An assessment, formal or informal, should address the organizational, physical, and psychosocial environments of the long-term care facility, including its philosophy, staffing patterns, emphasis on personalization, environmental features, staff attitudes, and activity programming (see Rader, 1995, for a fuller description of the assessment process). This information should guide the therapist throughout the treatment process, but is especially important for developing Mobilize strategies. The Mobilize phase of treatment has two goals: activate the resident and activate the environment.

Activating the resident involves helping him make the positive changes that were identified during the preceding phases. The therapist helps the resident initiate and follow through on plans. Here the resident is *doing* what was previously *learned*. There may be many ways in which residents are prepared to take a more active role in promoting their own well-being, and in this phase of treatment the therapist helps launch these efforts. For instance, a resident who had many friends earlier in his life may express a desire to meet new people and develop more meaningful relationships in the nursing home. In the Empower phase of treatment the therapist and resident may have worked on identifying the qualities the resident seeks in a potential friend, exploring possible opportunities for meeting others, and engaging in social skills training for how to approach and get to know other residents in the nursing home. During the Mobilize phase of treatment the resident actively engages in efforts to reach out to others and develop new relationships. The therapist provides encouragement and support as the resident initiates these new behaviors, and failures and successes may be processed together.

The reality of life in an institution and life with cognitive impairment, however, is that residents often need assistance first to make and then to sustain beneficial changes. Moreover, with ongoing cognitive decline residents may not be able to initiate activities, recall therapeutic strategies, or organize their behavior in optimal ways. Consequently, the other task in this phase of treatment is to engage resources in the environment around the resident to compensate for declining abilities. These resources include family members (those living nearby as well as those farther away), peers and friends both inside and outside the institution, and staff at *all* levels in the institution. Staff involvement is perhaps the most important because of the large role staff plays in a resident's day-to-day life. Collaboration with staff may involve talking with them informally about the resident (while respecting confidentiality), including them in therapy sessions, providing education about dementia and depression, listening to their perspective on the resident, empathizing with the challenges of their job, and reinforcing their positive contributions to the resident's well-being.

As an example, the therapist and resident may have identified that attending religious services enhances the resident's sense of continuity and meaning in life, improves her mood, and provides an outlet for social interaction. However, the resident routinely forgets to attend and also needs physical assistance to reach the room where services are held. Mobilize interventions might involve enlisting the staff to remind the resident prior to services each week; informing the resident in writing when services are being held; requesting a volunteer to transport the resident if staff are not available to do so; or asking family members to visit at the time of the services so they can both remind and transport the resident. Ideally, these solutions will be written in the resident's care plan so that the intervention and persons responsible are communicated to all staff. Documentation also provides a basis for accountability.

Actively including family and staff in treatment efforts is different from the approach taken in some traditional psychotherapies, but it echoes the family-focused approaches adopted in the treatment of other disorders (e.g., McFarlane, 1997). Furthermore, this broad approach is essential to helping residents with cognitive impairment because the system in which residents live–the people and the place, at all levels–can be an important element in the onset of depression, just as it can be an important element in its relief.

By enlisting environmental resources, Mobilize efforts anticipate a time in the resident's life when the more insight-oriented and self-initiated efforts of the Restore and Empower phases might be less effective because of advancing cognitive impairment. Practices that are put into place during the Mobilize phase are meant to benefit the resident beyond the end of therapy. As treatment progresses in this phase, the therapist's role becomes less central in the change process and eventually may involve primarily monitoring, follow up, and interventions aimed more at the staff than the resident. It should be noted that these activities may no longer meet definitions for "psychotherapy" as stated by Medicare and other third-party payers, and therefore may not be reimbursable. In fact, reimbursement challenges brought to the fore the importance of objective evaluation and documentation of treatment effectiveness, which led to our efforts to manualize the treatment.

CONSTRUCTION OF THE TREATMENT MANUAL

The development of R-E-M treatment was undertaken by a core team of four clinical geropsychologists (the authors). We also relied on extensive input from a larger group of psychologists who provided psychotherapeutic services to older adults at the Philadelphia Geriatric Center (PGC). We held 16 focus groups with these psychologists in order to learn about their clinical experiences and obtain feedback on the theoretical propositions constructed by the core team. These semi-structured discussions included topics such as how to educate clients about psychotherapy, barriers and obstacles to effective treatment, techniques for working with older adults who have dementia, and strategies for interfacing with the long-term care system. We also discussed in detail the theoretical underpinnings of R-E-M treatment. After each focus group, the core team met to review discussions and clarify the theoretical basis of the treatment.

Meanwhile, we conducted an extensive literature review to locate previous work related to psychotherapy with older adults, psychotherapy for depression, psychotherapy outcomes, mental health issues in older adults, dementia, and nursing home environments. Treatment manuals used by other researchers also were reviewed (Gallagher & Thompson, 1981; Luborsky, 1984; Shear & Weiner, 1996; Teri, Logsdon, & Uomoto, 1991; Thompson, Gallagher-Thompson, & Dick, 1995; Weissman & Klerman, 1988). Sections of the first version of our treatment manual were circulated among all of the PGC geropsychologists, and they provided written feedback on the organization and content of each chapter.

When the focus groups and first version of the treatment manual were complete, we conducted a preliminary trial of the treatment (see below). At the conclusion of the trial we asked each participating clinician for feedback on the manual. We also distributed the manual to five geropsychologists at different sites across the country. A face-to-face meeting was held with three of these reviewers at the annual meeting of the Gerontological Society of America in 1999. The other two clinicians provided written feedback. Comments from all of those sources have been integrated into a second version of the treatment manual that consolidates some chapters and expands the examples and case vignettes. A draft of the 122-page treatment manual is available from the authors.

PRELIMINARY TREATMENT TRIAL

A pilot trial of R-E-M treatment was conducted with three nursing home residents with comorbid depression and dementia. Residents were approached about participation, provided with information about the project, and asked to sign an informed consent form. Verbal assent was obtained from a relative of the patient. (The ethical issues, including confidentiality, of doing psychotherapy with individuals who live in long-term care settings and individuals who have dementia are complex and beyond the scope of this article. Readers are referred to Kane and Caplan [1990] and Moye [2000] and, in this collection, three articles by Duffy, Norris, and Zehr). Exclusion criteria were as follows:

1. MMSE score less than 10,
2. medical status that would interfere with participation in 16 sessions of psychotherapy,

3. commencement of antidepressant medication less than four weeks prior to referral to the project.

Residents who had been on antidepressant medication longer than four weeks were included. Residents and their psychiatrist agreed to maintain the current dosage of antidepressant medications during the trial unless an adjustment was deemed necessary, in which case the resident would be dropped from the trial (but allowed to continue psychotherapy). No residents required adjustment to their antidepressant medications during their participation. Characteristics of the three residents who participated in the trial appear in Table 1.

A geriatric psychiatrist conducted structured diagnostic interviews (SCIDs) to confirm initial diagnoses made by a referring psychiatrist and psychologist. Qualified residents then were seen for 16 sessions of individual R-E-M psychotherapy (one resident was seen for two additional sessions to ease termination), usually twice per week for 20-30 minutes per session. Weekly group supervision was used to review progress in therapy, discuss the application of the treatment, and solicit therapists' suggestions about how the treatment might be modified. These sessions also provided an opportunity for peer supervision.

TABLE 1. Characteristics of Residents in the Treatment Trial

| Characteristic | Resident | | |
	#1	#2	#3
Age	93	85	90
Gender	Female	Male	Female
Race/ethnicity	White	White	White
Marital status	Widowed	Separated	Widowed
Education	High school	High school	High school
History of depression	No	No	Yes
Baseline diagnosis (from SCID)	1) Major depressive disorder 2) Dementia NOS	1) Major depressive disorder 2) Dementia of the Alzheimer's type	1) Major depressive disorder 2) Dementia due to multiple etiologies
Baseline MMSE	20/30	23/30	21/30
Termination diagnosis (from SCID)	1) Major depressive disorder 2) Dementia NOS	1) Dementia of the Alzheimer's type	1) Depression NOS 2) Vascular dementia
Termination MMSE	22/30	23/30	11/30

Assessments were performed at baseline, session #3, session #10, session #16, one month after termination, and two months after termination. Sessions 1, 3, 10, and 16 were videotaped to enable us to perform behavioral observations of affective expression in session and to allow the rating of treatment adherence/competence. Ratings of affective expression also were collected outside of these sessions (between 1-4 hours after each session) by behavioral observation of the residents in their rooms or on the nursing home unit. To incorporate multiple perspectives, assessment information was obtained from the therapists, the residents, and staff members. Assessments were wide ranging and included evaluations of mood, self-esteem, cognitive functioning, functional impairment, agitation, observed emotion, progress toward treatment goals, therapeutic alliance, and treatment adherence/competence. A select few of the measures are reported here.

Ratings of resident mood made by the psychiatrist on the Cornell Scale for Depression in Dementia (Alexopoulos, Abrams, Young, & Shamoian, 1988) appear in Figure 2, in which higher scores indicate more severe depression. For all three residents, scores decreased during the trial and were at their lowest point at termination. A slight increase in depressive symptoms was seen at follow-up, suggesting the importance of some form of continuation of treatment to prevent relapse (Fishback & Lovett, 1992). It should be noted that one resident still had symptoms sufficient to meet criteria for major depressive disorder at termination. This resident remained melancholic and pessimistic but was less self-derogatory at the end of treatment.

Figure 3 includes ratings of functional status made by the nurse manager on the Multi-Dimensional Assessment Instrument (MAI; Lawton, Moss, Fulcomer, & Kleban, 1982) on which higher scores signify greater functional impairment. Although we expected that improvement in mood might motivate residents to participate more actively in their self-care, this was not the case among these residents. Scores on the MAI did not change significantly during the course of treatment. Of course, R-E-M treatment is not designed to target functional abilities. Moreover, the MAI itself addresses objective capability (e.g., "Can the resident dress herself?"), not more subtle factors such as motivation (e.g., "Is the resident interested in getting dressed? Does she help with dressing tasks?") which might be more likely to be influenced by a psychological intervention. Still, that there was no decline in functional status might itself be considered a positive outcome (i.e., maintenance of abilities), although comparison with a control sample would be necessary to validate this claim.

FIGURE 2. Scores on the Cornell Scale of Depression in Dementia (Psychiatrist Rated)

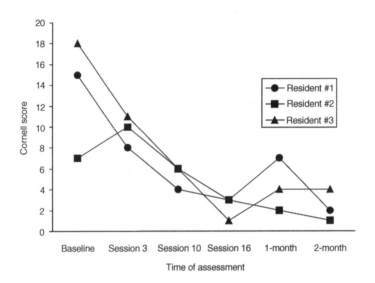

Ratings made by the nurse manager on the Activity Participation Scale (Van Haitsma, Lawton, Kleban, Klapper, & Corn, 1998) appear in Figure 4. Higher scores signify more frequent occupation and engagement in meaningful activity. Overall, participation increased during the course of treatment, although this trend was variable. Residents became more engaged in social and solitary activities and were less likely to sit alone in their room or sleep, although, as with mood, longer-term gains were inconsistent.

Therapist ratings of resident progress toward treatment goals appear in Figure 5. We used a goal attainment scaling approach (Kiresuk & Sherman, 1968) in which therapists and residents agreed on individualized treatment goals at the start of therapy and then periodically evaluated progress toward these goals. Because of their cognitive impairment the residents needed guidance in this process, but all were able to reach a consensus with their therapist about important goals. For example, resident #1 and her therapist agreed that one treatment goal would be to initiate at least three phone calls to her family or friends each week. Resident #3 and her therapist, in the context of addressing social isolation, decided that identifying people with whom she has enjoyable rela-

FIGURE 3. Scores on the Multidimensional Assessment Instrument (MAI; Nurse Rated)

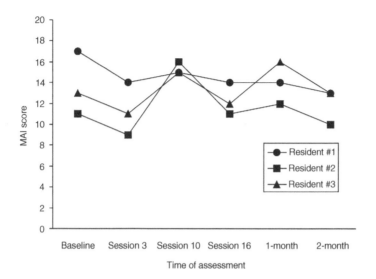

FIGURE 4. Scores on the Activity Participation Scale (APS; Nurse Rated)

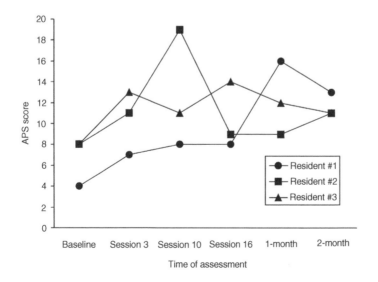

tionships would be one of her treatment goals. Therapists made ratings of progress at the end of each session on a seven-point scale ranging from -3 (severe decline, psychiatric hospitalization required) to $+3$ (extreme success, surpassing the treatment goals). Figure 5 includes the summed ratings made on the three treatment goals that were developed for each resident. For all residents we observed progress toward treatment goals. Near the end of therapy two of the residents experienced a slight decline in their progress, although they remained well in the "goal attained" range of the scale.

In the final figure, Figure 6, we provide some documentation of treatment adherence by showing the number of Mobilize interventions that were administered over the course of therapy, judged by a rater watching videotapes of the therapy sessions. As expected, Mobilize interventions increased in frequency during the therapy, reflecting the shift of therapeutic attention from relationship building to empowerment and then mobilization.

In summary, in this very preliminary trial of R-E-M treatment we observed some success at ameliorating depression among long-term care residents with dementia. More extensive evaluation is needed, particularly regarding the value of continuation treatment to prevent relapse. Nonetheless, this trial helped affirm the feasibility of the treatment, fo-

FIGURE 5. Therapist Ratings of Resident's Progress Towards Treatment Goals

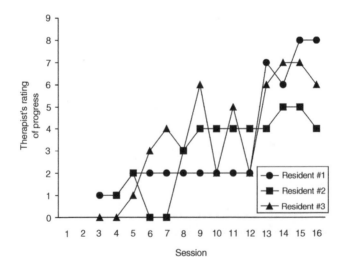

FIGURE 6. Frequency of Mobilize Interventions

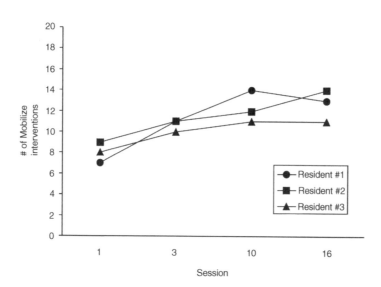

cus the theory behind the treatment, improve the treatment manual to make it more responsive to the needs of clinicians, and learn about the complexities of conducting a clinical trial. We hope to pursue a larger-scale evaluation of R-E-M treatment and are interested in collaborating with other clinicians and researchers.

CONCLUSION

Clinicians who work with older adults in long-term care settings know that residents, regardless of their cognitive status, often struggle with maintaining positive mood in the face of multiple losses and the realities of institutional living. Although practitioners recognize that psychotherapy is a useful component to a care plan, acknowledgement by administrators and reimbursement organizations of psychotherapy's benefits has been elusive. R-E-M psychotherapy is a new, manualized treatment especially suited to residents living in a long-term care setting who are diagnosed with dementia and depression. The treatment focuses on restoring residents' sense of self-esteem and dignity, empowering them to make positive changes in their lives, and mobilizing them and their care environment to support their long-term mental health. A preliminary empirical evaluation of the treatment provided encouraging results, and a larger trial with a revised and expanded treatment manual is being prepared. R-E-M offers promise as an effective psychotherapeutic treatment for long-term care residents with depression and dementia.

REFERENCES

Alexopoulos, G. S., Abrams, R. C., Young, R. C., & Shamoian, C. A. (1988). Cornell Scale for Depression in Dementia. *Biological Psychiatry, 23*, 271-284.

Baltes, M. M. (1988). The etiology and maintenance of dependency in the elderly: Three phases of operant research. *Behavior Therapy, 19*, 301-319.

Borson, S., & Fletcher, P. M. (1996). Mood disorders. In W. E. Reichman, & P. R. Katz (Eds.), *Psychiatric care in the nursing home* (pp. 67-93). New York: Oxford University Press.

Dobson, K. S., & Shaw, B. F. (1988). The use of treatment manuals in cognitive therapy: Experience and issues. *Journal of Consulting & Clinical Psychology, 56*, 673-680.

Feil, N. (1989). Validation: An empathic approach to the care of dementia. *Clinical Gerontologist, 8*, 89-94.

Feil, N. (1992). Validation therapy with late-onset dementia populations. In G.M.M. Jones, & B.M.L. Miesen (Eds.), *Care-giving in dementia: Research and applications* (pp. 199-218). London: Tavistock/Routledge.

Fielden, M. A. (1990). Reminiscence as a therapeutic intervention with sheltered housing residents: A comparative study. *British Journal of Social Work, 20*, 21-44.

Fishback, J. B., & Lovett, S. B. (1992). Treatment of chronic major depression and assessment across treatment and follow-up in an elderly female. *Clinical Gerontologist, 12*, 31-40.

Fisher, J. E., & Carstensen, L. L. (1990). Behavior management of the dementias. *Clinical Psychology Review, 10*, 611-629.

Floyd, M., & Scogin, F. (1998). Cognitive-behavior therapy for older adults: How does it work? *Psychotherapy, 35*, 459-463.

Folstein, M. F., Folstein, S. E., & McHugh, P. R. (1975). "Mini-Mental State": A practical method for grading the cognitive state of patients for the clinician. *Journal of Psychiatric Research, 12*, 189-198.

Frey, D. E., Kelbley, T. H., Durham, L., & James, J. (1992). Enhancing the self-esteem of selected male nursing home residents. *Gerontologist, 32*, 552-557.

Gallagher, D., & Thompson, L. W. (1981). *Depression in the elderly: A behavioral treatment manual*. Author: The University of Southern California Press.

Gallagher, D. E., & Thompson, L. W. (1983). Effectiveness of psychotherapy for both endogenous and nonendogenous depression in older adult outpatients. *Journal of Gerontology, 38*, 707-712.

Haley, W. E. (1983). Behavioral self-management: Application to a case of agitation in an elderly chronic psychiatric patient. *Clinical Gerontologist, 1*, 45-52.

Hausman, C. (1992). Dynamic psychotherapy with elderly demented patients. In G.M.M. Jones, & B.M.L. Bere (Eds.), *Care-giving in dementia: Research and applications* (pp. 181-198). London: Tavistock/Routledge.

Health Care Financing Administration: Medicare and Medicaid: Requirements for Long Term Care Facilities, Final Regulations. *Federal Register, 56*(187), 48865-48921, September 26, 1991.

Jones, S. N. (1995). An interpersonal approach to psychotherapy with older persons with dementia. *Professional Psychology: Research and Practice, 26*, 602-607.

Kane, R. A., & Caplan, A. L. (Eds.) (1990). *Everyday ethics: Resolving dilemmas in nursing home life*. New York: Springer.

Kasl-Godley, J., & Gatz, M. (2000). Psychosocial interventions for individuals with dementia: An integration of theory, therapy, and a clinical understanding of dementia. *Clinical Psychology Review, 20*, 755-782.

Katona, C. L. E., Hunter, B. N., & Bray, J. (1998). A double-blind comparison of the efficacy and safety of paroxetine and imipramine in the treatment of depression with dementia. *International Journal of Geriatric Psychiatry, 13*, 100-108.

Katz, I. R., Simpson, G. M., Curlik, S. M., Parmelee, P. A., & Muhly, C. (1990). Pharmacologic treatment of major depression for elderly patients in residential care settings. *Journal of Clinical Psychiatry, 51*, 41-47.

Kiresuk, T. J., & Sherman, R. E. (1968). Goal attainment scaling: A general method for evaluating comprehensive community mental health programs. *Community Mental Health Journal, 4*, 443-453.

Kitwood, T. (1998). *Dementia reconsidered*. Philadelphia: Open University Press.

Knight, B. G. (1996). *Psychotherapy with older adults*. Thousand Oaks, CA: Sage.

Lambert, M. J., & Bergin, A. E. (1994). The effectiveness of psychotherapy. In A. E. Bergin, & S. L. Garfield (Eds.), *Handbook of psychotherapy and behavior change* (pp. 143-189). New York: John Wiley & Sons.

Lappe, J. M. (1987). Reminiscing: The life review therapy. *Journal of Gerontological Nursing, 13*, 12-16.

Lawton, M. P., Moss, M. S., Fulcomer, M., & Kleban, M. (1982). A research and service oriented multilevel assessment instrument. *Journal of Gerontology, 37*, 91-99.

Lazarus, L. W., Groves, L., Gutmann, D., Ripeckyj, A., Frankel, R., Newton, N., Grunes, J., & Havasy-Galloway, S. (1987). Brief psychotherapy with the elderly: A study of process and outcome. In J. Sadavoy, & M. Leszcz (Eds.), *Treating the elderly with psychotherapy: The scope for change in later life* (pp. 265-293). Madison, WI: International Universities Press.

Lebowitz, B. D., Pearson, J. L., Schneider, L. S., Reynolds, C. F., Alexopoulos, G. S., Bruce, M. L., Conwell, Y., Katz, I. R., Meyers, B. S., Morrison, M. F., Mossey, J., Niederehe, G., & Parmelee, P. (1997). Diagnosis and treatment of depression in late life: Consensus statement update. *Journal of the American Medical Association, 278*, 1186-1190.

Lewinsohn, P. M., Steinmetz, J. L., Antonuccio, D., & Teri, L. (1984-1985). Group therapy for depression: The Coping with Depression course. *International Journal of Mental Health, 13*, 8-33.

Luborsky, L. (1984). *Principles of psychoanalytic psychotherapy: A manual for supportive-expressive treatment*. New York: Basic Books.

Luborsky, L., Mark, D., Hole, A. V., Popp, C., Goldsmith, B., & Cacciola, J. (1995). Supportive-expressive dynamic psychotherapy of depression: A time-limited version. In J. P. Barber, & P. Crits-Christoph (Eds.), *Dynamic therapies for psychiatric disorders (Axis I)* (pp. 13-42). New York: Basic Books.

Majeroni, B. A., & Hess, A. (1998). The pharmacologic treatment of depression. *Journal of the American Board of Family Practice, 11*, 127-139.

Marson, D. C. (1995). Modified self-management therapy for treatment of depression and anxiety in a nursing home resident. *Clinical Gerontologist, 16*, 63-65.

McAdams, D. P. (1993). *The stories we live by: Personal myths and the making of the self.* New York: William Morrow.

McFarlane, W. R. (1997). Fact: Integrating family psychoeducation and assertive community treatment. *Administration and Policy in Mental Health, 25*, 191-198.

Mega, M. S., & Cummings, J. L. (1996). Dementia. In W. E. Reichman, & P. R. Katz (Eds.), *Psychiatric care in the nursing home* (pp. 40-56). New York: Oxford University Press.

Molinari, V. (Ed.) (2000). *Professional psychology in long term care.* New York: Hatherleigh Press.

Moye, J. (2000). Ethical issues. In V. Molinari (Ed.), *Professional psychology in long term care* (pp. 329-348). Long Island City, NY: Hatherleigh Press.

Omer, H., & London, P. (1989). Signal and noise in psychotherapy: The role and control of non-specific factors. *British Journal of Psychiatry, 155*, 239-245.

Parmelee, P. A., Katz, I. R., & Lawton, M. P. (1989). Depression among institutionalized aged: Assessment and prevalence estimation. *Journal of Gerontology, 44*, M22-M29.

Parmelee, P. A., Katz, I. R., & Lawton, M. P. (1991). The relation of pain to depression among institutionalized aged. *Journal of Gerontology, 46*, P15-P21.

Parmelee, P. A., Katz, I. R., & Lawton, M. P. (1992). Depression and mortality among institutionalized aged. *Journal of Gerontology, 47*, P3-P10.

Perlmuter, L. C., & Eads, A. S. (1998). Control: Cognitive and motivational implications. In J. Lomranz (Ed.), *Handbook of aging and mental health: An integrative approach* (pp. 45-67). New York: Plenum.

Rader, J. (1995). Assessing the external environment. In J. Rader & E. M. Tornquist (Eds.) *Individualized dementia care: Creative, compassionate approaches* (pp. 47-82). New York: Springer.

Rattenbury, C., & Stones, M. J. (1989). A controlled evaluation of reminiscence and current topics discussion groups in a nursing home context. *Gerontologist, 29*, 768-771.

Reynolds, C. F. (1997). Treatment of major depression in later life: A life cycle perspective. *Psychiatric Quarterly, 68*, 221-246.

Reynolds, C. F., Frank, E., Perel, J. M., Imber, S. D., Cornes, C., Morycz, R. K., Mazumdar, S., Miller, M. D., Pollock, B. G., Rifai, A. H., Stack, J. A., George, C. J., Houck, P. R., & Kupfer, D. J. (1992). Combined pharmacotherapy and psychotherapy in the acute and continuation treatment of elderly patients with recurrent major depression: A preliminary report. *American Journal of Psychiatry, 149*, 1687-1692.

Sadavoy, J., & Robinson, A. (1989). Psychotherapy and the cognitively impaired elderly. In D. K. Conn & A. Grek (Eds.), *Psychiatric consequences of brain disease in the elderly: A focus on management* (pp. 101-135). New York: Plenum Press.

Schleifer, S. J., Keller, S. E., Bond, R. N., Cohen, J., & Stein, M. (1989). Major depressive disorder and immunity: Role of age, sex, severity, and hospitalization. *Archives of General Psychiatry, 46*, 81-87.

Shear, M. K., & Weiner, K. (1996). *Emotion focused treatment (EFT) for panic disorder.* Author: Department of Psychiatry, University of Pittsburgh School of Medicine.

Streim, J. E., & Katz, I. R. (1996). Clinical psychiatry in the nursing home. In E. W. Busse, & D. G. Blazer (Eds.), *The American psychiatric press textbook of geriatric psychiatry* (pp. 413-432). Washington: American Psychiatric Press.

Taragano, F. E., Lyketsos, C. G., Mangone, C. A., Allegri, R. F., & Comesana-Diaz, E. (1997). A double-blind, randomized, fixed dose trial of fluoxetine vs. amitriptyline in the treatment of major depression complicating Alzheimer's disease. *Psychosomatics, 38,* 246-252.

Teri, L., & Gallagher-Thompson, D. (1991). Cognitive-behavioral interventions for treatment of depression in Alzheimer's patients. *Gerontologist, 31,* 413-416.

Teri, L., Logsdon, R., & Uomoto, J. (1991). *Treatment of depression in patients with Alzheimer's disease.* Author: University of Washington School of Medicine.

Teri, L., Logsdon, R. G., Uomoto, J., & McCurry, S. M. (1997). Behavioral treatment of depression in dementia patients: A controlled clinical trial. *Journals of Gerontology, 52B,* P159-P166.

Teri, L., & McCurry, S. M. (1994). Psychosocial therapies. In C. E. Coffey & J. L. Cummings (Eds.), *The American Psychiatric Press textbook of geriatric neuropsychiatry* (pp. 662-682). Washington, DC: American Psychiatric Press.

Teri, L., & Reifler, B. V. (1987). Depression and dementia. In L. L. Carstensen & B. A. Edelstein (Eds.), *Handbook of clinical gerontology* (pp. 112-119). New York: Pergamon.

Teri, L., & Uomoto, J. (1991). Reducing excess disability in dementia patients: Training caregivers to manage patient depression. *Clinical Gerontologist, 10,* 49-63.

Teri, L., & Wagner, A. (1992). Alzheimer's disease and depression. *Journal of Consulting and Clinical Psychology, 60,* 379-391.

Thompson, L. W., Gallagher, D., & Breckenridge, J. S. (1987). Comparative effectiveness of psychotherapies for depressed elders. *Journal of Consulting and Clinical Psychology, 55,* 385-390.

Thompson, L. W., Gallagher-Thompson, D., & Dick, L. (1995). *Cognitive-behavioral therapy for late life depression: A therapist manual.* Palo Alto, CA: Older Adult and Family Center, Veterans Affairs Palo Alto Health Care System.

Tobin, S. S. (1999). *Preservation of the self in the oldest years.* New York: Springer.

Unterbach, D. (1994). An ego function analysis for working with dementia clients. *Journal of Gerontological Social Work, 22,* 83-94.

Van Haitsma, K. S., Lawton, M. P., Kleban, M., Klapper, J. A., & Corn, J. A. (1998). Methodological aspects of the study of streams of behavior in dementing illness. *Alzheimer Disease and Associated Disorders, 11,* 228-238.

Vittoria, A. K. (1998). Preserving selves: Identity work and dementia. *Research on Aging, 20,* 91-136.

Weissman, M. M., & Klerman, G. L. (1988). *Interpersonal counseling (IPC) for stress and distress in primary care settings.* Author.

Wragg, R. E., & Jeste, D. V. (1989). Overview of depression and psychosis in Alzheimer's disease. *American Journal of Psychiatry, 146,* 577-587.

Zweig, R. A., & Hinrichsen, G. A. (1996). Insight-oriented and supportive psychotherapy. In W. E. Reichman, & P. R. Katz (Eds.), *Psychiatric care in the nursing home* (pp. 188-208). New York: Oxford University Press.

Use of Positive Core Memories in LTC: A Review

Lee Hyer, EdD, ABPP
Steve Sohnle, PsyD
Dan Mehan, PhD
Amie Ragan, PhD

SUMMARY. We present a treatment for residents of LTC facilities, positive core memories (PCMs). Initially, we discuss memories at later life, research areas that have considered memory and memory repair at later life–issues of cognitive aging, reminiscence, self-defined memories (and other methods that highlight the PCM), memory repair methods, and the pragmatics of memory therapies that have been applied in LTC. We do this to highlight the PCM. We then present results of a small study on the use of PCMs. Finally, we endorse this form of therapy and place it in the context of treatment in LTC. In the appendix we present our treatment manual. *[Article copies available for a fee from The Haworth Document Delivery Service: 1-800-HAWORTH. E-mail address: <getinfo@haworthpressinc.com> Website: <http://www.HaworthPress.com> © 2002 by The Haworth Press, Inc. All rights reserved.]*

KEYWORDS. Positive core memories, reminiscence, long-term care, cognitive behavior therapy

---

Lee Hyer, Steve Sohnle, Dan Mehan, and Amie Ragan are affiliated with the University of Medicine and Dentistry of New Jersey.

[Haworth co-indexing entry note]: "Use of Positive Core Memories in LTC: A Review." Hyer, Lee et al. Co-published simultaneously in *Clinical Gerontologist* (The Haworth Press, Inc.) Vol. 25, No. 1/2, 2002, pp. 51-90; and: *Emerging Trends in Psychological Practice in Long-Term Care* (ed: Margaret P. Norris, Victor Molinari, and Suzann Ogland-Hand) The Haworth Press, Inc., 2002, pp. 51-90. Single or multiple copies of this article are available for a fee from The Haworth Document Delivery Service [1-800-HAWORTH, 9:00 a.m. - 5:00 p.m. (EST). E-mail address: getinfo@haworthpressinc.com].

INTRODUCTION

Mental health in long-term care (LTC) facilities has remained a challenge for healthcare providers. In fact, changes in the mental health care of residents of LTC facilities have altered measurably since OBRA-87 (Hawes et al., 1997). These changes have come in many forms, including the identification and typing of mentally ill residents (Phillips et al., 1997), improvements in psychotropic drug usage (e.g., Llorente et al., 1998), better management of dementia patients (Beck, 1996; Mintzer, 1995), endorsements on the importance of special care units (Frisoni, Gozzetti, Bignamini, Vellas, Berger, Bianchetti, Rozzini, & Trabucchi, 1998), an increased emphasis on quality of life (e.g., Binstock & Spector, 1997), and training of caregivers (e.g., Teri, 1999). Reviews too have noted many problems in LTC facilities, but also extol the promising direction and challenge (e.g., Beck, Rossby, & Baldwin, 1991; Lombardo et al., 1995; Mintzer, 1995).

Knowing that mental health services are essential to LTC, it would seem that more activity would have emerged on the care of these residents. In fact, little has been done to carefully apply psychological interventions in these settings. Five years after OBRA, only 19% (Smyer, Shea, & Streit, 1994) or 29% (Shea, Smyer, & Streit, 1993) of residents received mental health care at least once during their total length of stay in a nursing home. In a recent study of 899 such homes (Reichman et al., 1998), the need for and strengths of psychiatrists' services were assessed. In line with other studies, Directors of Nursing rated the need for such services as considerably greater than that actually provided. Conversely, it appears that when psychological or psychiatric interventions are applied, results are encouraging (e.g., Bakke et al., 1994; Rapp, Flint, Hermann, & Proulx, 1992).

In this paper we present a treatment for residents of LTC facilities and present data on a comparison evaluation. Our treatment addresses positive core memories (PCMs). To put this work in proper context, we first address the issue of memory at later life, what seems to be involved in memory repair, and consider "remembering" at later life in various forms. We then present results of a small study on the use of PCMs. Last, we discuss the need for this form of therapy and place it in the context of care in an LTC facility. In the Appendix we present our treatment manual.

Memory at Later Life

Remembering is best viewed as encompassing three steps: acquisition/encoding, retention or storage, and retrieval. Problems can occur at any of these phases (Loftus & Davies, 1984). Deptula, Singh, and Pomara (1993) noted that age-related decline is attributable to many factors, including cognitive loss, insufficient use of cognitive strategies, lack of practice in performing cognitive tasks, and decreased emotion.

As an overview, Schacter (1998) described seven "sins" of memory. Three of the sins included different types of forgetting. They are: *transience*, which involves decreasing accessibility of information over time; *absent-mindedness*, which includes inattention and shallow processing (which contributes to poor future recall); and *blocking* which refers to the temporary inaccessibility of information that is stored in memory. The next three involve *inaccuracy*, misattribution involving the attribution of a memory to an incorrect source; *suggestibility*, referring to the implanting of memories as a result of leading questions or a poor context; and *bias*, which refers to retrospective distortions and unconscious influences that are related mostly to current knowledge. Last, there is *persistence*. These are events that we cannot forget. Over the years memory can be "abused" by any of these. Older people abuse them all.

The autobiographical memory by itself is not well studied (Brewer, 1986). Despite this, the extant research on autobiographical memories suggests that recall is highly prone to both error or bias (Litz et al., 1996). We know, for example, that recollections are not simply a direct retrieval of information from a decaying archive. Memory degrades with time. Later memory relies on heuristic strategies to reconstruct recalled events. Recall for particular episodes can be disrupted by interference from other similar events that occur perhaps before or after the episode and by important schemata that may describe a prototypical class for the event (for example, medical event). Memories also are distorted by post-event information and by the extent to which events are rehearsed (Loftus & Davies, 1984). Additionally, memories are also altered by the respondent's preconceived notions about the event or by their attempts to salvage self-esteem by creating a similarly coherent and consistent narrative. It seems best to conceive of memory as a process, as reconstructive, and as not reproductive.

That said, most autobiographical memories for major life events are relatively accurate (Hyer & Sohnle, 2001). Among the elderly, events such as marriages, deaths, births, holidays, injury and illness, education, family, war, love, love affairs and recreation sports are remembered with relative authenticity (Cohen & Faulkner, 1989). Current findings suggest that highly salient or stressful events may be recalled more accurately than information associated with laboratory studies of memory (Goodman, Hirschman, Hepps, & Rudy, 1991). It has been shown also that "reconstructions" of major personal events represent "relatively minor editorial revisions that bring the past more in line with a person's current self-image" (Ross & Conway, 1986, p. 139). The "fundamental integrity" of most major autobiographical recollections is the rule (Barclay, 1986). It may be that what a person remembers depends on existing mental schema. Once a particular event is integrated under the existing mental schemes, some distortion occurs as the schema alters the memory to fit its needs. Degradation then occurs only to a small extent with normal aging.

Memory at later life for normal aging is often seen as impoverishment, beset with an over-generalized coding proclivity, sometimes lack of effort or distraction. Problems, however, involve the working memory and the problems in retrieval, other memory tasks or storage problems. When forced to engage in elaboration or semantic processing of information during the study phase of the free-recall task, the performance of normal elderly adults, but not that of dementia patients, is even enhanced (Craik & Rabinowitz, 1984; Schacter, 1987). This finding suggests that severe episodic memory impairment of dementia is not primarily due to difficulties in retrieving information but rather reflects a deficit in consolidation or storage.

In addition, there is little evidence that people with diagnosable psychological disorders are more likely to experience memory distortions than other people. It appears that confidence in one's memories is moderately related to demonstrated accuracy of recall. This may be related to health problems–associated with higher levels of memory complaints and problems (Cutler & Grams, 1988). Overall a partial reconstructive perspective of autobiographical memory is more accurate than the espousal of either literal reproduction or substantial alterations in adult memories of childhood events. We mention too that research ("fuzzy trace theory"), which has demonstrated that "gist" memories and "verbatim" memories are functionally independent and have different properties, may ultimately have an impact on how autobiographical memory is conceptualized (Reyna, 1995; Reyna & Brainerd, 1995).

People who are depressed may be an exception. Depressed people have recall processes that are askew. A systematic bias is evidenced by depressed patients who consistently overestimate the occurrence of negative events, often in a summary fashion. Difficulties in retrieving specific autobiographical memories also may contribute to emotional disturbance in several ways (Williams, 1992). Depressed patients cannot retrieve specific memories about themselves, for example, and often experience difficulty benefiting from cognitive therapy because of the emotional quality of these autobiographical memories. An inability to retrieve specific positive memories may even blunt positive affect (Rubin, 1986). Interestingly, it has been reported (Schacter, Kihlstrom, Kihlstrom, & Berren, 1989) that autobiographical memories are difficult to retrieve only in depressed patients with histories of abuse and not in those without history of abuse.

Finally, it must not be forgotten that the unburdening of a memory is always a function of the psychosocial and cultural influences as much or more than of storage and retrieval systems. The person who listens and the cultural context make a difference in the story told. In essence, the autobiographical memory is imperfect and involves a "constant process of selection, revision, and reinterpretation" (Brewin, Andrew, & Gotlib, 1993, p. 85). (See Table 1 for a summary of issues of memory at later life as well as the autobiographical memory.)

FACTS OF THE AGING MEMORY

Decline of Functional Memory:

- Working memory can be a problem as processing speed slows.
- Memory is a process–a combination of stored facts and imaginings. It is constructed rather than reproduced.
- Problems of retrieval are evident in normal aging.
- Recall of a given event ("target event") is obscured by interference from similar events occurring since the target (unique events are recalled more readily and accurately).
- Schemas play a role in "deciding" what is remembered.
- Objective facts are stored better than subjective ones.
- Recollection is not simply decaying material.
- Although not necessarily accurate, once formed, memories are hard to eliminate.
- Inaccuracy is both random and systematic (as in a systematic bias with depressed people).

Facts of the Autobiographical Memory:

- Memories for major life events are relatively accurate.
- Metacognition, the awareness of cognitive functioning, remains intact.

TABLE 1. Study Groups

SUBJECT	Diagnosis	Age	Months in Home	POMS Pre Test	POMS Post Test	Mood Scale Pre Test	Mood Scale Post Test
			PCM GROUP				
P1	Dep	69	24	77	−9	9	0
K	Dep	81	37	43	47	7	5
P2	Dep	90	42	123	17	14	4
G	Adj	78	103	31	−3	8	6
C	Adj	79	66	33	12	3	2
B1	Adj	81	31	12	−4	2	0
K	Dep	76	16	74	18	11	3
B2	Adj	76	18	19	–	4	–
S	Adj	84	17	17	14	7	2
K	Dep	83	16	42	37	8	5
			CONTROL GROUP				
D	Dep*	74	49	42	46	9	12
B1	Adj**	79	35	5	4	2	3
V	Adj	81	24	10	13	1	0
R	Adj	84	12	–	−14	–	5
E.	Dep	75	11	76	−10	8	4
F	Dep	68	22	101	77	12	13
J.	Dep	77	45	114	127	8	13
W1	Adj	78	68	6	1	3	4
W2	Dep	73	62	58	45	8	9
W3	Adj	85	42	9	12	2	1
B2	Dep	84	32	96	93	12	15
S	Dep	71	19	61	20	3	0

* Major Depression ** Adjust Disorder

- There is little evidence that even people with diagnosable psychological disorders are more likely to experience memory distortions than other people.
- The age at which an event occurs, its intensity (affective), complexity and distinctive features influence the construction of a memory.
- Emotion appears to facilitate the accuracy of recall of central details. High emotion appears to slow forgetting.

REMEMBERING AT LATER LIFE

We address several features of remembering at later life. Memory is often a critical source of information about self. It is also a form of therapy. Knight (1986) points out: "All psychotherapy involves some elements of life review" (pp. 127-8). Bengston, Reedy and Gordon (1985) see as an essential task of old age the preservation of a coherent, consistent self in the face of loss and the threat of loss. These authors suggest that, because human resources are so scant and the task is so pressing, life review primarily is used to create an image intended to be believed, a myth to achieve a feeling of stability, justifying the narrator's life. For these authors typically the older person becomes the protagonist in a drama that is worth telling or having lived for. Fact and fantasy commingle in life review (Lewis, 1973). This has been labeled narrative truth (Hermans & Hermans-Jansen, 1995).

We highlight several renditions of "positive" life review offerings as lead-in to our method. We also consider memory work in nursing homes and highlight the group work in this setting.

REMINISCENCE

For over three decades reminiscence and life review have been applied to older populations. This approach has also been used in many venues by many sorts of professionals including educators and community education workers (Duffin, 1992; Lawrence and Mace, 1992) and oral historians (Samuel, 1975; Thompson, 1988; White, 1980), to name two. Additionally, several writers have recently suggested that men and women communicate and tell stories differently (Gray, 1992; Tannen & Aries, 1997). Theories that provide understanding for the use of reminiscence as a therapeutic technique have largely evolved from Erikson

(1982) or Butler (1963). In fact, Butler extended Erikson's views by postulating that reminiscing is a way of achieving ego integrity. Several studies have extended Butler's ideas about life review: the relationship between chronological age and talk about the past (e.g., Marshall, 1980, 1986), the link between reminiscence and life review (e.g., Coleman, 1974), and the benefits of reviewing the past (e.g., Wallace, 1992).

Unfortunately, studies conducted on the efficacy of reminiscing as a therapy have yielded conflicting results; some promising (e.g., Fry, 1983), some less so (Parsons, 1983), and some mixed (Sherman, 1981). For the most part studies have found some positive effect of the use of reminiscence in socialization but not for others, as in self-esteem (Cook, 1991).

Remembering also seems related to diagnosis. The relationship between depression and reminiscence results in more negative memories (e.g., Segal, Williams, & Teasdale, 2001), and those with anxiety interrupt the reminiscing and have fewer positive memories (Hyer & Sohnle, 2001). Additionally, personality can be a mediator in the expression of reminiscence. In an early paper Fry and Ogston (1971) found a "delicate balance" with the personality traits of sentience and openness and the use of reminiscence. Molinari et al. (in press) too found that older people who were more extraverted had higher openness, and older people who were more open indulged in more problem solving. In another study Cully, LaVoie, and Gfeller (2001) assessed 77 older adults on the relationship between frequency and functions of reminiscence, personality styles, and psychological well-being. Canonical correlation analysis indicated that individuals with negative psychological functioning reminisce as a way to refresh bitter memories, reduce boredom, and prepare for death. Conversely, those individuals high on extraversion and openness reminisce for purposes of teaching and conversing.

Reminiscence and life review share some similarities. Both involve memory and recall, are characterized by a free-flowing process, can access happy or sad memories, and are implemented predominantly with the elderly. Both can be therapeutic. They are distinct in that life review is a more integrity-seeking process–one that is more intense, focuses on issues across the life span, is a more psychoanalytically-based theory, involves a more active role on the part of the clinician, and often targets painful memories and issues. The focus is usually internal, and integrity is the desired outcome.

Reminiscence is not just remembering. Webster (see Molinari) identified several components of reminiscence: boredom reduction, death preparation, identity/problem solving, intimacy maintenance, bitterness revival, and teach/inform. Viney (1993) also speculated on the types of remembering. He held that elders' stories were in three dimensions–self-limiting, self-empowering, and age-related. Perhaps the most accepted taxonomy of reminiscence is that given by Wong and Watt (1991). They distinguish six different forms of reminiscence: integrative, instrumental, narrative, transmissive, escapist and obsessive. Greater amounts of integrative and instrumental reminiscence characterized people (in their study) who were better adjusted. The former conveys a sense of meaning and coherence to the life-story. The latter recalls past attempts to cope with difficult situations and thus may contribute to an enhanced subjective perception of control. The less well-adjusted people were characterized by greater amounts of obsessive reminiscence. Molinari and Reichlin (1985) place life review in a context of mourning within a stage model (reorganization of relationship to lost others; obsessive recounting and reiteration; reflection on self-absorption; and the end result, learning to relinquish what has been lost).

Evidence exists that integrative reminiscing increases during transitions, bereavement, and medical setbacks (e.g., hospitalization) (Rybarczyk & Bellg, 1997). Integrative reminiscence is not necessarily natural and most often requires encouragement. When it does occur, it is appealing and probably helpful for the person: "Narration confers spellbinding power on older people" (Garland, 1994, p. 23).

Reminiscence seems to be a naturally flowing event for older people that often can be utilized to place memories in the context of the total person. Often this is for pleasure, to experience and enhance self-image. It can also be for self-understanding. If older people are offered more opportunity to shape the content and process of their reminiscing, at least some may choose very different events and activities from those available in a pre-packaged form. Fry (1983) conducted such an experiment. As a result of adopting a more reflexive and open approach to the selection of reminiscence content, it is possible that older people may come to radically different conclusions both about which past experiences they regard as important and also about the sense they now make both of their history and their present lives.

Reminiscence is satisfying then in itself without necessarily leading to psychological insight. Stories help everyone to develop and maintain a sense of identity, provide everyone with guidance by which to live, enable everyone to place order on the sometimes chaotic events, and give everyone more power than they might otherwise have. Additionally as we noted above, the very processes characteristic of life review are found in psychotherapy.

Additionally, in old age the keeper of the archives can suspend reality requirements just long enough to make it work. Reality can be bent because "who would know." Older people, for example, often see themselves in over-valued views: The family was not always that good; the 15-year-old was not that graceful; the house not that nice. If very old age is reached, truth is altered in even different ways. The old-old tend to give up the quest for a youthful self-concept: They feel old, become less introspective, and focus on the practicalities of death. The old-old change the idea of being old to one of being a person, about which there are many things, including life's accomplishments. And, across all this time, the state of self follows health status: All things being equal, if you are healthy and active, so are your memories.

There are skeptics. In general, the application of memory work in this way has been criticized for:

1. a lack of clarity on how to apply procedures;
2. over-reliance on clinical judgment of how to use it;
3. little scientific validity;
4. limited utility in handling specific problems (such as adapting to organic dysfunction);
5. a lack of clarity about how this therapy might benefit persons with reactive depression, or conflict with other therapies.

In one important study Coleman (1994) studied older people and identified two verbal and two non-verbal groups. Of the two verbal groups, the first group enjoyed talking and were well adjusted. For them creative reminiscence was easy. The second group were the compulsive reminiscers. This group talked a lot but often brooded and were very troubled. The task of their therapy was to see (in a cognitive behavioral way) how justified and rational the past was. In the two non-verbal groups, one of these saw no value in talking. They were simply too busy. It was viewed as best to leave this group alone because they were well adjusted. The fourth group, on the other hand, did not want to reminisce because the past was so bad. These were chronically depressed. Again, the use of grief therapy and perhaps cognitive behavioral therapy can be applied to these people. Many people in later life do not normally talk: A life review is also hard work.

Older adults then review a greater number of life events than younger adults. They do this for more "mature" reasons. They desire to be heard, perhaps to alter previous experiences, but mostly to "tell it again." This is good news for therapists.

LIFE EXPERIENCE INTERVIEW

Rybarczyk and Bellg (1997) noted what has been clear for many clinicians, the difference between a narrative and reminiscence (facilitative) approach. Where the narrative approaches are used almost exclusively by psychotherapists, primarily allied health professionals working with older adults use reminiscence. Reminiscence therapists work within an existing life story, to help the client get new perspectives on current issues or to facilitate the integration of unresolved past events and choices. Narrative therapists focus on changing or "rewriting" dysfunctional stories about the self. Narrative therapists often address parts of the life story that deal with those aspects of the self. Reminiscence workers address positive aspects of the individual's life story, focusing on the past exclusively.

Rybarczyk and Bellg (1997) advocated two approaches with memories. In one, the "counselor" takes on a primarily supportive role, approaching the older adult as a "wise teacher" (Burnside, 1978) and focusing mainly on rose-colored memories. Choosing what to emphasize is the point at which narrative therapists attempt to intervene. This life experience interview (LEI) is based on the premise that the positive feelings elicited by simple reminiscing will effectively counteract anxiety triggered by a stressful situation. The LEI covers topics that frequently evoke positive emotions, such as childhood activities, family traditions, adventures in adolescence and early dating experiences. No direct effort is made to guide the interviewee toward remembering events that relate to successful coping. The goal of reminiscence interviewing is not to gather information but to create a positive psychological experience for the storyteller. To put this more succinctly, "The process is more important than the product" (Rybarczyk & Bellg, 1997).

The other approach is more active. The therapist plays a more active role in trying to help the client integrate memories into a cohesive and positive life story. Reminiscence is stretched, focusing on challenges successfully met, underscoring the strengths and resources used to meet those challenges, and summarizing key lifelong attributes at the close of the interview. The overall goal is to increase interviewees' awareness of their coping strengths and resources by directing them to recall past successes in meeting life's challenges. Rybarczyk and Bellg (1997) endorsed such an approach at least 25% of the time. Regardless of the approach, results were very encouraging for patients on medical units (Rybarczyk & Bellg, 1997). Subjects who participated in either of the two reminiscence interviews experienced a decrease in anxiety after the interview, compared with an increase in anxiety among the subjects who received the present-focus interview or no interview. Life event interviews led to substantial reductions in the anxiety that patients commonly experience when facing an invasive medical procedure and were as effective as the relaxation techniques and interventions widely used in health care settings to alleviate stress. Finally, when an interview focuses on past experiences of successful coping, it leads to a positive change in the patient's appraisal of his or her coping abilities and resources.

SELF DEFINING MEMORY

Self defining memories (SDMs) (Singer & Salovey, 1993) are not the structural factors of memory but are key episodes in the person's life, the declarative and episodic memories of the self. They are central to one's past, interpretation of the present, and possible predictions of the future. They represent two ends of the narrative continuum, that part that preserves the affective immediacy of the moment and the one that subserves the power of the summarized account.

SDMs then are prototypical and exemplify the person. These memories are a blend of summary/single event memory, a blend of abstraction and immediacy, a blend of reason and emotion, centrally located in the psychic structure of the person's life as to represent the person in a single event. Through this integration of both the single event and the summarized memory, the purpose and meaning of the person is fleshed out. They represent what Loevinger (1976) and McAdams (1993) noted as the highest stage of ego development. They are the most representational meaning in self definition the person has about themselves. Singer and Salovey (1993) note:

> In rare moments in our lives during a long intimate conversation with someone from whom we seek understanding or validation . . . as part of a . . . group or after an excruciating painful defeat or loss, we might step back and demand such narrative unity from our memory. What each of these moments has in common . . . is a commitment to articulate one's knowledge of one's self, to ask and attempt to answer the question 'who am I.' (p. 160)

Singer and Salovey (1993) believe then that each person carries around a unique collection of autobiographical memories, a sort of carousel of slides of the most important personal memories of life, witnessed by their vividness and intense affect. These memories are snapshots that represent core slides to which people return repeatedly. In a moment they convey representation and instantiation. These images crystallize characteristic interests, motives, and concerns of the individual into a short hand moment. Recently, Singer (2001) noted that SDMs are most characteristic when integrated into the personality or schema of the person. These memories contain many false recollections and embellishments, thereby not having to pass the test of historical truth.

IMPORTANCE AND CONSISTENCY OF THE LIFE STORY

Story repair or story enhancement is based on a few basic assumptions:

1. that development of identity involves the construction of a life story;
2. that psychopathology is caused by or the result of life stories gone awry;
3. that psychotherapy is primarily an exercise in "repairing stories" (Howard, 1991).

If so, potential changes in human existence may be connected to our memories. We are what we remember ourselves to be.

We are meaning-making beings, striving to punctuate, organize and anticipate the interactions with the world. People construe meaning, organized around a core set of assumptions, which both govern the perception of life events and organize behavior in relation to these. These are almost "choiceless events" in a choosing environment. Therefore, account making, the telling and knowing of our stories, allows us to know again our own issues and obtain social validation. Thomas Moore (1994) noted: "Storytelling is an excellent way of caring for the soul. It helps us see the themes that circle in our lives, the deep themes that tell the myths we live. It would take only a slight shift in therapy to focus on the storytelling itself rather than on its interpretation."

McAdams (1984, 1985, 1987, 1990, 1993, 1996) views the life story as an internalized and evolving narrative of the self that incorporates the reconstructed past, perceived present, and anticipated future. It can be seen as the core self. For a given person, the life story is the narrated product of the characteristic way in which the person arranges and reacts to life and creates themes. It confers unity and purpose by constructing a more or less coherent, followable, and vivifying story that integrates the person into society in a productive and generative way. The person then has a purposeful self-history that explains how time connects (within the person), yesterday, today and tomorrow. The fact that storied accounts are embedded in the discourse of everyday life does not mean then that these stories are ephemeral.

Additionally, the life story seems to mimic what we know about change across the life span, constancy and change. Gerontologists have been concerned with such issues as the stability of change in the self-concept. Caspi and Roberts (1999) indicated that there is both homotypic continuity and heterotypic continuity, both genotype and phenotype consistency of the person across the years. Bengston, Reedy and Gordon (1985) concluded from their review of studies of the relationship between aging and the self-concept that most aspects of the self-concept show substantial stability in structure and mean levels of positive and negative attributes. That the self-concept remains stable as individuals age is substantiated by a number of investigators (McCrae & Costa, 1988; Ryff, 1991). Ryff (1989), for example, used a cross-sectional design, and found that older people rate themselves as being comparable to or better than younger people on most of her aspects of well-being. Furthermore, she reported that elderly subjects' actual and ideal selves approximated each other more closely than younger individuals' selves.

The focus on life also shifts over time. Older people appear to be generally satisfied at later life in terms of most dimensions of the self. Self integration becomes transformational as the life course transits (at later life) to generativity. Like a legal reading of the U.S. Constitution, the self changes ever so slightly over time to meet the needs of the new time. The structure of the self, then, is not predetermined or simply passed down from one generation to the next. This is why the autobiographical memory is so important. It is by the story, the storied self, that the clinician can understand what the individual is like, who they are as people. The person eventually arrives at a self, more or less in final form, through the synthesis of contradictory identifications and greater individualization, and through the turbulence of adolescence, through the transition periods of adulthood, through middle-life and eventually into older age.

MEMORY IN LTC FORMAT

Nursing homes have a tradition in group activities, such as remotivation and reminiscence. Lichtenberg and Duffy (2000) noted that group therapy works very well in LTCs. They noted that the logistics are relatively easy to arrange, that groups are welcomed by residents as interesting activities, and that they serve as "vital settings" to nourish individual friendships. Groups can be used with Alzheimer's patients (Reichlin, 1999), around special themes such as men's issues (Sprenkel, 1999), women's issues (Crose, 1999), and reminiscence (Molinari, 1999). They are also well adapted to using expressive therapy methods, such as art (Hanser, 1999) and music (Weiss, 1999).

Addressing a nursing home population, Molinari (1999) noted that life review is an active grappling with the past. This is a special form of reminiscence that has an evaluative component. It is both intrapersonal and interpersonal. He outlined a group format for the application of reminiscence. He suggested that the clients should be verbal, motivated, psychologically introspective, and not be in an acute crisis. By implication the patient cannot be compromised cognitively. Sessions should be weekly, 60-90 minutes. Closed groups are preferred. It is most helpful to have a topic for each session. The first session should have a set agenda in which the leader instructs the group about differences between life review and reminiscence. Members should be asked to prepare for each session. The leader should be ready to empower the content and not the process of the group. The leader should also be ready to distract clients who are negative responders. If the person becomes mired in depressive recriminations (that positive experiences cannot be elicited), the facilitator should alter the treatment. In fact, a "reminiscence crisis" can ensue which may need to subside before the therapy can continue.

At its base the goal of reminiscence is to deconstruct an individual's perspective on life into a more positive and coherent narrative emphasizing strengths, successes, and lessons learned. It is intended to integrate disparate aspects of the self, to assist in current problem solving, and to bequeath a legacy. This can be performed in LTC in a group format.

CONCLUSION

There are many unanswered questions about the autobiographical memory. How does the narrative assert an influence in the coding, storage, and retrieval of data, at any moment in time but also across the life-span? In fact, the issue is really "how does the aging process influence self and vice versa." How this occurs is unknown; that it does is indisputable. Interestingly, results of research have yet to show whether a person's developmental stage contributes to specific types of problems, such as memory loss or damage to the self-concept (Cole & Putnam, 1992; Kendall-Tackett et al., 1993).

We note too that the efficacy of remembering as it applies to psychotherapy has mixed reviews. It does seem to have a favorable influence in terms of increased self-esteem, reduced agitation, and higher ego-integrity (Taft & Nehrke, 1990). It has also been found to be ineffective but benign where more substantive outcomes are applied. However this is viewed, the individual does something that can be important. He/she assesses the past to achieve a better understanding of self and to establish a sense of meaning for one's life. Often it is to solve present problems and cope with losses in the current situation (Sherman, 1991). It can be said that there is something in the memory that facilitates change. Often too, this is not the case and the memory creates problems. This occurs in the minority of occasions, however.

COGNITIVE BEHAVIOR THERAPY (CBT) AT LATER LIFE

During the past 20 years the use of cognitive behavioral therapy (CBT) has proven effective with later life depression (Beutler et al., 1987; Gallagher & Thompson, 1981, 1982; Hyer, Swanson et al., 1990; Hyer, Swanson, & Lefkowitz, 1990; McCarthy, Katz, & Foa, 1991; Thompson, Gallagher, & Breckenridge, 1987) and anxiety (Scogin, Rickard, Keith, Wilson, & McElreath, 1992). Treatment gains have also been maintained (Gallagher-Thompson, Hanley-Peterson, & Thompson, 1990). The same result applies (but to a lesser extent) with interpersonal psychotherapy (Reynolds et al., 1999).

Early (e.g., Garfield, 1978; Smith et al., 1980) and more recent (e.g., Gallagher-Thompson & Thompson, 1995; Gatz, 1994; Gatz, Popkin, Pino, & VandenBos, 1985; Knight, 1996; Schramke, 1997) reviews also indicate that psychotherapy in general with older people is effective. This applies to several pathological areas (see Zeiss & Steffen, 1996), combined with medication (Gerson et al., 1999; Thompson, Gallagher, Hansen, Gantz, & Steffen, 1991), or applied to more difficult problems (Hanley-Peterson et al., 1990; Thompson, Gallagher, & Czirr,

1988). Interestingly, these encouraging findings apply to older adults with cognitive decline (Snow et al., 1999; Wetherell, 1998).

More recent reviews have focused on depression. In their narrative review of six cognitive and behavioral therapies on depressed elderly, Morris and Morris (1991) indicated that older adults could benefit from these treatments. Robinson et al. (1990) in their review on the efficacy of psychotherapeutic treatment for depression found for a high effect size (d = .73, N = 37). Scogin and McElreath (1994) conducted a meta-analysis of 17 studies on the efficacy of psychosocial treatments for geriatric depression. The overall effect size was notable (d = .78, N = 23). Effect sizes above about .6 indicate that the mean treated client was better off than 75% of the clients in control conditions. This result is in accordance with other reviews (Smith et al., 1980; Engels et al., 1993; Prioleau et al., 1983).

In one important review Engels and Vermey (1997) conducted a meta-analysis of 17 studies on the efficacy of nonmedical (psychological) treatments for depression in the elderly. Results revealed that treatment was more effective than placebo or no treatment. Effects were equal for mild and severe depression and proved to be maintained over time. The mean effect size (d = .61) was adequate. Results apply less to group therapy (Smith et al., 1980; Robinson et al., 1990; Scogin et al., 1992).

A series of studies by Gallagher and Thompson (Gallagher & Thompson, 1981, 1982; Thompson, Gallagher, & Breckenridge, 1987) are especially important because treatments were carefully outlined, procedures manualized, patients randomized, measures specified, and patients followed for a year. The CBT elements that represent the core of the approach to therapy and are presumably some of the reasons for its demonstrated effectiveness are as follows: collaborative therapeutic relationship, a focus on a small number of clearly specified goals, emphasis on change, psychoeducational, length of therapy contracted and linked to goals, agenda set at each meeting, skill training (cognitive, behavioral, and interpersonal), and health status. Additionally, moderating conditions exist. Factors that may contribute negatively to treatment outcome include the extent to which symptoms are endogenous rather than reactive, the presence of a personality disorder, severity of PTSD/depression at the onset of treatment, patient expectancies or commitment for change, and the patient's role in the development of the therapeutic alliance (Gallagher & Thompson; 1983; Gaston, Marmar, Thompson, & Gallagher, 1988; Gaston, Marmar, Gallagher & Thompson, 1989; Marmar, Gaston et al.).

PCM STUDY

A small study on PCMs (positive core memories) in a CBT (cognitive behavioral therapy) format was conducted. We applied a 12 session group therapy to residents of an LTC facility.

Subjects

We selected 24 consecutively referred residents for psychological care. Referrals were made as a result of team meetings consisting of a social worker, physician, nurses, CNAs, and rehabilitation medicine personnel. All residents were having problems in the facility. The average age was 75, time in the home was 40 months, and the diagnoses were either major Depressive Disorder or Adjustment Disorder as a result of depression or anxiety. There were no differences between the groups on these indices (see Table 1).

There were 12 members in the control group that were tested pre or post: there were 10 members of the PCM group. Two members of the PCM group elected not to partake: two members also did not receive the POMS at the beginning of the treatment. There is various missing data for the control group also. Reasons for the missing data ranged from brief hospitalizations, flu, home visits, and in one case, a quarantine. One member of the PCM group died at the end of the group and could not be re-tested.

Residents were randomly separated into two groups. The PCM group received a 12-session treatment that focused on positive core memories. The control group received standard milieu therapy that included psychopharmacological treatment or the usual activities of the LTC facility, or both. No psychotherapy was given to that group.

Measures

The residents were given the POMS (Profile of Mood Scale) (McNair, Lorr, & Droppleman, 1992) and the Mood Scale (short form of the Geriatric Depression Scale). They were given these pre- and post-therapy. The POMS was given because it subserves different mood areas (tension-anxiety, anger-hostility, vigor-activity, fatigue-inertia, confusion-bewilderment). We used a composite score for the pre- and post-test. The Mood Scale is a 15-item short form of the GDS. Both scales have been used on various populations and have acceptable psychometrics.

Treatment

The PCM treatment is a structured therapy that attempts to optimize 1-3 positive core memories and apply these in the person's day-to-day life. A manual was used to elicit the PCMs, massage these and develop coping mechanisms (see Appendix).

In brief, the group had 12 sessions.

Session 1:   introduction and testing
Sessions 2-4:   identification of 1-3 PCMs
Sessions 5-10: consolidation of PCMs in the day-to-day events
Sessions 11-12: termination and relapse considerations

The key intervention involved the group facilitators obtaining and elucidating PCMs from each participant. When one or two were found that met the criteria (see Appendix), it (they) was used as the central feature of the therapy for that person. Lessons from the memory were extracted and they were applied to the daily activities of the resident. Positive coping strategies were developed.

RESULTS

Because of the small numbers, missing data, and skewed distribution of the data, we calculated a Wilcoxon Signed Rank Test on pre-test POMS and post-test POMS scores for both the control and the experimental groups. This test was not significant for the control group. However, the test was significant for the experimental group. These results indicate that POMS scores did not change significantly in the control group. In contrast, POMS scores were reduced from pre-test to post-test in the experimental group, suggesting that the PCM treatment affected mood states positively.

Similarly, the Wilcoxon Sign Test was applied to pre-test and post-test Mood Scale scores for both the control and the experimental groups. As before, this test was not significant for the control group. However, the test was significant for the experimental group. These results indicate that depression level as measured by the Mood Scale did not change significantly in the control group, but was reduced from pre-test to post-test in the experimental group. This suggests that the PCM treatment was effective in reducing depressive symptoms.

More directly, it can be seen that in the PCM group only one subject got worse (and that was only by a small amount) on the POMS. This was in contrast to the control group where four subjects declined over time. On the Mood Scale, seven declined in the control group; no one got worse in the PCM group. Additionally, subjects were universally satisfied with the PCM group, whether due to attention or the effects of the treatment. A case is presented at the end to explicate the process of the PCM therapy.

CONCLUSION

Mental health needs are modal in LTC settings. Research has shown that they are essential for the care of residents, that these needs are special, and that they are wanting (Borson, Reichman et al., 2000). Unfortunately, we do not yet know with any certainty what constitutes the best care at what cost for what residents. We do not yet know how to match residents with good care.

This review and study attempted to highlight and emphasize the importance of autobiographical memory in LTC. This may be an activity that can make a difference in the quality of life. Zarit, Dolan, and Leitsch (1998) remind us that the real task in the care of a resident in an LTC facility is one that builds on the competencies of the resident with a supportive, yet challenging environment that maximizes the potential for prolonged functioning. "Excess disability" can be the norm in many facilities; the application of "psycho"-therapies may be reconsidered. The application of the PCM may especially be apt. This review is suggestive of this.

The application of the PCM met many of the concerns outlined by Molinari regarding care in an LTC facility. The method was in a group format, was structured with active therapists, identified "memories" that were enjoyable and easy to rediscover. Residents were encouraged to be verbal, were motivated, and were encouraged to be psychologically introspective. The focus was both intrapersonal and interpersonal. Several of the members also had minor cognitive problems and did well.

In addition, many of the features of previously studied memory methods were in place. Memories were identified and had many of the characteristics of SDMs, self-defining memories. Narrative repair occurred in several cases, even with the "good" memories. When negative memories were in evidence, the resident was able to "repair" these with the PCM rules. PCM queries assisted in the formation and identification of the person, the agent of the PCM. About this process, David Gutmann says:

> Through reminiscence, older persons may creatively revisit their past to conform to some sustaining personal myth; by finding or constructing the threads that connect the current self with some

past, idealized self, they can overcome the devastating experience of discontinuity and self, they can overcome the devastating experience of discontinuity and self-alienation. (1990, p. 43)

One other feature of reminiscence was in evidence also. There was an integrative quality to the reminiscing. Eventually most residents realized a sense of meaning and coherence to the life-story. They were able to see that past attempts at coping with problems, for example, "really" created a sense of control. For the most part memories were enjoyable by themselves. Additionally, in this study the core features of CBT were in place. Residents "felt" safe and motivated in this collaborative process. The therapists were active and stayed on task. Assimilative queries were the norm as the agency of the person was unearthed.

Theories of memories (e.g., Adler, 1927) place emphasis on individual memories at the center of the understanding of the life goals and the central conflicts of the person. The addition here is that the autobiographical memory or everyday memory is also important in the understanding and meaning of the person in the context of their life. Recent data are suggesting that both the explication of positive memories change in well-being. This may result in the formation of a more coherent narrative that both provides integration and improves working memory (Carpenter, 2001). This may be especially important at later life and for frail elders. Here we saw that the positive memories can be influential in mood.

Treatment studies are often difficult in LTC facilities as the residents are frail and the staff is reluctant to assist to partake. The brief study had many limitations. It was a study on a sample of convenience with small numbers. It was held in one setting and had no attention control. It also had missing data.

That said, every effort was made to conform to the treatment protocol and the treatment was provided in a "real world" setting. The measures appeared relevant and the participants became involved and enjoyed the experience. The application of this method was appealing to the therapists also.

From a critical perspective, the issue is raised as to how did these memories translate into better moods. In fact, Molinari and Reichlin's (1985) questions have not yet been answered: What is the optimal time, ideal frequency of sessions, type of content? What processes lead to what kind of desirable (or undesirable) outcome? How do older people benefit? Does the nature of life review vary according to age? How is life review experienced from the client's perspective? How does life review affect reactions to ongoing problems? Is reminiscence important in the process of aging?

Waxing poetic, it may be said that one's memories may indeed be one's poetry. They are "the thick autonomy of memory . . . not easily penetrable by the direct light of consciousness; resistant to conceptual understanding; sedimented in layers; and having 'historical depth' " (Casey, 1999). This is an immersion in the temporal, meaningful environment. Memory is not confinement of information within the person. For Casey, memory is already everywhere: "Memory is . . . more porous than enframing."

In effect, the memory is the person, especially in an LTC facility. The "mind" does not capture memories by internalizing exact replicas of experienced events. Rather, people find themselves surrounded by layers of meaning, awareness, and reinterpretation that are affected by social and cultural constructions. Casey also spoke of memory as commemoration, the act of intensified remembering. Commemoration signifies solemnity and seriousness, the importance and centrality of certain memories. It is a purposeful, transformative process. It is more than "doing again": It is "remembering through." Memory is a process. Memory then is best thought of in this sense as a verb, not a noun, reconstructive, not reproductive. At a higher level, memory is a symphony of meaning seeking. Robert Kegan (1989) in *The Evolving Self* writes: "The activity of being a human being is the activity of meaning making. This lasts until death."

Answers to critical issues remain in doubt. But, as the understanding of LTC issues evolves, chiefly the clarification of critical issues or best practices regarding psychotherapy or quality of life, perhaps this study will give pause on the use of an easily accessible and natural aspect of being–the memory. Indeed, whatever one's view, the use of memory or life review is part of every psychotherapy.

REFERENCES

Adler, A. (1933). The earliest memories of childhood. *Internationale Zeitschrift Fuer Individual-Psychologie, 11*, 81-90.

Arbuthnott, K. & Arbuthnott, D. (1999). The best intentions: Prospective remembering in psychotherapy. *Psychotherapy 36*(3), 247-256.

Bakke, B., Kvale, S., Burnes, T., McCarten, J., Wilson, L., Maddox, M., & Cleary, J. (1994). Multicomponent interventions for agitated behavior in a person with Alzheimer's disease. *Journal of Applied Behavioral Analysis, 27*, 175-176.

Barclay, C. R. (1993). Remembering ourselves. In Graham M. Davies & Robert H. Logie (Eds.), *Memory in everyday life. Advances in psychology, 100* (pp. 285-309). Amsterdam, Netherlands: North-Holland/Elsevier Science Publishers.

Beck, C., Rossby, L., & Baldwin, B. (1991). Correlates of disruptive behavior in cognitively impaired elderly nursing home residents. *Archives of Psychiatric Nursing, 5*(5), 281-291.

Bengston, V. L., Reedy, M. N., & Gordon, C. (1995). Aging and self-conceptions. In J. E. Birren & K. W. Schaie (Eds.), *Handbook of the psychology of aging.* New York: Van Nostrand Reinhold.

Bengtson, V. L. & Schaie, K. W. (Eds). (1999). *Handbook of theories of aging.* New York: Springer.

Beutler, L.E., Scogin, F., Kirkish, P., Schretlen, D., Corbishley, A., Hamblin, D., Meredith, K., Potter, R., Bamford, C.R., & Levenson, A.I. (1987). Group cognitive therapy and alprazolam in the treatment of depression in older adults. *Journal of Consulting and Clinical Psychology, 55,* 550-557.

Binstock, R. H. & Spector, W. D. (1997). Five priority areas for research in long-term care. *Health Services Research, 33*(5), 715-730.

Borson, S., Reichman, W. E., Coyne, A. C., Rovner, B., & Sakauye, K. (2000). Effectiveness of nursing home staff as managers of disruptive behavior: Perceptions of nursing directors. *American Journal of Geriatric Psychiatry, 8*(3), 251-253.

Brewin, C. R., Andrews, B., & Gotlib, I. H. (1993). Psychopathology and early experience: A reappraisal of retrospective reports. *Psychological Bulletin, 113*(1) 82-98.

Brink, T. (1979). *Geriatric psychotherapy.* New York: Human Sciences Press.

Burnside, I. (1996). Life review and reminiscence in nursing practice. In J. E. Birren & G. M. Kenyon (Eds.), *Aging and biography: Explorations in adult development.* (pp. 248-264). New York: Springer Publishing Co., Inc.

Carpenter, S. (2001). A new reason for keeping a diary. *Monitor on Psychology, 32*(8), 68-70.

Casey, J. (1999). *The half-life of happiness.* New York: Vintage.

Caspi, A. & Roberts, B. W. (1999). Personality change and continuity across the lifetime. In L. A. Pervin & O. P. John (Eds.), *Handbook of personality: Theory and research, 2nd ed.* (pp. 300-326). New York: Guilford.

Clarke, K. M. (1996). Change processes in a creation of meaning event. *Journal of Consulting & Clinical Psychology, 64*(3), 465-470.

Cohen, G. & Faulkner, D. (1989). The effects of aging on perceived and generated memories. In L. W. Poon & D. C. Rubin (Eds.), *Everyday cognition in adulthood and late life.* (pp. 222-243). New York: Cambridge University Press.

Cole, P. M. & Putnam, F. W. (1992). Effect of incest on self and social functioning: A developmental psychopathology perspective. *Journal of Consulting & Clinical Psychology, 60*(2), 174-84.

Coleman, P. G. (1994). Reminiscence within the study of ageing: The social significance of story. In J. Bornat (Ed.), *Reminiscence reviewed: Perspectives, evaluations, achievements* (pp. 8-20). Bristol, PA: Open University Press.

Cook, E. (1991). The effects of reminiscence on psychological measures of ego integrity in elderly nursing home residents. *Archives of Psychiatric Nursing, 5,* 292-298.

Craik, F. I. & Rabinowitz, J. C. (1985). The effects of presentation rate and encoding task on age-related memory deficits. *Journal of Gerontology, 40*(3), 309-315.

Crose, R. (1999). Addressing late life developmental issues for women: Body image, sexuality and intimacy. In M. Duffy (Ed.), *Handbook of counseling and psychotherapy with older adults* (pp. 57-76). New York: Wiley.

Cully, J. A., LaVoie, D., & Gfeller, J. D. (2001). Reminiscence, personality, and psychological functioning in older adults. *The Gerontologist, 41*(1), 89-95.

Deptula, D., Singh, R., & Pomara, N. (1993). Aging, emotional states, and memory. *American Journal of Psychiatry, 150(3),* 429-34.

Duffin, P. (1992). *Then and now: A training pack for reminiscence work.* Manchester: Gatehouse Books.

Engels, G. I., Garnefski, N., & Diekstra, R. F. W. (1993). Efficacy of rational-emotive therapy: A quantitative analysis. *Journal of Consulting & Clinical Psychology, 61*(6), 1083-1090.

Engels, G. I. & Vermey, M. (1997). Efficacy of nonmedical treatments of depression in elders: A quantitative analysis. *Journal of Clinical Geropsychology, 3*(1), 17-35.

Erikson, E. (1975). *Life history and the historical movement.* New York: Norton Press.

Frisoni, G. B., Gozzetti, A., Bignamini, V., Vellas, B. J., Berger, A. K., Bianchetti, A., Rozzini, R., & Trabucchi, M. (1998). Special care units for dementia in nursing homes: A controlled study of affectiveness. *Archives of Gerontology & Geriatrics, 6,* 215-224.

Fry, P. S. (1983). Structured and unstructured reminiscence training and depression among the elderly. *Clinical Gerontologist, 1*(3), 15-37.

Fry, P. S. & Ogston, D. G. (1971). Emotion as a function of the labeling of interruption-produced arousal. *Psychonomic Science, 24*(4), 153-154.

Gallagher, D. E., & Thompson, L. W. (1982). Treatment of major depressive disorder in older adult outpatients with brief psychotherapies. *Psychotherapy: Theory, Research & Practice, 19*(4), 482-490.

Gallagher, D. E., & Thompson, L. W. (1983). Effectiveness of psychotherapy for both endogenous and nonendogenous depression in older adult outpatients. *Journal of Gerontology, 38*(6), 707-712.

Gallagher, D. E., Thompson, L. W., & Peterson, J. A. (1981-1982). Psychosocial factors affecting adaptation to bereavement in the elderly. *International Journal of Aging & Human Development, 14*(2), 79-95.

Gallagher-Thompson, D., Hanley-Peterson, P., & Thompson, L. W. (1990). Maintenance of gains versus relapse following brief psychotherapy for depression. *Journal of Consulting & Clinical Psychology, 58*(3), 371-374.

Gallagher-Thompson, D. & Thompson, L. W. (1995). Psychotherapy with older adults in theory and practice. In B. M. Bongar & L. E. Beutler (Eds), *Comprehensive textbook of psychotherapy: Theory and practice. Oxford textbooks in clinical psychology,* Vol. 1. (pp. 359-379). New York, NY: Oxford University Press.

Garfield, S. L. (1957). *Introductory clinical psychology: An overview of the functions, methods, and problems of contemporary clinical psychology.* NY: Macmillan.

Garland, J. (1987). Working with the elderly. In J. S. Marzillier & J. Hall (Eds.), *What is clinical psychology?* Oxford medical publications (pp. 163-188). Oxford, England UK: Oxford University Press.

Gaston, L., Marmar, C. R, Gallagher, D., & Thompson, L. W. (1989). Impact of confirming patient expectations of change processes in behavioral, cognitive, and brief dynamic psychotherapy. *Psychotherapy, 26*(3), 296-302.

Gaston, L., Marmar, C. R., Thompson, L. W., & Gallagher, D. (1988). Relation of patient pretreatment characteristics to the therapeutic alliance in diverse psychotherapies. *Journal of Consulting & Clinical Psychology, 56*(4), 483-489.

Gatz, M. (1994). Application of assessment to therapy and intervention with older adults. In M. Storandt & G.R. VandenBos (Eds.), *Neuropsychological assessment of dementia and depression in older adults: A clinician's guide.* Washington, DC: American Psychological Association.

Gatz, M., Popkin, S., Pino, C., & VandenBos, G. (1985). Psychological interventions with older adults. In J. E. Birren & K. W. Schaie (Eds.), *Handbook of the psychology of aging* (2nd ed.) (pp. 755-788). New York: Van Nostrand Reinhold.

Gendlin, E. T. (1991). On emotion in therapy. In J. D. Safran & L. S. Greenberg (Eds.), *Emotion, psychotherapy, and change* (pp. 255-279). New York: Guilford Press.

Gerson, S., Belin, T.R., Kaufman, A., Mintz, J., & Jarvik, L. (1999). Pharmacological and psychological treatments for depressed older patients: A meta-analysis and overview of recent findings. *Harvard Review of Psychiatry, 7*(1), 1-28.

Gonccalves, O. F. (1994). Cognitive narrative psychotherapy: The hermeneutic construction of alternative meanings. *Journal of Cognitive Psychotherapy, 8*(2), 105-125.

Goodman, G. S., Hirschman, J. E., Hepps, D., & Rudy, L. (1991). Children's memory for stressful events. *Merrill-Palmer Quarterly, 37*(1), 109-157.

Grams, A. E. & Cutler, S. J. (1992). Predictors of self-reported problems of confusion among the aged. *International Journal of Aging & Human Development, 35*(4), 287-304.

Gutmann, D. (1990). Psychological development and pathology in later adulthood. In R. A. Nemiroff & C. A. Colarusso (Eds.), *New dimensions in adult development.* (pp. 170-185). New York, NY: Basic Books, Inc.

Haight, B. K. (1992). The structured life-review process: A community approach to the aging client. In G. M. M. Jones & B. M. L. Miesen (Eds.), *Care-giving in dementia: Research and applications* (pp. 272-292). London: Tavistock/Routledge.

Hamerman, D. (1998). Aging: A global theme issue. *Journal of the American Geriatrics Society, 46*(5), 656-667.

Hanley-Peterson, P., Futterman, A., Thompson, L., Zeiss, A.M., Gallagher, D., & Ironson, G. (1990). Endogenous depression and psychotherapy outcome in an elderly population [abstract]. *Gerontologist, 30,* 51A.

Hanser, S. B. (1999). Using music therapy in treating psychological problems of older adults. In M. Duffy (Ed.), *Handbook of counseling and psychotherapy with older adults* (pp. 197-213). New York: Wiley.

Hawes, C., Morris, J. N., Phillips, C. D., Fries, B. E., Murphy, K., & Mor, V. (1997). Development of the nursing home Resident Assessment Instrument in the ISA. *Age and Ageing, 26-S2,* 19-25.

Hermans, H. J. M. & Hermans-Jansen, E. (1995). *Self-narratives: The construction of meaning in psychotherapy.* New York: Guilford.

Howard, G. (1991). Culture tales: A narrative approach to thinking, cross-cultural psychology, and psychotherapy. *American Psychologist, 46,* 187-197.

Hyer, L. & Sohnle (2001). *Trauma among older people: Issues and treatment.* Philadelphia, PA: Brunner/Routledge.

Hyer, L. & Summers, M. (1995). An understanding of combat trauma at later life. *VA Merit Review.* Augusta, GA.

Hyer, L., Swanson, G., Lefkowitz, R., Hillesland, D., Davis, H., & Woods, M. (1990). The application of the cognitive behavioral model to two older stressor groups. *Clinical Gerontologist, 9*(3/4) 145-190.

Kegan, R. (1989). *The evolving self: Problem and process in human development.* Boston: Harvard University Press.

Kendall-Tackett, K. A., Williams, L. M., & Finkelhor, D. (1993). Impact of sexual abuse on children: A review and synthesis of recent empirical studies. *Psychological Bulletin, 113*(1), 164-180.

Knight, B.G. (1996). *Psychotherapy with older adults* (2nd ed.). Newbury Park, CA: Sage.

Lewis, M. I. & Butler, R. N. (1972). Why is women's lib ignoring old women? *Aging & Human Development, 3*(3), 223-231.

Lichtenberg, P. A. & Duffy, M. (2000). Psychological assessment and psychotherapy in long-term care. *Clinical Psychology: Science and Practice, 7,* 317-328.

Litz, B.T., Weathers, F. W., Monaco, V., Herman, D. S., Wulfsohn, M., Marx, B., & Keane, T. M. (1996). Attention, arousal, and memory in posttraumatic stress disorder. *Journal of Traumatic Stress, 9*(3).

Llorente, M. D., Olsen, E. J., Leyva, O., Silverman, M. A., Lewis, J. E., & Rivero, J. (1998). Use of antipsychotic drugs in nursing homes: Current compliance with OBRA regulations. *Journal of the American Geriatrics Society, 46*(2), 198-201.

Loevinger, J. (1976). Origins of conscience. *Psychological Issues, 9* (4, Mono 36), 265-297.

Loftus, E. F., & Davies, G. M. (1984). Distortions in the memory of children. *Journal of Social Issues, 40*(2), 51-67.

Lombardo, N. B. E., Fogel, B. S., Robinson, G. K., & Weiss, H. P. (1995). Achieving mental health of nursing home residents: Overcoming barriers to mental health care. *Journal of Mental Health & Aging, 1*(3), 165-211.

Marmar, C. R., Gaston, L., Gallagher, D., & Thompson, L. W. (1989). Alliance and outcome in late-life depression. *Journal of Nervous & Mental Disease, 177*(8), 464-472.

Marshall, V. (1980). *Last chapters: A sociology of aging and dying.* Belmont, CA: Wadsworth.

Marshall, V. (1986). *Later life: The social psychology of aging.* Beverly Hills: Sage.

McAdams, D.P. (1993). *The stories we live by: Personal myths and the making of the self.* New York: Morrow.

McAdams, D.P. (1996). Personality, modernity, and the storied self: A contemporary framework for studying persons. *Psychological Inquiry, 7*(4), 295-321.

McCarthy, P., Katz, I., & Foa, E. (1991). Cognitive-behavioral treatment of anxiety in the elderly: A proposal model. In C. Saltzman & B. Lebowitz (Eds.), *Anxiety in the elderly: Treatment and research* (pp. 197-214). New York: Springer.

McCauley, R. N. (1998). Walking in our own footsteps: Autobiographical memory and reconstruction. In U. Neisser & E. Winograd (Eds.), *Remembering reconsidered: Ecological and traditional approaches to the study of memory:* Emory symposia in cognition, 2 (pp. 126-144). New York: Cambridge University Press.

McCrae, R.R. & Costa, P.T., Jr. (1990). *Personality in adulthood.* NY: Guilford Press.

McNair, D. M., Lorr, M., & Droppleman, L. F. (1992). Profile of mood states revised. San Diego, CA: Educational and Institutional Testing Service.

Mintzer, J. E., Brawman-Mintzer, O., Mirski, D. F., & Barkin, K. (2000). Anxiety in the behavioral and psychological symptoms of dementia. *International Psychogeriatrics, 12*(11), 139-142.

Molinari, V. (1999). Using reminiscence and life review as natural therapeutic strategies in group therapy. In M. Duffy (Ed.), *Handbook of counseling and psychotherapy with older adults* (pp. 154-165). New York: Wiley.

Molinari, V. (Ed.). (2000). *Professional psychology in long-term care: A comprehensive guide*. New York: Hatherleigh Press.

Molinari, V., Cully, J., Kendjelic, E., & Kunik, M. (2001). Reminiscence and its relationship to attachment and personality in geropsychiatric patients. *International Journal of Aging and Human Development, 52*(2), 173-184.

Molinari, V. & Reichlin, R. E. (1985). Life review reminiscence in the elderly: A review of the literature. *International Journal of Aging & Human Development, 20* (2), 81-92.

Moore, T. (1994). *Care of the soul*. New York: Free Press.

Morris, R.G. & Morris, L.W. (1991). Cognitive and behavioral approaches with the elderly. *International Journal of Geriatric Psychiatry, 6*, 407-413.

Nichols, C. (1991). *Manual for the assessment of core goals*. Palo Alto: Consulting Psychologists Press.

Pennebacker, J. & Francis, M. (1996). Cognitive, emotional, and language processes in disclosure. *Cognition and Emotion, 10*, 601-626.

Prioleau, L., Murdock, M., & Brody, N. (1983). An analysis of psychotherapy versus placebo studies. *Behavioral & Brain Sciences, 6*, 275-310.

Rantz, M. J. F. (1993). Analysis of changes in chronically confused nursing home residents' status subsequent to OBRA 87 implementation. *Dissertation Abstracts International, 53*(12-B), 6226.

Rapp, M. S., Flint, A. J., Hermann, N., & Proulx, G. (1992). Behavioural disturbances in the demented elderly: Phenomenology, pharmacotherapy and behavioural management. *Canadian Journal of Psychiatry. 37*(9), 651-657.

Reichlin, R. E. (1999). Integrated group approaches with the early stage Alzheimer's patient and family. In M. Duffy (Ed.), *Handbook of counseling and psychotherapy with older adults* (pp. 166-181). New York: Wiley.

Reichman, W. E., Coyne, A. C., Borson, S., Negron, A. E., Rovner, B. W., Pelchat, R. J., Sakauye, K. M., Katz, P., Cantillon, M., & Hamer, R. M. (1998). Psychiatric consultation in the nursing home: A survey of six states. *American Journal of Geriatric Psychiatry, 6*(4), 320-327.

Reyna, V. F. (1995). Interference effects in memory and reasoning: A fuzzy trace theory analysis. In F. N. Dempster & C. J. Brainerd (Eds.), *Interference and inhibition in cognition* (pp. 29-59). San Diego, CA: Academic Press, Inc.

Reyna, V. F. & Brainerd, C. J. (1995). Fuzzy-trace theory: Some foundational issues. *Learning & Individual Differences, 7*(2), 145-162.

Reynolds, C. F., Frank, E., Perel, J. M., Imber, S. D., Cornes, C., Miller, M. D., Mazumdar, S., Houck, P. R., Dew, M. A., Stack, J. A., Pollock, B. G., & Kupfer, D. J. (1999). Nortriptyline and interpersonal psychotherapy as maintenance therapies for recurrent major depression: A randomized controlled trial in patients older than 59 years. *Journal of the American Medical Association, 281*(1), 39-45.

Robinson, L.A., Berman, J.S., & Neimeyer, R.A. (1990). Psychotherapy in the treatment of depression: A comprehensive review of controlled outcome research. *Psychological Bulletin, 108*, 30-49.

Ross, M. & Conway, M. (1986). Remembering one's own past: The construction of personal histories. In R. M. Sorrentino & E. T. Higgins (Eds.), *Handbook of motivation and cognition: Foundations of social behavior* (pp. 122-144). New York: Wiley.

Rubin, D. C. (1986). *Autobiographical memory.* New York: Cambridge University Press.

Rybarczyk, B. & Bellg, A. (1997). *Listening to life stories: A new approach to stress intervention in health care.* New York: Springer.

Ryff, C. D. (1989). Happiness is everything, or is it? Explorations on the meaning of psychological well-being. *Journal of Personality & Social Psychology, 57*(6), 1069-1081.

Ryff, C. D. (1991). Possible selves in adulthood and old age: A tale of shifting horizons. *Psychology & Aging, 6*(2), 286-295.

Samuel, R. (1975). *Village life and labour.* London: Routledge and Kegan Paul.

Schacter, D. L., Kihlstrom, J. F., Kihlstrom, L. C., & Berren, M. B. (1989). Autobiographical memory in a case of multiple personality disorder. *Journal of Abnormal Psychology, 98*(4), 508-514.

Schramke, C. (1997). Anxiety disorders. In P. Nussbaum (Ed.), *Handbook of neuropsychology and aging* (pp. 80-97). New York: Plenum.

Scogin, F. & McElreath, L. (1994). Efficacy of psychosocial treatments for geriatric depression. *Journal Consulting and Clinical Psychology, 62*(1), 69-74.

Scogin, F., Rickard, H.C., Keith, S., Wilson, J., & McElreath, L. (1992). Progressive and imaginal relaxation training for elderly persons with subjective anxiety. *Psychology and Aging, 7,* 419-424.

Segal, Z. V., Williams, J. M. G., & Teasdale, J. D. (2001). *Mindfulness-based cognitive therapy for depression: A new approach to preventing relapse.* New York: Guilford.

Shea, D. G., Smyer, M. A., & Streit, A. (1993). Mental health services for nursing home residents: What will it cost? *Journal of Mental Health Administration, 20*(3), 223-235.

Sherman, E. (1981). *Counseling the aged: An integrative approach.* New York: Free Press.

Sherman, E. (1991). *Reminiscence and the self in old age.* New York: Springer Publishing Company.

Singer, J. (2001). "Examining the integrative function of self-defining memories." Presentation at the 109th Annual Meeting of the American Psychological Association, San Francisco (Aug 25, 2001).

Singer, J. A. & Salovey, P. (1993). *The remembered self: Emotion and memory in personality.* New York: The Free Press, MacMillan, Inc.

Smith, J. & Baltes, P. B. (1997). Profiles of psychological functioning in the old and oldest old. *Psychology & Aging, 12*(3), 458-472.

Smith, M.L., Glass, G.V., & Miller, T.I. (1980). *The benefits of psychotherapy.* Baltimore, MD: Johns Hopkins University Press.

Smyer, M.A., Shea, D. G., & Streit, A. (1994). The provision and use of mental health services in nursing homes: Results from the National Medical Expenditure Survey. *American Journal of Public Health, 84*(2), 284-287.

Spreen, O. & Strauss, E. (1998). *A compendium of neurological tests: Administration, norms and commentary.* New York: Oxford Press.

Sprenkel, D. G. (1999). Therapeutic issues and strategies in group therapy with older men. In M. Duffy (Ed.), *Handbook of counseling and psychotherapy with older adults* (pp. 214-227). New York: Wiley.

Taft, L. B. & Nehrke, M. F. Reminiscence, life review, and ego integrity in nursing home residents. *International Journal of Aging & Human Development, 30*(3), 189-196.

Tannen, D. & Aries, E. (1997). Conversational style: Do women and men speak different languages? In M. R. Walsh (Ed.), *Women, men, & gender: Ongoing debates* (pp. 79-100). New Haven, CT: Yale University Press.

Tedeschi, R.G. & Calhoun, L.G. (1995). *Trauma and transformation growing in the aftermath of suffering.* Thousand Oaks, CA: Sage Publications, Inc.

Teri, L. (1999). Training families to provide care: Effects on people with dementia. *International Journal of Geriatric Psychiatry, 14*(2), 110-116.

Thompson, L. W., Gallagher, D., & Breckenridge, J. S. (1987). Comparative effectiveness of psychotherapies for depressed elders. *Journal of Consulting & Clinical Psychology, 55*(3), 385-390.

Thompson, L.W., Gallagher, D., & Czirr, R. (1988). Personality disorder and outcome in the treatment of late-life depression. *Journal of Geriatric Psychiatry, 21,* 133-146.

Thompson, L.W., Gallagher, D., Hanser, S., Gantz, F., & Steffen, A. (1991, November). *Comparison of desipramine and cognitive/behavioral therapy in the treatment of late-life depression.* Paper presented at the meeting of Gerontological Society of America, San Francisco.

Turner, B. F., Tobin, S. S., & Lieberman, M.A. (1972). Personality traits as predictors of institutional adaption among the aged. *Journal of Gerontology, 27*(1), 61-68.

Verwoerdt, A. (1987). Psychodynamics of paranoid phenomena in the aged. In J. Sadavoy & M. Leszcz (Eds.), *Treating the elderly with psychotherapy: The scope for change in later life* (pp. 67-93). Madison, CT: International Universities Press, Inc.

Viney, L. L. (1993). *Life stories: Personal construct therapy with the elderly.* Chichester, England UK: John Wiley & Sons.

Wallace, B. (1992). Reconsidering the new life review: The social construction of talk about the past. *The Gerontologist, 32,* 120-125.

Webster, J. D. (1997). The Reminiscence Functions Scale: A replication. *International Journal of Aging and Human Development, 44,* 137-148.

Weiss, J. C. (1999). The role of art therapy in aiding older adults with life transitions. In M. Duffy (Ed.), *Handbook of counseling and psychotherapy with older adults* (pp. 182-196). New York: Wiley.

Wetherell, J. L. (1998). Treatment of anxiety in older adults. *Psychotherapy, 35*(4), 444-458.

White, J. (1980). *Rothschild buildings: Life in an east end tenement block 1887-1920.* London: Routledge and Kegan Paul.

Williams, J. M. G. (1992). Autobiographical memory and emotional disorders. In S. A. Christianson (Ed.), *The handbook of emotion and memory: Research and theory* (pp. 451-477). Hillsdale, NJ: Lawrence Erlbaum Associates, Inc.

Wong, P.T. & Watt, L.M. (1991). What types of reminiscence are associated with successful aging? *Psychology and Aging, 6,* 272-9.

Zarit, S.H., Dolan, M. M., & Leitsch, S. A. (1998). Interventions in nursing homes and other alternative living settings. In I. H. Nordhus & G. R. VandenBos (Eds.), *Clinical geropsychology* (pp. 329-343). Washington, DC: American Psychological Association.

Zeiss, A. M. & Steffen, A. M. (1996). Interdisciplinary health care teams: The basic unit of geriatric care. In L. L. Carstensen & B. A. Edelstein (Eds.), *The practical handbook of clinical gerontology.* (pp. 423-450). Thousand Oaks, CA: Sage Publications, Inc.

APPENDIX
PCM MANUAL

Procedure

The treatment is administered in a twelve-session group format. With the facilitator's assistance and encouragement, each participant identifies at least one but preferably two or three *positive core memories (PCMs),* which serve as focal points. The PCMs become the basis for myriad "learnings" or life lessons that transcend the specific event. Facilitators (and other participants) find practical or meaningful roles for these learnings in their current experience. An objective measure(s) is used both as an adjunct to the diagnostic process and as a baseline to evaluate the treatment.

Key Activities

Session 1

- Introduction of facilitator(s).
- Introduction of participants.
- Description of the method, expectations.
- Explain and secure commitments regarding confidentiality, mutual respect, etc.
- Respond to questions, concerns.
- Completion of baseline measure(s).

Sessions 2-4

- Identification of PCMs (at least one–attempt 2 or 3).
- Ask for the PCM in as much detail as possible (surrounding events, people involved, challenges, obstacles overcome).
- Encourage participant interaction (many will identify strongly with others' PCMs–This can help each person appreciate his or her own PCM more deeply).
- Assist those having difficulty generating memories. Facilitators may have to "mine" participant narratives (often with the help of other participants) to identify the PCM.
- Encourage "homework" assignment of continuing to generate PCM possibilities after sessions 2 and 3.

Sessions 5-10

- Ask participants to describe how the life lessons and other learnings involved in the PCMs are still present, how they affect their *current experience* (how is the PCM alive in them today?).
- As with identifying PCMs, participant interaction is very helpful here.
- Encourage narratives about how the PCM and related memories or learnings emerged at different times and in different places over the years.

Sessions 11 and 12

- Administer post-test.
- Termination process. Consolidate what has been learned.
- For issues not resolved/resolvable–assess tolerance for lack of closure, ambiguity. Integrate this with PCM (draw strength from PCM for ongoing struggles).
- Discuss relapse and encourage residents to reach out (to predesignated staff) for assistance if this occurs.
- Ask for feedback on the process.
- Consider "booster" session at one month.

Session 13

- Optional "booster" session.
- Determine if residents are still accessing PCMs.
- Ask for feedback on the process.

Principles for PCM

- Affect tolerance and resource building.
- Should negative memories result, the therapist can alter the memory.
- Establishing a coping contract (REAS method).

Some rules:

- Get the story out in chronological order.
- Be reflexive and non-reflexive.
- Centered in the moment, the present including affective experience.
- Reinforce/validate the continuity, stability of the self.
- Respect cognition–allow room for the thoughts.
- While focusing on the present, keep a positive eye to the future.

Last resort:

* Change the memory: Re-construct the construction.

Preliminaries

Two levels of problems are identified, one for coping and stabilization and one for growth. A "bad" memory may be stuck, preventing the processing of information. Residents then would have problems with affect tolerance. In the beginning then, the therapist needs a way to manage affect tolerance and assist in resource instillation.

Affect tolerance involves coping with affect, containing excitement, defending against shame. It leads directly to dissociation. Resources, on the other hand, are already present. So the therapy is not an "installation" so much as it is an enhancement of extant but dormant skills.

Affect Tolerance

Key question: "Can you handle/cope with this emotion?"

The resident who can differentiate emotions from one another and can trust them has an advantage. If this skill is lacking, then affect will cause problems. One troubling problem more associated with aging is ontological insecurity. This is a more global form of anxiety in which the person's sense of coherence and intactness as a functioning self is threatened. In this experience there is an experience of threat and vulnerability to basic self-organization. When this threat to basic self-organization occurs, affect tolerance or the ongoing supportive quality of the therapeutic bond is crucial in helping the person to affirm a sense of self and internalize the therapist's support.

There are several techniques of affect tolerance. This involves coping with affect, containing excitement, defending against shame. Other coping strategies involve distancing, suspending the emotion, freezing the feeling, and placing these in a box or safe place.

Resource Building

Key question: "What do you need to make this work?"

Here the therapist ensures the patient has coping resources. That is, the strategies are best developed through an understanding of the personality.

Example: An Avoidant personality can be taught that the deficient trust can be overcome by recalling the time when they were able to be trusting and be rewarded for it.

Distinguish between present "Now" resources and "Then" resources.

Now resources:

1. How would the client prefer to be acting?
2. What are goals for the future?
3. What is called for now in the day-to-day functions of living?
4. What metaphors, images, symbols, stories are available to represent the resource?
5. Who is the key mentor/model of the person?
6. Can you use prayer?
7. What about music, novels, etc.?
8. What about a positive goal state or future self?

Then resources:

1. Embryonic resources for change?
2. What were the damages with caretakers (parents)?
3. What are the missing resources for each personality?
4. What metaphors, images, symbols, stories are available to represent the resource?
5. What about generic issues of safety, trust, self-esteem, independence, intimacy and power?

ADDITIONAL GUIDELINES FOR PCM

The therapist should attempt to make the past vivid and the story personal. In approaching the PCM, it is important to remember that memories can be changed, especially at later life, through words.

Once the client becomes engaged in the process, focus on two tasks:

- Ask questions.
- Make facilitating comments pursing the process goals outlines below. When the patient fails to take cues to follow up on pleasant experiences, the interviewer can change the topic to a positive one.

Negative memories: Acknowledge these briefly and then redirect the interview toward something positive. The same is true if the patient becomes tearful, as happens on occasion. The interviewer should acknowledge the tears by offering support, give the resident a moment to recover, and then, with the permission of the resident, move to the meaning of the memory.

The most effective way to encourage reflection is to reinforce the resident. The interviewer can give reinforcement by showing increased interest, by nodding, or simply by asking the participant to elaborate further. Reflection can also be facilitated by questions that are provocative and stimulating.

The final few minutes (of a memory) can be used to summarize the strengths and resources that have emerged from the life story.

1. Get the story out in chronological order.

Key question: "What happened?"

(Introduce the process. Example from Rybarczyk and Bellg 1997):

> You've lived a pretty long life, and you must have some wonderful memories. There have been many moments that you have an experience that has been so much a part of you as to be defining, perhaps where you lived and what you did, interactions with your children, or a long intimate conversation with someone. No doubt you have stepped back and thought of this. What each of these moments has in common is that they attempt to answer the question, "Who am I."

> Reminiscing about early life gives real pleasure and puts people in a good frame of mind–which would be very helpful for somebody having difficulties. This may really help people get through problem times. I think people's lives are very interesting, and I would enjoy it if you want to go into detail about things you like to remember.

> For today with me the idea is to talk about your life and to begin, more or less, at the beginning. It seems to work better to do it chronologically, starting with the very earliest memories, and it doesn't really matter how far we get. What are some of your earliest memories?

Guided imagery can also been helpful. Several exercises may be particularly helpful for clients who have difficulty in "switching on" to life review.

Older clients, however, may have difficulty achieving clarity of the image. The therapist may have to suggest more detail in setting the scene than is the case with younger persons. Retaining an imagined scene may also be more difficult. Breaking the scene down into smaller parts (as was done with the sample hierarchy described in this section) may help.

Once the PCM is stated, the therapist can ask: "What was it like for you to tell this story?" The client is asked only to comment on the *process* of the story-telling. This leads into the other rules.

2. Be reflective.

Key question: "What does this story mean to *you*?"

The client both experiences and reflects on the experience. This is the observing ego, needed for perspective in therapy. This is, of course, reflexivity, a dialectical approach helping the person examine the self from multiple perspectives. The essential feature of the treatment is discovery.

These probes can facilitate this experience:

- Can you get a broader sense of that feeling?
- Can you stop and sense the meaning of that feeling?
- What is that feeling?
- What is that "sore spot" up against?
- Can you get in touch with the whole issue?
- What say do you have over those feelings?
- What word/image/metaphor goes with that?
- What's in the way of this being okay?
- What is the worst of this?
- What are you all about?
- How are you stuck?
- Just sit quiet, clear a space and see what else is there.
- Be friendly to yourself, create a space.
- Let your body tell you what all that feeling is about.

3. Be nonreflexive: Present centered/use affect.

Key question: "Can you stay with that: Experience that feeling?"

This, of course, is the other side of the reflexivity task. Residents can get stuck in the past. Processing the past involves more than remembering or re-experiencing. By making the past present, a new re-experience, a new texture evolves. Memory exists in present consciousness. Keep a present focus. Attend to current feeling, sensations, and thoughts. Facilitate experiential processing rather than conceptual processing. It is not insight into abstract patterns of behavior across situations, such as "rebelling against authority," or "pushing people away when they get close," that is searched for in therapy. Rather it is the re-experience of a concrete, particular instance that is sought after.

By exploring a particular situation as completely and fully as possible, people access fundamental models of the world, the models responsible for their experience of self. It is these holistic models, not conceptual meanings, that need reorganizing.

Affect is a barometer for immediacy. Affect recruits cognitions. With the mere identification of the emotion the therapist assists the person in the understanding and accepting conflict.

Fully experiencing a single moment of an event will bring forth all the elements of the actual experience from memory. So the task is to keep the patient in the present. The mindfulness of the present is necessary and sometimes sufficient for change.

4. Validate the stability of the self.

Key question: "How does this reflect YOU?"

The clinician can celebrate the positive, listen and enjoy. This involves making vivid the notion that "This really was you!" Attend to issues of the past and present that are empowering to the self.

Some examples:

- "You've always been a resourceful person."
- "You were willing to make a lot of sacrifices to achieve your goals."
- "You really stand up for yourself when you need to."
- "You seem to be very good at making adjustments."
- "Your family really stuck together."
- "The work ethic was very important to you."
- "You have been good at finding creative solutions to things."
- "Your willpower got you through again."
- "Your sense of humor served you well."
- "You seem to have had lots of love in your life."

5. Respect cognition.

Key question: "Are you looking at the whole picture?"

- What evidence do you have to support this thought?
- Is there any other way to see this, an alternate explanation?
- What is the best/worst possible outcome of this?
- Are you underestimating or overestimating your responsibility or influence in this?
- Are you ignoring the positive aspects or discounting your ability to deal with it?
- What does this memory say about who you are?

The therapist can make cognitions more focused or more expanded.

- Focusing: "Tell me more about that."
- Expanding: "When were you not that way?"

Through this process, the person becomes open to other possibilities. A change in thinking regarding a memory is similar to the cognitive therapy process, where clients modify beliefs and schema. This means that the therapist focuses first on cognitions.

6. Look to the future/generativity.

Key question: "How will others benefit (have they benefited) because of you?"

Stories are the most important components in this therapy. They help develop and maintain a sense of identity. Initiate a generativity script, one that emphasizes continued growth and development throughout the life span. "You did this," and "You will leave that" are empowering phrases. People really do change by life review.

7. "Last Resort": Change the memory if necessary.

Key question: "Can we switch gears? Please share that good time you had when . . ."

Final points:

- While unusual, it is possible that some residents will not produce any PCMs. Often the judicious use of time as well as a therapeutic foraging in the past is required.
- PCM is contraindicated with psychotic or recently psychotic individuals, those experiencing a pathological grieving. The highly depressed patient also can be a problem.
- In most circumstances, the therapist can usually elicit a PCM and this can serve as the foundation for change.

The Coping Contract

The resident is asked to:

- Identify the important learnings from the PCM for day-to-day living.
- Isolate current problems and insert a coping method to assist.

One method that has been helpful is *REAS*.

> *Recognize*: "This is the problem. I have learned from my PCM. I can do this."

*E*valuate: Objective measure (e.g., scaling device).
*A*ct: Relaxation, thinking, active coping, DO something.
*S*upport self: Access other people or favorite places, things, activities.

In sum, restructuring reality with PCMs is done simply with clinical interest in the new memory itself. This interest is of course one that ushers in even more positive epiphanies of the memory.

CASE

Mr. P is a 75-year-old white male who has been in the LTC facility for over four years. He has COPD, renal failure (on dialysis), and assorted minor problems. He was married and later divorced. He has two children who are supportive. He worked as a bus driver for over 40 years. He was in the service in 1942-45. He experienced combat but does not feel that this is a current problem.

He does not enjoy the nursing home. He has problems with several residents and at least one staff member. He also resents his physical condition (limitations) and is given to complaining. He meets DSM criteria for recurrent major depression. He is currently on no psychiatric medications. He reports no memory problems, has a Mini Mental State Examination (MMSE) of 27 and a Beck Depression Inventory (BDI-II) of 18. He was referred to the PCM group having been among the 24 who were referred for therapy.

> PCM: I was 17 and I was going nowhere. The baseball team, the Giants, asked me to come for a tryout. I was so excited and came to the field most willingly. There were several ballplayers there and I felt funny. I was there in camp for two weeks. I realized that this was not for me. At first this was a terrible disappointment. I only realized that this was not my life. I went home and soon met my wife. WW-II was already in progress.

PCM Procedures

Preliminaries

Despite the negative quality of the memory, there was no need for affect tolerance or resource procedures. He was in control and clear-minded about his memory and life.

Rules

1. Get the story out in chronological order.

Key question: "What happened?"

This was done smoothly. When asked: What was it like for you to narrate this story, Mr. P indicated that he had not told this story for some time and it felt good, "like it was waiting."

2. Be reflective.

Key question: "What does this story mean to *you*?"

This too was eventful. He indicated that he realized that he was his own man and that he was on his way. This had been more of a bad fantasy than a positive experience. The illusion of his being a baseball player was in fact what had stopped him. He was now able to get on with his life. He felt confident.

3. Be nonreflexive: Present centered/use affect.

Key question: "Can you stay with that: Experience that feeling?"

He noted that he was puzzled by his reaction. He realized that this was more important that he originally thought. He believed that this was one of the most important moments in his life.

4. Validate the stability of the self.

Key question: "How does this reflect YOU?"

He believed that he was a more assured man now and that he could know where he was going. In a strange way this failure made him aware that he could do other things and could be content at them. He was now his own man.

5. Respect cognition.

Key question: "Are you looking at the whole picture?"

- What evidence do you have to support this thought?
- Is there any other way to see this, an alternate explanation?
- What is the best/worst possible outcome of this?
- Are you underestimating or overestimating your responsibility or influence in this?
- Are you ignoring the positive aspects or discounting your ability to deal with it?
- What does this memory say about who you are?

Little in the way of assimilative queries was required. He quickly realized that he was onto something and that he needed to reflect on these.

When asked about the best outcome, he noted that it was liberating for him.

6. Look to the future/generativity.

Key question: "How will others benefit (have they benefited) because of you?"

He noted that he led a good life. Now things were "bad." He felt that he was a good father and that he had been fair and positive with people. He now had to challenge himself with his new problems.

Coping Contract

Mr. P indicated some triggers for depression–looking at himself and feeling like he was dead. He also became angry with others. So he decided:

R: Recognize his triggers and feelings.
E: Scale this 1-10 and monitor.
A: The learning was that he was his own man and he can handle anything. He would visualize himself during the PCM.
S: He would support himself by going for coffee with friends.

Disruptive Behavior:
Systemic and Strategic Management

Michael Duffy, PhD, ABPP

SUMMARY. Disruptive behavior in nursing home residents such as noncompliance, aggression, demanding and dependent behavior, and wandering consumes an inordinate amount of administrative and staff time. Frequently, staffs behave in a reactive manner that exacerbates symptoms. This chapter argues for a nonreactive approach that views disruptive behavior from a systemic perspective. This in turn leads to more strategic solutions that better fit the complex forces that shape the behavior. At times these solutions are counterintuitive. Clinical situations discussed include demanding behavior, hypochondriacal behavior and dementia. *[Article copies available for a fee from The Haworth Document Delivery Service: 1-800-HAWORTH. E-mail address: <getinfo@haworthpressinc.com> Website: <http://www.HaworthPress.com> © 2002 by The Haworth Press, Inc. All rights reserved.]*

KEYWORDS. Disruptive behavior, combativeness, noncompliance, strategic management

Disruptive behavior, more than any other problem behavior, is likely to draw a *reactive* response, even from professional and experienced

---

Michael Duffy is affiliated with the Counseling Psychology Program at Texas A&M University.

Address correspondence to: Michael Duffy, Counseling Psychology Program, Department of Educational Psychology, Texas A&M University, College Station, TX 77843.

[Haworth co-indexing entry note]: "Disruptive Behavior: Systemic and Strategic Management." Duffy, Michael. Co-published simultaneously in *Clinical Gerontologist* (The Haworth Press, Inc.) Vol. 25, No. 1/2, 2002, pp. 91-103; and: *Emerging Trends in Psychological Practice in Long-Term Care* (ed: Margaret P. Norris, Victor Molinari, and Suzann Ogland-Hand) The Haworth Press, Inc., 2002, pp. 91-103. Single or multiple copies of this article are available for a fee from The Haworth Document Delivery Service [1-800-HAWORTH, 9:00 a.m. - 5:00 p.m. (EST). E-mail address: getinfo@haworthpressinc.com].

therapists. It is the nature of disruptive behavior to disrupt, to unbalance, to cause crisis. Indeed, in some cases, such effects may be the precise *purpose* of disruptive behavior. The symptoms of disruptive behavior usually create a sense of *urgency*–of the need for immediate and oftentimes unreflective action on the part of the helper. When the intervention is unreflective, it is often ineffective in solving the problem; it may indeed escalate the situation and increase a sense of loss of control both on the part of the client and of the therapist.

In fact, it is especially important to be *nonreactive* to disruptive behavior and to search for the sometimes less than obvious set of forces, and, therefore, solutions that might apply. In nursing homes disruptive behavior takes many forms: noncompliance with medical procedures, physical assaults, demanding and dependent behavior, sexual acting out, aggressive or anti-social acts, persistent psychosomatic symptoms, wandering, inappropriate toileting, etc. This chapter will address several of these problems in case examples.

A SYSTEMIC VIEW OF BEHAVIOR

A systems view of these behaviors involves seeking to identify the sometimes complex set of forces that may give meaning to these behaviors. It frequently also can mean that the solution may take less than obvious forms and be nontraditional. So, for example, the depressed older resident might be best treated by a telephone conference with an absent adult child with whom there is unfinished business. Or, improving the nursing staff's physical care management techniques might best treat the aggressive dementia patient. Symptomatic behavior is not always as it appears to be, and coming to appreciate the dynamic or phenomenological *meaning* of a particular behavior can more effectively guide a strategic solution to the problem.

The recent emphasis on DSM Axis I symptomatic problems within the field of psychology and psychotherapy has given rise to an overly simplistic understanding of behavior. Related to this is the relative ignoring of Axis II personality and sub-clinical temperamental problems that in most cases accompany symptomatic behavior. Even experienced clinicians may be tempted to assume that *everything that looks the same is the same*. An example of this tendency is to miss the various meanings of depression and anxiety. Although DSM IV treats depression in a fairly monolithic manner, in fact there may be a variety of meanings for a symptom pattern that looks identical or "almost identical" on the surface. While depressive symptoms may look the same across patients and therefore treatment is assumed to be the same, many therapists recognize that this is not the case. The treatment of depressive symptoms will vary considerably depending on the particular meaning of depression in the patient. For example, a situational/reactive depression will be treated quite differently from a depression involving a narcissistic or sociopathic dejection occasioned through loss of a significant relationship. Or, the treatment of a complicated bereavement due to traumatic loss of spouse will be different from a vegetative depression associated with a biologically-oriented disorder.

However, what is true of depression can be *reversed in the case of anxiety*: while anxiety symptoms take on a surprising array of symptomatic patterns, they may share a basic dynamic meaning. I have found that in dealing with a variety of different anxiety symptoms such as specific phobias, test anxiety, performance anxiety, obsessive and compulsive symptoms, etc., the underlying phenomenological condition is frequently quite similar, and the common features can often be best described under the rubric of generalized anxiety. So, in the case of *depression*, often *what looks the same is indeed quite different;* in the case of *anxiety*, *what looks different may be quite similar* in the internal world of psychological meaning. Anxiety, while taking many different forms, can in fact represent a quite similar internal state of destabilization.

From the contrariwise examples given above, it becomes clear that many diagnostic and treatment situations are *counterintuitive*. Indeed, it may be the case that one of the primary effects of professional training is to help move the trainee from an intuitive understanding of human behavior to a counterintuitive position. For example, even though the intuitive reaction to distress in a client is to *reassure* them that all will be well, we are well aware that, upon some reflection, such reassurance is rarely effective. In fact, the counterintuitive stance will allow the person to express their worst fears and will usually lead to a more helpful outcome. In my experience of training paraprofessionals, I have found this above example to be of great importance. The volunteers naturally begin their work as helpers from an intuitive position, that "nice is best," and only gradually begin to adopt a more complex understanding that persons are best helped by being allowed to completely express their negative feelings about a situation. In a parallel example, our clients are rarely talked out of their *guilt feelings* by a reassuring posture, which attempts to convince them "not to feel guilty." Again, it is more helpful to take a counterintuitive position, which is to allow the client to explore fully the degree of their guilt. This approach frequently results in a more objective evaluation of guilt and frequent reduction of inappropriate and irrational guilt feelings.

STRATEGIC APPROACH TO CHANGE

A *systemic understanding* of behavior will frequently lead to a particular strategic approach to dealing with the problem. One example is the different strategic approaches one might use in working with the symptoms of depression. In one case, the depressive symptoms may be a relatively straightforward reactive *expression* of stress or loss in the person's life. In another case, the person's symptoms may be better described within a personality or temperamental approach that is captured in the current concept of "depressive personality" (Millon, 1990). In other words, the depressive behavior serves not only to signal distress but has a *purposive* element and is designed to influence the behavior of other persons. So, for example, a tendency to depressive self-pitying behavior will have a distinctive effect on surrounding relationships, initially producing "sympathetic" behavior and then eventually producing "avoidant" behavior on the part of perspective helpers. As is typical of dysfunctional personality adjustment, the symptom initially "works well"; producing sympathy that insures its repetition. Then, of course, the helpers get "burnt out" and leave, thus insuring eventual failure of the symptom to achieve its goal.

Each of these two depression scenarios, based on a systemic understanding of their different meanings, will lead to different strategic approaches. In the first case of straightforward reactive depression, the helper will no doubt be involved in physical, cognitive, and affective remedies to reduce the depressive symptoms. In the second case, based more on personality disposition and adjustment, the helper will also need to deal with personality and interpersonal dynamics in psychotherapy. If this is not done, then the depressive symptoms are likely to be resistant to change. Of course, it is critical to remember that these two scenarios do not represent an "either/or situation"; the symptoms of depression can have *both* meanings and need depressive symptoms to be relieved through aggressive treatment. A similar error of this type is to assume that when a borderline patient is depressed, there is no reason to treat the depression. In fact, borderline patients get depressed. Aggressive symptom treatment is also particularly necessary in geriatric depression, which may not be as amenable to spontaneous remission as depression in younger adults. However, to miss the personality features in some depressions can impede success. Conversely, when we occasionally find, for example, that the depression is resistant to antidepressive medication or cognitive and physical intervention strategies, this is a good time to explore the Axis II dimensions of the problem.

THE TACTICS OF CHANGE

The third level of understanding the systemic approach to the management of disruptive behavior is the specific *tactics* that are suggested by a systemic understanding. This can be illustrated by a case of depression in the nursing home. Depression may at times result from a "narcissistic dejection" on the part of an older adult who has lost contact with an adult child with whom unfinished business exists. On the basis of a lifelong codependent and perhaps symbiotic relationship with the child, the parent is thrown into a dejected and depressed state of mind when the adult child becomes disconnected and fails to meet the parent's emotional needs. In a world in which women are expected to be completely altruistic and nurturant, this type of narcissistic loss situation is often hidden, and this is especially so in the nursing home context where family members are relatively unknown. Therapeutic interventions derived from a symptomatic understanding of the depression will frequently be unsuccessful in helping the older adult who seems to resist all forms of symptom relief. In a nursing home world where "activities programming" is the universal therapeutic panacea for emotional problems (Maddox, 964), no one knows their limitations better than the activities director. In such a case the understanding of the narcissistic loss and failed relationship aspect of the depression will provide a systemic understanding that will lead to a more accurate therapeutic strategy. It is clear that the solution to the depressive state will involve some form of family intervention or therapy. A systemic family intervention thus becomes the strategic approach for dealing with depression in this case. The next stage will involve the specific tactics of change designed to implement the strategy. Sometimes this will involve ongoing family therapy but very frequently, given the relationship described above, a series of more brief focused interventions will be suggested. For example, if the absent adult child is at a great distance from the parent, it may be possible to engage the therapeutic use of phone calls, letters, audio letters, or an occasional intensive therapy session (Duffy, 1986). Thus, we see that a systemic understanding of the depression leads to a strategic approach designed to be more sensitive to the situation, which leads to a specific set of tactics that are well adjusted to the reality of the relationship. This approach also requires a good deal of flexibility and responsiveness to changing situations (Greenleaf, 1997).

What follows is a series of case situations, which illustrate a systemic, strategic, and tactical approach to dealing with disruptive behaviors in the nursing home context.

DEMANDING BEHAVIOR

The general public seems very sensitive to and critical of the situation of unanswered call bells in nursing homes. They may be much less familiar and sympathetic to the plight of understaffed and poorly paid nursing home caregivers dealing with sometimes very demanding nursing home residents. Again, demanding behavior may be relatively similar at a behavioral or symptomatic level, but may involve a variety of more subtle psychological meanings. On the one hand, demanding behavior may represent the relatively straightforward reciprocal reactivity between a resident who has a legitimate feeling of being neglected, with a staff person who feels increasingly "beaten on." In another situation, demanding behavior may represent a more pervasive aspect of characterological behavior related to more long-term personality adjustment. Again, the intuitive and naturalistic reaction to demanding behavior is initially to respond with sympathy and attention, eventually to be followed by the tendency to avoid this resident and their "endless series of requests and demands." This natural and intuitive response behavior is best replaced by a counterintuitive understanding of the interaction. From a counterintuitive point of view, the more a caregiver avoids interaction with the resident, the more persistent will the requests become, so that a vicious circle of reciprocal behavior becomes more and more recalcitrant. A counterintuitive approach to such a situation, based on a systemic and strategic approach, is to psychologically *approach* rather than avoid. Put in a practical and specific way, it can take up to twenty annoying minutes to *avoid* contact with a particularly demanding resident; it may take only one minute to make a *psychological connection* with that person. The strategy is to move *towards* versus away from *psychological connection* with the patient. When a patient begins to make demanding gestures (and this is particularly true in the characterological patient), it becomes important to act against the *intuitive reaction of escape* and to move toward the patient. Frequently, this move in relatively short time will reverse the reciprocal cycle of mutually defeating behavior. As the pattern is changed, the resident will then frequently feel attended to and the demanding behavior will reduce. Further, it may be helpful as a tactic to anticipate the resident's needs and to contact the resident *before* the request (demand) has been made. In the context of general therapy, it can be helpful to extremely dependent patients who make frequent and intrusive out-of-session contact to make an occasional and unexpected phone call to them! This anticipates and precludes the inevitable and unwanted contact that the patient may make. It will also reduce the "testing behavior" as the patient contacts us to reassure themselves (ineffectively!) that we (still) care!

DEPENDENT BEHAVIOR

In a similar way, extremely dependent behavior can be disruptive for caregivers. Again, an intuitive approach to such behavior on the part of many helpers and nursing home staff is to attempt to get the older resident to move in the direction of more autonomous behaviors using rewards, constraints, or even at times inappropriate negative behavior. If these various approaches meet with little success, again, it will be helpful to adopt a more complex strategy that involves a counterintuitive approach to working with dependent behavior. Practically, this means, it is usually more effective to strategically *allow* dependent behavior rather than to dissuade the resident. Clients who perceive the comfort of being allowed to psychologically *approach* and "depend on the caregiver" will frequently reduce their anxious and urgent need to "cling."

When we look at the natural developmental sequence in the development of independence and autonomy we find that "being allowed to cling" is the best precursor for the development of a healthy autonomy. The child who is allowed to depend is able to develop the ego integrity that permits autonomy.

However, the intuitive instinct to "escape" dependent behavior is so strong even in professional helpers, that learning to "tolerate" dependency becomes a very useful issue in both clinical and paraprofessional training in the nursing home staff. Of course, the "proof of the pie is in the eating" and nursing home staff must be allowed to test out this counterintuitive approach for themselves, and with time will be able to evaluate its effectiveness.

HYPOCHONDRIACAL BEHAVIOR

Hypochondriacal behavior can be extremely invasive for busy nursing home staff. Again, the initial reaction of helpers to hypochondriacal behavior is initially one of sympathy and attention. Only after continued attempts to treat and reduce the apparent medical problems do the help-ers–both nursing home staff and physicians–begin to suspect that all is not as it seems to be. At this point, medical caregivers frequently move into an "all-or-nothing," "either/or" position. Having deduced that the behavior has no linear medical cause, the conclusion is reached that it is "purely psychological." The attempt is then made to convince the resi-dent that they have no need to be concerned about the medical condi-tion; by so doing, they succeed in communicating to the resident that he/she should not be worried or concerned about their health and, con-sequently, do not need doctor's visits. This message, of course, falls on deaf ears, and leads to a failure in heightened anxiety in the relationship between the patient and the caregiver. The usual result of this approach is the increase in hypochondriacal behaviors to the resultant frustration of both patients and health care providers. Attempts are now made to limit the patient's contact with the providers. This is, in turn, perceived by the resident as rejecting and discounting behavior and leads to the typical vicious circle of hypochondriacal behavior with which we are so familiar.

A counterintuitive strategy for treating hypochondriacal behavior is one of *acceptance* of the patient's frame of reference as *phenomenologically meaningful* and then to *continue psychological contact*. In this scenario, the caregiver and physician refrain from pushing the patient away and, in fact, suggest that ongoing attention for the medical problem is neces-sary–which indeed it is. Again, this is a counterintuitive response and requires some training and practice. In this case, the physician, for exam-ple, will provide regular medical attention and suggest regular visits to the physician's office. These visits are prescribed authoritatively (and therefore not resented) and for specific and manageable periods of time. This "moving toward" the patient psychologically reduces the degree of pressure and frustration felt by the physician and at the same time allevi-ates the dependency needs of the patient. In this way, the hypochondriacal behavior will reduce as the patient reduces in anxiety and agitation.

NARCISSISTIC BEHAVIOR

Narcissism is a close relative of some of the above problems but has its own specific meaning and character and can be extremely disruptive in the daily life of a nursing home. Anyone who has worked in nursing homes and conducted psychotherapy groups will be conscious of the inevitable presence of one or two residents who are distinct in their narcissistic demand to be the center of attention. Indeed, it seems that such narcissistic entitlement is even more rampant in nursing homes than in general clinical populations. It is interesting that narcissistic personality disorder seems to survive into late life. While we have become aware that many personality problems, such as sociopathy and antisocial behavior tend to ameliorate with the passage of time and development, narcissistic traits seem to have great resilience and survive healthfully into late life! Again, it is predictable that the initial posture of the helper towards narcissistic resident is to be sympathetic toward the resident's needs. As the behavior increasingly reveals its self-preoccupation, the helper becomes increasingly disenchanted and loses the felt willingness to help, often avoiding the resident. In working with narcissistic temperament and behavior, it is important to quickly develop *empathy* for the narcissistic behavior. For example, it seems reasonable that persons who have distinct narcissistic entitlement are those who have been indulged and "spoiled" during their formative years. In fact, however, the reverse is usually the case. While the narcissistic person may have been indulged with physical resources, they almost uniformly have experienced emotional deprivation. The developmental dynamics of narcissism point to an ineffective nurturance which has left the person still in an emotional "feeding frenzy" in which other persons serve as "resources." The narcissistic person is at a primitive level in the development of a healthy sense of self, and thus other persons are predominantly resources for their perceived needs. This represents a more empathic view of the person's experience and can allow the caregiver or therapist to be "present" to this person without inordinate frustration. This counterintuitive therapeutic posture allows the therapist to be clear about the limits of their involvement, to feel psychologically free and "in charge of" the case and therefore to be able to work with this person without a reactive sense of annoyance. In turn, this allows the therapist (and/or caregiver) to assertively and pleasantly address the unreasonable bids for attention.

BEHAVIOR OF DEMENTIA PATIENTS

Demented behavior in nursing homes takes several forms from aggressive behavior to wandering to inappropriate toileting, etc. Given the nature of cognitive damage involved in dementia, it is not surprising that a systemic understanding of the nature of these behaviors points to a relatively primitive and simple organization. The meaning of such behaviors is largely understood at the neurological and behavioristic level rather than at the level of complex psychological cognitive dynamics. This underlines the fact that seeking the systemic meaning of a behavior does not necessarily invoke complex, psychodynamic processes. Indeed, a therapist is wise to seek a parsimonious meaning for any given symptomatic pattern, rather than have a predetermined theoretical "set" as to the meaning or purpose of any given behavior. While behaviorist principles, in general, have seen some decline in the field of psychotherapy, they have become emphasized again in therapies with dementia patients. The use of stimulus manipulation techniques (Hussian, 1986) for example, have helped to curtail difficult and disruptive behaviors such as wandering and disruptive toileting. In the case of wandering behavior, while passive restraints have become a useful therapeutic method, stimulus manipulation can also work effectively. This might involve, for example, placing large visible grids around the exit from nursing homes and training the demented resident, through associated verbal cues, to avoid crossing these grids. Similarly, inappropriate toileting behavior may be helped with providing large stimuli/cues to direct toileting behavior toward the bathroom.

Dealing with aggressive behavior in dementia patients requires a more calibrated approach. Close inspection of the interactions that lead up to aggressive behavior suggests two possibilities. One possibility is that on occasion demented behavior can be inherently aggressive in type and psychopharmacological intervention may be appropriate. Another possibility is that the aggressive behavior of demented patients is a product of the reciprocal interaction that occurs between themselves and caregivers. A typical example follows. As a psychological consultant I was called into a nursing home to evaluate a resident who had (non-lethally) stabbed a nurse with a fork. Interestingly, the staff had prepared the resident well for my psychological assessment (likely hoping that an evaluation of dementia would produce a referral to another facility!). In fact, this serendipitous occurrence helped diagnose the problem. During the period of time the staff had remained "hands off" the resident in order to produce a calm that would facilitate psychological assessment, they stumbled onto the solution to the problem! The resident was quite calm and cooperative during the psychological and cognitive assessment, and it became clear that the incident with the fork had occurred when a staff member had attempted to direct the resident away from a dangerous area of the nursing home. They had probably done so in a directive and physically authoritative manner that produced an aggressive reaction from the resident. A systemic understanding of a situation like this leads to a strategic position of being more "passive" toward movement in a demented resident. While the intuitive instinct of the caregiver is to direct and physically lead the resident away from the danger, a more effective tactic is somewhat the reverse of this. In working with dementia patients, rather than use physical touch to constrain or direct the person, it frequently helps for the helper simply to hold out an "invitational" hand toward the resident, encouraging them to make physical contact. My experience of this strategy suggests that touch becomes an almost magnetic force, which leads the resident to reach for the hand of the caregiver. This reverses the dynamics that have led to oppositional and aggressive behavior and tends to produce a more collaborative behavior on the part of the demented patient.

DEPRESSIVE BEHAVIOR

Depressive behavior which is unyielding and leads to lack of involvement in prescribed nursing home activities, such as social activities and health care, can cause disruption and consume inordinate amounts of time and attention. As mentioned earlier, understanding the dynamic meaning of such symptom patterns will help to design strategic and tactical solutions. Another example from geriatric practice will emphasize the danger of relying on symptom profiles as a sole basis for diagnosis. An unhappy spouse referred her older husband who had a long-term problem of intractable and recurring depression lasting most of their marriage. He described his symptoms as "unbearable" and leading him to the depths of despair, for which he apologized profusely to his wife. Long-term treatment with antidepressive medication seemed to have brought little relief to him or to their marriage. A consultation with a psychiatrist colleague suggested the presence of a Bipolar II disorder, instead of a major depression. However, both I, as the psychotherapist, and the psychiatrist also recognized a pervasive personality disorder, histrionic personality with narcissistic traits, which emerged in both clinical interviews and psychological assessment. While more appropriate psychopharmacological treatment helped alleviate the depressive symptoms, most gains in psychotherapy and in marital counseling came from a better understanding of his manipulative interpersonal style. While the presence of a significant personality problem does involve some diminution of responsibility in dysfunctional behavior, the patient in this case was able to respond to therapeutic challenges and to accept a more instrumental role in managing his life and marriage (Friedman, 1989).

Another important dimension of depressive behavior is that it may represent two psychological positions that are polar opposites. Sometimes depression is a signal of the *beginning* of a psychological problem; at other times depression is a signal of the movement towards *recovery*. The distinction between these two meanings of depressive symptoms is critical in developing a therapeutic strategy and related tactics. In the life of a relatively engaged, social, and interactive resident the sudden appearance of depressive symptoms may signal the need to investigate events or occurrences in the patient's life such as loss and grieving. However, in other cases the situation is reversed. I recall several years ago working with a hypochondriacal patient in the manner described earlier in this paper. The initial condition of the patient was extreme agitation, which settled down into a pervasive hypochondriacal manner of dealing with the residents, staff, and physicians. Using the approach outlined earlier, the hypochondriacal symptoms and agitation diminished in a few weeks. However, on a subsequent visit, the nursing home van driver informed me that he had recently taken my client to the hospital because of the onset of severe depression. This led me to assume that I had missed some important dynamics in understanding this case. Fortunately, at that time I was reading some material that suggested that depression can be both the "entry" and the "exit" to more serious psychological problems (Verwoerdt, 1987). While depression is among the most painful of disorders and one of the most disruptive, it is not necessarily the most serious of disorders. The logic of the situation appeared to be as follows: my patient's hypochondriasis essentially involved an avoidant psychological state in which physical symptoms were substituted for a direct experience of loss and hopelessness and lack of nurturance she was experiencing. The onset of depressive symptoms, rather than signaling the failure of therapy, in fact signaled the progression from the avoidant hypochondriacal state to a more direct and therefore painful depression in which she began to acknowledge and face the feelings that were involved. Thus, this patient began to experience a depression that was the beginning, rather than the end, of *movement toward health*. Such understanding of the meaning of symptoms once again indicates the importance of definition in our systemic understanding of symptomatic behavior. Predictably, my patient became less depressed, as well as less hypochondriacal and eventually was able to engage in residential life and activities in a healthy, non-symptomatic manner.

CONCLUSION

The various clinical situations described above were provided to illustrate the need for a systemic and strategic understanding and approach to working with problems. These elements, in turn, enable the therapist to design specific techniques or tactics which are most likely to be accurate and effective in reducing the symptomatic behavior and, hopefully, the underlying psychological situation or condition. It therefore becomes a principle of psychotherapeutic practice that "not all is what it seems to be" and the solutions to common problems often follow counterintuitive directions.

REFERENCES

Duffy, M. (1986) The techniques and contexts of multigenerational family therapy. *Clinical Gerontologist*, 5(3/4), 347-361.

Friedman, S. (1989) Brief systemic psychotherapy in a health maintenance organization. *Family Therapy*, 16(2), 133-144.

Greenleaf, E. (1997) Locus and communication. *Journal of Systemic Therapies*, 16(2), 144-172.

Hussian, (1988) Modification of behaviors in dementia via stimulus manipulation. *Clinical Gerontologist*, 8(1), 37-43.

Maddox, G.L. (1964) Disengagement theory: A critical evaluation. *Gerontologist*, 4, 80-82.

Millon, T. (1990) *Toward a New Personology*. New York, NY: John Wiley and Sons, Inc.

Verwoerdt, A. (1987) The psychodynamics of paranoid phenomena. In J. Sadovoy and M. Leszcz (Ed.), *Treating the Elderly with Psychotherapy*. Madison, CT: International University Press Inc.

SECTION TWO: MULTIDISCIPLINARY AND SYSTEMIC ISSUES

Family Work in a Long-Term Care Setting

Suzann M. Ogland-Hand, PhD
Margaret Florsheim, PhD

SUMMARY. Following placement of a relative in a nursing home, many family members maintain an active caregiving role. Families are often an invisible force in long-term care settings. Although they do not live or work inside the facility, their influence on resident and staff functioning is profound. Psychologists working in long-term care settings are frequently asked to intervene around issues involving family members. Understanding the interactive nature of problems both within and between the resident, the family, the staff, and the larger community facilitates the development of successful psychological interventions.

    This article presents the psychologist's use of a systemic approach in guiding interventions with families of long-term care residents. Com-

Suzann M. Ogland-Hand is affiliated with Pine Rest Christian Mental Health Services, Grand Rapids, MI. Margaret Florsheim is affiliated with Palo Alto VA Health Care System, Palo Alto, CA.

This article is based on a paper presented at the 102nd Annual Meeting of the American Psychological Association, Los Angeles, CA, August 15, 1994.

[Haworth co-indexing entry note]: "Family Work in a Long-Term Care Setting." Ogland-Hand, Suzann M., and Margaret Florsheim. Co-published simultaneously in *Clinical Gerontologist* (The Haworth Press, Inc.) Vol. 25, No. 1/2, 2002, pp. 105-123; and: *Emerging Trends in Psychological Practice in Long-Term Care* (ed: Margaret P. Norris, Victor Molinari, and Suzann Ogland-Hand) The Haworth Press, Inc., 2002, pp. 105-123. Single or multiple copies of this article are available for a fee from The Haworth Document Delivery Service [1-800-HAWORTH, 9:00 a.m. - 5:00 p.m. (EST). E-mail address: getinfo@haworthpressinc.com].

mon concerns are reviewed, including family members' adjustment to long-term care placement and the challenges between families and staff. Case examples are used to illustrate these concerns and challenges. The use of a systemic model in family work in long-term care settings is described, and then illustrated with a case example. This case is presented to highlight the interactive nature of problems that can arise between staff and families, the impact of these problems on resident care, as well as the utility of systemic conceptualization in guiding family interventions in long-term care settings. *[Article copies available for a fee from The Haworth Document Delivery Service: 1-800-HAWORTH. E-mail address: <getinfo@haworthpressinc.com> Website: <http://www.HaworthPress.com> © 2002 by The Haworth Press, Inc. All rights reserved.]*

KEYWORDS. Long-term care, systems conceptualization, treatment of family members

Following placement of a relative in a nursing home or assisted living facility, many family members maintain an active caregiving role. While many family members continue their unexpected career in caregiving (Aneshensel, Pearlin, Mullan, Zarit & Whitlatch, 1995), families are often a seemingly invisible force in long-term care. Although they do not live or work inside the facility, their influence on resident and staff functioning is profound. Psychologists can influence family well-being in long-term settings (Qualls, 2000). In this setting, psychologists are often asked to intervene around a variety of family problems (Cauffield, Moye & Travis, 1999; Cohn, 1988; Cohn & Jay, 1988; Harahan, 2001; Hartz & Splain, 1997; O'Dowd & Gomez, 2001; Sidell, 1999; Whitlatch, Feinberg & Stevens, 1999; Zarit, 1996). Understanding the interactive nature of problems both within and between the resident, the family, and the staff facilitates the development of successful psychological interventions.

CONCERNS INVOLVING FAMILY MEMBERS: ISSUES WHERE PSYCHOLOGISTS ARE ASKED TO INTERVENE

Identifying and describing specific concerns of family and long-term care staff can be a helpful first step towards problem-solving. The following is a description of common issues involving family members of nursing home residents where psychologists are often asked to intervene. This list is not meant to be exhaustive, but to represent a sampling of common concerns presenting themselves to psychologists consulting in long-term care. Identifying and normalizing such concerns for both nursing home staff and family members can be a useful first step toward changing problematic patterns of communication between these groups.

Adjustment to Placement

The placement of a family member into a long-term care facility may precipitate a family crisis. A family's difficulties discussing placement may lead to a crisis versus planned decision for placement. Discussing options for long-term care may not be communicated among all family members. Sometimes when placement occurs, family members are not in agreement.

Case example: Tom, a caregiver, tells the psychologist how guilty he feels placing Anne, his wife of 45 years, in the nursing home. However, since Anne's second stroke, Tom can no longer manage her care at home. He states this decision has been particularly difficult because his son and daughter repeatedly remind him of their belief that it is a family's duty to care for each other. Tom's adult children, however, are not involved in Anne's day-to-day care. Tom has tried to tell his children that he is unable to handle their mother's daily care. Tom still questions whether he made the right decision. He feels guilty and depressed, and unsupported by his children.

A brief assessment indicates that Tom is moderately depressed. As the psychologist and Tom discussed how to proceed, they identified Tom's depression as a primary problem, with the lack of communication with his children, as well as Anne's decline, as likely primary contributors to his symptoms.

Family Role Adjustments

The role shifting that can occur within a family as they adjust to illness and placement can be difficult, especially for those with engrained beliefs about those roles.

Case example: Bob and Emma, an older couple, had traditional roles in their marriage. Bob was the "head" of the family, and Emma supported his decisions. After Bob's severe left-sided stroke left him aphasic, Emma became his primary caregiver and assumed many of the roles that formerly belonged to Bob, roles which were new for her and about which she felt a lack of confidence. Bob was frustrated at his loss of functioning and decreased ability to communicate with others. After Bob's placement, Emma frequently took him on outings, which in a dramatic way displayed the other shifts in their roles: now Emma was driving the car, and Bob was the passenger. On these trips, Bob would attempt to direct Emma's driving: he would point for her to switch lanes or grunt directions for her to pass cars, and one time even grabbed the wheel from her as she was entering the freeway. While Emma was scared, frustrated and angry, she was unsure how to handle this situation, as well as other role-shifts within their relationship.

An assessment with the psychologist indicated that Emma was moderately depressed. Together, Emma and the psychologist identified treatment targets. One problem was Emma's inexperience with being more assertive and active in her interactions with Bob. A second problem was Emma's significant grief and shock about Bob's decline since his stroke, which resulted in significant changes in their lifestyle (their difficulty communicating with each other, her having to become a decision-maker, and his subsequent nursing home placement). A third concern identified was Emma's acknowledged skill deficits for some of the new tasks she had assumed in response to Bob's health decline.

Case example: Henry has always relied on Linda to manage their home and their three teenage children. Since Linda developed an early-onset dementia, his life became a nightmare. After Linda's placement, Henry was faced with the responsibility of managing the household, a responsibility he had never had before. He was feeling overwhelmed and unsure of himself. During an assessment with the psychologist, he voiced his fears for the future, and his difficulty knowing how to address these issues with his children. In a family meeting with Henry and his children, they all voiced sadness and grief at Linda's decline and prognosis. Together, they identified problems of coping with Linda's decline, and working together to address tasks of managing their house and family.

Family Involvement After Placement of Resident

Family members' involvement with a relative following long-term care placement may undergo adjustments. Some family members have difficulty deciding how frequently to visit. Frequently, family members are unclear how to be involved after placing their loved one in a nursing home. Sometimes they aren't sure how to interact with the person, or even how to visit someone when they have been providing direct care in the past. Psychologists may point out how common confusion is for families after placement, normalizing their experience. Most family members welcome advice on how to have productive and enjoyable visits.

Case example: Sam and Evelyn had been married for 45 years. Evelyn's illness became so debilitating that she required nursing home care. Sam had devoted the past 12 years to caring for his wife. However, once she was placed, he didn't know what to do with his time and became depressed. A brief assessment with the psychologist indicates that Sam is severely depressed. Problems for treatment included grief and lack of identification of potentially pleasurable activities. Treatment targets surrounded grief work, identification of pleasant events, and increasing Sam's involvement in enjoyable activity on a daily basis.

Sexual Issues

Placement in a skilled nursing home often involves loss of privacy and corresponding adjustments in expressions of intimacy. Most room assignments require adjusting to the needs of a roommate. If the sexual relationship between a couple was positive prior to placement, the couple may miss the sexual aspect of their relationship. Not knowing how to interpret the distance that is created between them after placement, residents may raise concerns that their spouse is having an affair. Or, the resident could end up in bed with another person, perhaps purposefully, or because the resident is quite demented. The resident and the caregiver may have strong reactions to these situations that need to be discussed and clarified.

Case example: Eldon, a 64-year-old man, lives in assisted living following a stroke. He says that prior to his placement, he and his wife enjoyed an active sexual relationship. Eldon, due to financial limitations, is assigned to share a room with another resident and misses expressions of physical intimacy that he previously enjoyed with his wife. During a brief assessment, both Eldon and his wife identified feeling saddened by the loss of physical intimacy. Lack of privacy in the shared room was identified as the primary cause of this change. Treatment involved strategies to arrange for this couple to have private time together in the assisted living setting.

Long-Standing Marital/Family Conflict

Some persons placed in nursing homes come from families with long-standing conflict. Chronic conflict may exist within a marriage, the entire family, or with specific family members. Interestingly, some family relationships with a high level of conflict actually improve following placement due to the distance that now exists between family members.

Case example: An elderly couple with long-standing marital conflict report that following the nursing home placement of the wife, they are experiencing reduced conflict and enjoying biweekly visits.

Case example: Mitch and Helen describe a long-term history of marital conflict, with frequent, loud arguments. After Mitch's placement in the nursing home, their marital conflict continued. Staff and residents complain about loud shouting matches between the couple occurring during the wife's visits.

As the psychologist met with the couple for an assessment, she determined that both were distressed about the nonproductive nature of their conflicts, with both Mitch and Helen expressing that they did not feel "heard" by the other. Following this meeting, the couple agreed to work with the psychologist on improving marital communication.

Family Members with Their Own Psychopathology

Psychological symptoms or disorders in the long-term care resident's spouse or children are often unexpected and difficult for staff and others to handle.

Case example: The alcoholic son of a 101-year-old nursing home resident frequently is intoxicated during visits to his mother. During his visits, the son was loud and belligerent, frequently complaining to staff about his mother's grooming. Nursing staff complained about the son's behavior to the consulting psychologist.

During the assessment, the 77-year-old son voiced that his mother seemed generally well cared for, but was concerned that her hair and fingernails were often long. The son then tearfully admitted to multiple recent losses, including his wife of 45 years who had died 2 years ago suddenly of a heart attack. He stated that he didn't know how he would cope with his mother's death when it occurred, because he already felt so alone. He admitted to using alcohol to cope with feelings of loneliness and grief, and after some discussion with the psychologist agreed that his alcohol use was a problem.

Treatment included connecting the son with cosmetology services at the nursing home to arrange regular hair cuts and manicures for his mother. The son was also, over time, connected with a range of community resources to address his drinking problem, build a positive support system, and address his losses more adaptively.

Case example: Nancy resides in assisted living, and her husband Bob has a history of manic depressive illness. During manic phases of his illness, he comes in to the assisted living facility and becomes publicly demanding and histrionic with staff regarding his wife's care. His emotional displays upset and frighten staff.

The psychologist provided the staff with education about bipolar disorder, and what to expect during varying times of that illness. The psychologist also met with Bob to evaluate his need for further treatment.

Adherence to the Treatment Plan

Adherence to the plan of care is difficult for some families. For example, it is not uncommon for diabetic residents to have family members who bring them candy. Other families, because of personal and family dynamics, may have difficulty knowing what their limits are regarding care for a family member visiting home, which can also impact adherence to the treatment plan.

Case example: Bill has lived in a nursing home since his second stroke. Nursing home staff have worked hard to encourage Bill to actively participate in his daily care as much as he is able. Bill's wife, Carol, visits Bill daily and during visits caters to his every wish, including feeding Bill although he is physically capable of feeding himself.

An assessment with Carol determined that Bill's decline had taken a toll on Carol. While she was not depressed, she was frustrated with the reality that she could not alter Bill's medical situation, and she struggled with feelings of helplessness. Carol saw feeding Bill as one way to "do something" for him. In a quarterly treatment planning meeting, the psychologist helped Carol and the rest of the treatment team clarify these issues, and worked toward a mutuality agreeable resolution.

Goals/Treatment Implementation

Sometimes conflict exists between staff and family surrounding implementation of treatment goals for the resident. This can be framed as "who should do what?" (Bonder, Miller, & Linsk, 1991). Sometimes staff doesn't have the resources for treatment that is indicated. It's not necessarily that the staff members are bad or uncaring, but just limited in their resources. At the same time, family members of residents may have limited resources as well: they may live too far away to be involved in daily care, and may not be able to afford hiring someone to provide these services. Clear communication between staff and family can clarify expectations and limits regarding the subdivision of these tasks.

Case example: Sarah, a nursing home resident, had advanced Parkinson's disease, and received regular physical therapy, including stretching and range-of-motion to maintain flexibility and her limited mobility. Sarah's husband and daughter insist she participate in rigorous physical therapy exercises. Staff members view the family's goals as unrealistic.

During an assessment with the psychologist, Sarah's husband and daughter were each tearful and sad about the long decline they had observed in Sarah. Treatment for their grief and depression followed.

Case example: An ethical issue involves declining health status of a resident, Gertrude, who develops terminal cancer after having multiple small strokes. Her husband doesn't want her bothered, stating "why don't you just make Gertie happy." Staff's position is to keep her as mobile as possible, get her out of bed, and to maintain the functioning that remains.

During an assessment with the psychologist, Gertie's husband voices that she was always the light of his life. Since her nursing home placement, he visits daily, and does all he can to make her comfortable and contented. He does not appear to have any untreated mental health problems. After her diagnosis of untreatable cancer, he feels he made peace with her impending death, and "just wants her to be happy." With some support from the therapist about her approaching death and what he has been experiencing, the psychologist is then able to provide him with some education. He is able to listen and understand that even though Gertie isn't expected to live for another year, her last months and days will be easier on her if she maintains her mobility and flexibility until later into her disease course.

End-of-Life Decisions

End-of-life care decisions may be difficult for family members to consider or to discuss with each other. For the spouse, it may be too upsetting to even think about life without their partner, and staff may feel very uncomfortable continuing raising the issue. Conflict may exist between the couple regarding code status or the withholding or withdrawing of life sustaining treatments, such as artificial nutrition and hydration.

Case example: Dave reschedules several meetings with the nursing home team staff to discuss his wife's increasing swallowing difficulties associated with her progressing Huntington's disease. In an assessment with the psychologist, he finally admits that he avoids these discussions due to his difficulties acknowledging his wife's decline. Treatment for his depression and grief is able to begin.

Case example: Barbara had been married to Sam for over 50 years. Sam had been living in the nursing home since his second stroke. He now had developed cancer, and the physician stated Sam had at most one year left. In a medical emergency, Sam does not want any extraordinary measures taken to save his life, advocating a do not resuscitate (DNR) code status order, while Barbara wanted every measure taken to save Sam's life. Barbara was very sad about losing Sam, and also had fears of the financial impact of Sam's death on her. She had been relying on Sam's pension ever since he had retired, and once he dies, she fears she will become impoverished. Staff members at the nursing home acknowledge the conflict between Barbara's realistic financial concerns and her husband's care wishes.

Abuse: Financial, Physical, Psychological

Sometimes staff must deal with physical, financial or psychological abuse issues. For example, a resident might become a potential victim of financial abuse when his wife dies, and another family member with ulterior motives gets the resident to sign over power-of-attorney.

Case example: John, a resident in assisted living, reports that his woman friend, Dorothy, is pushing for marriage. John receives a large pension, and staff at the assisted living facility suspect Dorothy has motives of financial gain. The psychologist meets with John, who acknowledges that he does not want to marry Dorothy. He reports that he likes being able to provide Dorothy with cash gifts at his discretion, and identifies that he wishes to maintain control over his finances. Connecting John with an attorney allows him to make adjustments in his will consistent with his wishes.

Case example: Joe has Parkinson's disease and lives in the nursing home. His wife, Caroline, becomes verbally abusive due to her own distress over Joe's appearance and speech changes. Joe drools and has reduced speech volume. Nursing home staff witness Caroline yell at Joe during a visit, "Stop mumbling!" Later, the resident's roommate reports seeing Caroline slap Joe.

The psychologist meets with Caroline and determines she has developed panic disorder and depression, and is embarrassed about how her own behavior has changed since Joe's decline. Caroline admits to expressing frustration toward her husband on more than one occasion in verbally and physically abusive ways. Together with the psychologist she agrees to contact local adult protective services, who collaborate with the psychologist to connect Caroline with appropriate mental health services.

Summary

Psychologists providing consultation to long-term care are frequently asked to intervene with concerns involving family members of residents. These concerns may be associated with family adjustments occurring as a result of nursing home placement, may reflect communication difficulties and/or psychopathology that may pre-exist within the family, or may arise from communication difficulties that exist between family members and long-term care staff.

CHALLENGES FOR PSYCHOLOGISTS IN A LONG-TERM CARE SETTING

Psychologists working with families in the context of a long-term care setting may face multiple challenges in implementing effective interventions. The following section outlines some of these for consideration in providing psychological consultation to nursing homes.

Consultant Role: No Ongoing Relationship with Staff

Many psychologists in long-term care settings are consultants, having limited time to spend on relationships with staff, or not even having the opportunity to observe interactions between staff and family. Reimbursement restrictions may limit a psychologist's opportunities to observe patient/family/staff interactions. Having an ongoing relationship with staff facilitates the staff feeling supported and understood in their work demands with both residents and family members. Developing such ongoing relationships over time is essential to effective interventions in long-term care settings. This requires patience, as well as willingness to spend time on the unit that may not initially appear to be patient-related or even reimbursable in the private sector.

"Do Something About This Family"

Referrals generated by nursing home staff are frequently framed as staff requests to "do something about this family." Having a systemic perspective suggests that multiple parties, including staff, contribute to difficult interactions. Likely, staff members do not initially view themselves as part of the dysfunctional system. To solicit staff's observations about their own contributions requires that the psychologist is seen in a constructive and supportive role. It is critical for the psychologist to elicit the staff support in this process, as well as to identify staff's contribution to the problem in a way that they don't feel blamed.

Multicultural Background of Staff and Families

Long-term care staff members are often multicultural. The different cultural backgrounds of staff can pose a challenge to psychological intervention. Staff members are likely to hold strong beliefs about families and family involvement in care. These expectations are frequently not articulated and may not be readily understood by the psychologist, who may represent yet a different cultural background. Such verbally unexpressed expectations are often behaviorally expressed in ways that make staff and family interactions complicated to decipher. It is incumbent upon the psychologist to be sensitive to cultural and ethnic differences of families and nursing home staff, and to facilitate the articulation of these strongly held beliefs.

Change in Family System Over Time

By the time the psychologist sees the long-term care resident, health status may have dramatically altered his/her behavior so that it is hard to understand how the person functioned in the family prior to illness. The resident may not be able to provide historical information, and family members may have their own distorted views. Gathering historical family information can be a challenge. However, this historical data is essential because it provides a perspective on how interactions in the family have or have not changed in response to illness and long-term care placement.

Ethical Issues

While psychologists are called in to aid in various situations, this in itself can be a challenge because the family may not be the identified patient. Questions arise regarding how to share information. Charting can also be a complicated ethical issue. Psychologists need to chart about family involvement in a way that is helpful to the staff, yet with sensitivity to the confidentiality needs of family members. (See Norris's article in this series.)

Time Factor

Key members of the family or the staff may not be available at the same time. Frequently the whole family is not available, due to work schedules, and/or family members living out of the area. This can be a challenge because the key people that impact the system are needed for changes to occur.

Staff availability can also be a challenge. Nursing staff work different shifts and sometimes key staff are not available. This can be a challenge because the psychologist may not be around when important events occur. Further, different shifts have different workloads and experience different resident/family problems. For example, staff working evening shifts may have problems with residents sun-downing, while day shift staff may face difficulties getting residents ready for daily appointments. Family visits may occur during specific shifts. The importance of making oneself available to different shifts is critical for effective psychological intervention in long-term care.

Psychologists: A Balancing Act

Balancing between participant and observer may be difficult for the psychologist involved in long-term care. On the one hand, it's important for the psychologist to be accepted and to be a part of the nursing home system, while at the same time, in order to formulate effective interventions, it's important for the psychologist to maintain the more objective perspective of an observer.

Summary

As noted above, psychologists working in long-term care settings can experience challenges developing effective relationships with family and staff necessary to implement appropriate systemic interventions. In order to develop constructive partnerships with all parties involved, psychologists need sensitivity, flexibility and creativity.

INTERACTIONAL MODEL OF SYSTEMIC COMMUNICATION: A CASE EXAMPLE

The following case example will be used to illustrate the use of an interactional model of communication. This model will be used to clarify the systemic nature of many family concerns in skilled nursing facilities and its utility in formulating practical interventions.

Case Example

Neil Adams, a frail 75-year-old depressed male with 20-year history of Parkinson's disease, is a resident of the Shady Oaks Nursing Home where he has lived for the past four years. He has been married to his wife, Joyce Adams, for the past 40 years. The head nurse referred Joyce to the psychologist, and reported that while Joyce comes frequently to Shady Oaks, she "doesn't know how to provide emotional support to her husband. She isn't loving to him in a way that he needs. She can't just sit with him." Joyce was also described as demanding and critical of staff and as always bothering staff about things. The psychologist was asked to "fix Joyce."

Interactional Model of Systemic Communication

Using a systemic case conceptualization, the problem is seen as lying within the interaction of the long-term care staff, the resident and family, not just within one party; this means that each party has responsibility for contributions to the difficult interactions. So, in the case example, instead of viewing Joyce as the problem that needs to be fixed, systemic theory suggests that an interactional difficulty likely exists between Joyce and the staff, i.e., the problem is contained in their interaction.

One way to examine the interactions between members of a system is to diagram how the behavior of one party affects the experience, thoughts and feelings of the other person, which in turn impacts the other person's experience, thoughts and feelings, and so on (see Figure 1). White's (1993) model is a helpful one to explain how interactions between parties can get bogged down. To explain this case, this model is particularly useful for three reasons. First, the model clarifies the interactional nature of communication, i.e., how the behavior of one party is experienced by the other, which in turn impacts the second party's behavior. Second, the model highlights the circularity of dysfunctional interactions, i.e., how the patterns of communication can become self-reinforcing and redundant. Finally, this way of understanding interactional patterns can also identify multiple points of intervention. Interventions can then be geared to changing any point, and instituting change at any point in the cycle will shift the interaction.

Assessment of the Problem

To obtain more information, the psychologist met separately with Joyce and with the staff. As the psychologist met with Joyce, she learned that Joyce saw her role as being an advocate for her husband's care. Joyce voiced specific incidents she had had with staff that left her feeling unhappy. She had repeatedly tried to raise concerns with staff about her husband's care, but she always heard the staff put her concerns back on her. For example, when Joyce asked about Neil's dental care, she reported staff would state to her, "Why don't you pick up a toothbrush and brush them yourself?"

The psychologist also felt that grief and loss were issues for Joyce, noting that within their 40-year marriage, half of it had been spent adjusting to Neil's continued decline from Parkinson's. Joyce admitted feeling sad as she watched her husband slowly decline, and sometimes when she left Shady Oaks, she would feel sad and tearful for hours at home. Joyce said it was difficult to visit Neil, and because of her sadness, she only felt able to come in for brief visits. Joyce also described perceiving the staff's reactions to her questions (e.g., "Why don't you pick up a toothbrush . . .") as not only misunderstanding her role as caregiver to her husband, but also not taking responsibility for their jobs as care providers. This perception by Joyce led her to feel angry towards staff and concerned about the adequacy of their care to her husband, further fueling her feelings of guilt about his placement.

FIGURE 1. Model of Interactional Communication

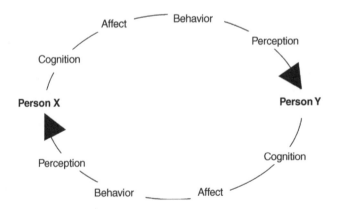

In order to gather more information about the staff's contributions to the interaction, the psychologist met with staff briefly during shift change report. Staff labeled Joyce as "a pain in the neck" because they perceived her as critical and demanding of them. They felt the only time they heard from Joyce was when something was wrong. Staff also perceived Joyce's complaints as being indirect. Instead of asking staff to brush her husband's teeth, staff described Joyce saying, "Don't my husband's teeth look disgusting?" As a result, staff labeled Joyce as "devious" and "manipulative." They also labeled her as "uninvolved" because they perceived Joyce as not providing emotional support to her husband. On her visits, for example, all she did was to escort her husband on quick walks around the courtyard, and then leave; she didn't sit with him and hold his hands the way other caregivers did with their spouses.

Case Conceptualization

To begin to fill in the interactional model, it is helpful to begin with an instance where problematic communication occurs (see Figure 2). In this case, the *behavior* or action that we observe is Joyce speaking to a staff member about her husband's teeth saying, "Don't my husband's teeth look disgusting?" Staff's *perception*, what they see and hear, are Joyce's whiny voice, her indirect criticism, and her multiple questions and demands.

Staff's *thoughts* are then that she is devious and manipulative; she'll never be happy no matter what we do; her demands are unreasonable–we've got 50 residents to care for, not just her husband; and she doesn't understand us.

Staff *feel* angry, unappreciated, overworked, and overwhelmed. In response, staff state to Joyce, "Why don't you pick up a toothbrush and brush his teeth yourself?" In turn, Joyce *hears* the staff's curt replies, notes they sound irritated, sees them as rushed, and perceives that staff cut her questions off. She *thinks* they don't take my concerns seriously; they are placing all the responsibility on me; they'll never be satisfied with what I do; they don't want to take care of Neil; and they don't want my input. As a result, she feels frustrated, unappreciated, and angry. In turn, she only interacts with staff when there is a concern focusing on negatives. She decides to no longer attend quarterly care plan meetings, further engraining the staff's beliefs that she is "uninvolved."

Intervention

This example illustrates an interaction based on several cycles of nonproductive communication, which served to further engrain the be-

FIGURE 2. Model of Interactional Communication: Case Example

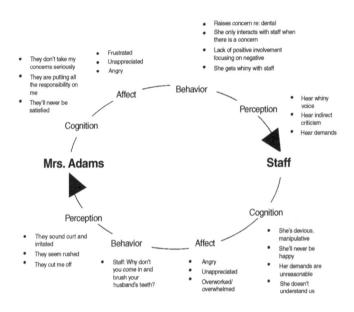

liefs each party had about the other. As with many cycles of nonproductive communication, communication worsened. Joyce, frustrated at not getting her needs met, called in authority figures to back her up. She complained to the nursing supervisor, who told staff it *was* staff's responsibility to provide Neil's dental care, and Joyce took Neil to the dentist, who prescribed a twice a day dental rinse. This action by Joyce further engrained the staff's beliefs that she was devious and manipulative.

As in any interactional system, nonproductive communication patterns can develop. It's important at this point to note that the actions or interventions that took place from the authority figures–the nursing supervisor and the dentist–focused solely on this issue of the teeth brushing. They addressed the *content* of this particular issue, but not the unproductive *process* that was going on between staff and Joyce. Given that these interventions didn't address the systemic process issues between staff and Joyce, other problems are likely to occur following this same nonproductive interactional pattern. Further, it's important to note that in this situation, it is not that either the staff or Joyce was having unreasonable requests, but the nonproductive interactions between them were serving only to engrain distorted perceptions and beliefs of the other.

Thus, interventions from the psychologist in the system must address the process of what is going on between the two parties. In this interactional systemic model, interventions can occur at any point and on multiple levels. In this case example, several interventions were made. Interventions were geared primarily in shifting Joyce's behavior, which resulted in shifts in staff behavior as well, and ultimately shifts in the perception, thoughts and feelings of both parties.

First, it was decided that the caregiver, the resident, and the staff would be better served by having a weekly check-in, initiated by Joyce, with one nursing staff, so she could briefly receive an update regarding Neil's medical care, and could discuss her concerns and questions. The psychologist's hope was that as time passed, occasionally Joyce might not have any complaints regarding Neil's care; then this weekly check-in could also provide a pleasant interaction between Joyce and a staff member where they could begin to develop a different type of relationship with each other. This might shift Joyce from avoiding staff contact, to having more frequent positive contact.

Additionally, the psychologist met individually with Joyce to provide support and address problematic communication with staff. The psychologist let Joyce know how well the staff responded to positive feedback about their work with residents, and encouraged more positive interactions with staff. So the shift was from Joyce giving negative feedback to Joyce giving both positive and negative feedback.

The psychologist also suggested to Joyce that she let staff know some of her feelings about watching her husband gradually deteriorate, in hopes that the staff would develop some empathy for the losses she was experiencing. This was important to help shift the staff's perceptions from "She's a manipulative and devious person–and has always been," to understanding the fact that Joyce was grieving over Neil's decline and feeling a loss of control over making any impact on her husband's illness.

Shifting Joyce's perceptions of staff was important as well, so that Joyce might begin to recognize staff members were sometimes overwhelmed with the demands of their jobs when she spoke to them.

Joyce and the psychologist also worked to clarify Joyce's communication towards staff, so they would clearly hear her limits. That is, if staff was enlisting Joyce's involvement in providing Neil's dental care, she needed to be clear with them what her limits were regarding each specific issue. For example, in the past she may have stated, "Don't you think it's easier for you to do his dental rinse than it would be for me to take 30 minutes each way to drive here and back!" It would be helpful if she could be more direct and clear, "I understand you may not be able to provide twice daily dental rinses for Neil, but I'm not able to do it either. I would be able to do that on Monday mornings, but that's all. What shall we do about this problem?" By Joyce increasing the directness of her communication, staff shifted their cognitions from "Joyce is devious," to "Joyce is being more direct and clear about her limits."

Finally, since spending time "just sitting" with Neil for one or two hours continued to cause Joyce emotional pain, at the encouragement of the psychologist, she decided she would hire a paid attendant who could develop a companion-type relationship with him. This helped the staff see Joyce as concerned about her husband's emotional needs.

As a result of these multiple interventions on multiple levels, the staff and the caregiver's relationship improved. The staff's perception of Joyce shifted, and she became more open about giving them positive feedback, sharing some of her feelings regarding her husband's decline, as well as being more clear about her limits, and following through with the weekly check-in with the assigned nursing staff.

CONCLUSION

Long-term care facilities provide a complex and rich environment where systemic interventions can provide long-lasting change. Problems involving patient, family and staff interactions are frequently embedded in many referrals for psychological intervention in nursing homes. Multiple opportunities, as well as challenges, exist for psychologists doing family work in long-term care settings. Interventions to address systemic issues within long-term care can ultimately be effective in promoting broad change and enhancing functioning.

REFERENCES

Aneshensel, C. S., Pearlin, L. I., Mullan, J. T., Zarit, S. H., & Whitlatch, C. J. (1995). *Profiles in caregiving: The unexpected career.* Academic Press: San Diego, CA.
Bonder, B. R., Miller, B., & Linsk, N. (1991). Who should do what?: Staff and family responsibilities for persons with Alzheimer's disease in nursing homes.*Clinical Gerontologist, 10*(4), 80-84.

Cauffield, C. A., Moye, J., & Travis, L. (1999). Long term marital conflict: Antecedents to and consequences for discharge planning. *Clinical Gerontologist, 20* (2), 82-86.

Cohn, M. D. (1988). Consultation strategies with families. In M. A. Smyer, M. D. Cohn, & D. Brannon (Ed.), *Mental health consultation in nursing homes* (pp. 168-191). New York, NY: New York University Press.

Cohn, M. D. & Jay, G. M. (1988). Families in long-term-care settings. In M. A. Smyer, M. D. Cohn, & D. Brannon (Ed.), *Mental health consultation in nursing homes* (pp. 142-168). New York, NY: New York University Press.

Harahan, M. F. (2001). New paradigms for guiding research, interventions and policies for family caregivers. *Aging & Mental Health, 5* (S52-S55).

Hartz, G. W. & Splain, D. M. (1997). *Psychosocial intervention in long-term care* (pp. 165). New York, NY: Haworth Press.

O'Dowd, M. A. & Gomez, M. F. (2001). Psychotherapy in consultation-liaison psychiatry. *American Journal of Psychotherapy, 55*(1), 122-132.

Qualls, S. H. (2000). Working with families in nursing homes. In V. Molinari (Ed.), *Professional psychology in long-term care* (pp. 91-112). New York, NY: Hatherleigh Press.

Sidell, N. (1999). The experience of community-dwelling spouses of nursing home users: Marital satisfaction, coping and mental health. *Clinical Gerontologist, 21*(1), 57-60.

White, B. B. (1993, Fall). Integrating gender and systems: A gendered social contextual model for systemic couple's therapy. Unpublished manuscript.

Whitlatch, C. J., Feinberg, L. F., & Stevens, E. J. (1999). Predictors of institutionalization for persons with Alzheimer's disease and the impact on family caregivers. *Journal of Mental Health & Aging, 5*(3), 275-288.

Zarit, S. H. (1996). Interventions with family caregivers. In S. H. Zarit, & B. G. Knight (Ed.), *A guide to psychotherapy and aging* (pp. 139-159). Washington, DC: American Psychological Association.

Pleasant Events-Based Behavioral Intervention for Depression in Nursing Home Residents: A Conceptual and Empirical Foundation

Suzanne Meeks, PhD

Colin A. Depp, MA

SUMMARY. In this theoretical/review article, we set forth a conceptual model and empirical evidence as the foundation for a behavioral intervention in nursing homes involving pleasant events. The risk for depression is nearly twice as great among nursing home residents as it is for community-residing elders, with up to 50% of nursing home residents affected by significant depressive symptoms. Although we now have a good understanding of the epidemiology and manifestations of depression in late life, and are beginning to apply effective treatments to some groups of elders, the benefits of the past decade of research have yet to reach the frailest elders living in nursing homes. The health and cognitive multiple comorbidity of this population makes treatment extremely

Suzanne Meeks and Colin A. Depp are affiliated with the University of Louisville.

Address correspondence to: Suzanne Meeks, PhD, Department of Psychological and Brain Sciences, University of Louisville, Louisville, KY 40292 (E-mail: smeeks@louisville.edu).

The authors are indebted to several people who have commented on earlier forms of the rationale presented herein, including George Niederehe, Kimberly Van Haitsma, Stanley A. Murrell, and Janet Woodruff-Borden. Most particularly, the authors thank Linda Teri for her ground-breaking work, feedback, and encouragement.

[Haworth co-indexing entry note]: "Pleasant Events-Based Behavioral Intervention for Depression in Nursing Home Residents: A Conceptual and Empirical Foundation." Meeks, Suzanne, and Colin A. Depp. Co-published simultaneously in *Clinical Gerontologist* (The Haworth Press, Inc.) Vol. 25, No. 1/2, 2002, pp. 125-148; and: *Emerging Trends in Psychological Practice in Long-Term Care* (ed: Margaret P. Norris, Victor Molinari, and Suzann Ogland-Hand) The Haworth Press, Inc., 2002, pp. 125-148. Single or multiple copies of this article are available for a fee from The Haworth Document Delivery Service [1-800-HAWORTH, 9:00 a.m. - 5:00 p.m. (EST). E-mail address: getinfo@haworthpressinc.com].

challenging. The behavioral model we describe is based on the work of Lewinsohn and others. The intervention would adapt work already completed by Teri and her colleagues with elderly dementia patients and their families. We make specific recommendations concerning adapting this treatment approach to nursing homes, and evaluating its effects. *[Article copies available for a fee from The Haworth Document Delivery Service: 1-800-HAWORTH. E-mail address: <getinfo@haworthpressinc.com> Website: <http://www.HaworthPress.com> © 2002 by The Haworth Press, Inc. All rights reserved.]*

KEYWORDS. Nursing homes, depression, behavioral therapy

INTRODUCTION

Depression in long-term care is a significant public health issue. Approximately 1.4 million older Americans reside in nursing homes (National Center for Health Statistics, 1997). Although this represents only a small percentage of all older adults, this medically frail group of elders absorbs a disproportionate share of health care dollars. In addition to medical frailty, this population of elders is at high risk for depression. In their update of the 1991 NIH Consensus Statement on depression in late life, Lebowitz and his colleagues (1997) pointed out the need for treatments that are tailored to meet the needs of elders with significant disability or physical illness. While research on depression and treatments for depression in late life have begun to proliferate, empirically-supported treatment models that are specifically appropriate for elders in long-term care are lacking. The purpose of the present article is to lay an empirical and conceptual foundation for a behavioral approach to treating depression in long-term care.

Epidemiology of Depression in Long-Term Care

Major depression is nearly twice as prevalent in nursing homes as it is among community dwellers, with estimates ranging from 6-25% (Ames, 1990, 1992; Burns et al., 1988; German, Shapiro, & Kramer, 1986; Katz & Parmelee, 1997; Kim & Rovner, 1995; Strahan & Burns, 1991), as compared to community estimates of 2-8% (Regier et al., 1988). Variations in prevalence estimates are due primarily to differing assessment methods (Masand, 1995), but the differential prevalence is clear regardless of the estimates used. Perhaps even more striking are the rates of minor depression and sub-syndromal depressive symptoms, which affect up to 50% of nursing home residents (Kim & Rovner, 1995; Samuels & Katz, 1995; Parmelee, Katz, & Lawton, 1992). Minor depression and depressive symptom elevations are clear risk factors for major depression (Howarth, Johnson, Klerman, & Weissman, 1992; Mossey, 1997; Parmelee et al., 1992), and are also associated with poorer recovery from illness and injury, greater functional impairment, and higher use of health care services (Fries et al., 1993; Mossey, 1997). Incidence rates for depression in nursing homes also are elevated, suggesting that even those who are admitted to nursing homes without depression may be at greater risk of developing depression once there (Katz, Lesher, Kleban, Jethanandani, & Parmelee, 1989; Katz & Parmelee, 1997).

An indicator of the clinical significance of depression is the need for increased nursing care. Depression among those in residential care is related to decreased cognitive status, functional capacity, clinician-rated health, and pain (Katz & Parmelee, 1997). Fries et al. (1993) found that the diagnosis of depression was related to greater use of nursing time, even when impairment in activities of daily living (ADL) was statistically controlled. Depression may increase mortality in nursing homes, even controlling for dementia (Katz et al., 1989; Rovner et al., 1991; Shah, Phongsathorn, & George, 1993), through loss of appetite and resulting poor nutrition, immune system deficiency, loss of parasympathetic tone (Masand, 1995), or an association with cardiovascular disease (Musselman, Evans, & Nemeroff, 1998; Wulsin, Valliant, & Wells, 1999). Depression also increases the possibility of passive and active suicidal behaviors (Reynolds et al., 1998; Wulsin et al., 1999). Depression in nursing homes may therefore not only complicate medical treatment but also may endanger the lives of residents who suffer from it.

Dementia and depression are highly comorbid in nursing home residents. Dementia affects up to 67% of nursing home residents (Magaziner et al., 1996; Rovner et al., 1990). Depression is a significant complicating factor in dementia (Teri & Wagner, 1992; Meyers, 1998; Wragg & Jeste, 1989). The co-existence of the two disorders has been associated with more readmission days, more inpatient psychiatric days, and more nursing home admissions than found in patients with only one of the disorders (Kales, Blow, Copeland, Kammerer, & Mellow, 1999). Depression may increase agitation and aggression in patients suffering from dementia (Lyketsos et al., 1999), so both the amount of care and the stress on the caregiver are likely to be high. It is therefore important that treatments for depression in nursing homes are applicable to those residents with significant cognitive impairment.

Because the majority of depressive syndromes found in nursing homes will not be full-blown major depression (MDD), the clinical significance of minor and sub-syndromal depressions is also important. Data suggest that depressive symptoms persist across several assessment periods, even among people improving from MDD (Ames, 1992; Katz & Parmelee, 1997). In fact, among medical patients in hospitals sub-syndromal depressive symptoms increase the risk for MDD, with poorer recovery from illness and injury, greater functional impairment, and higher use of health care services (Blazer, Hughes, & George, 1987; Blazer & Williams, 1980; Kennedy et al., 1989; Lyness, King, Cox, Yeodiono, & Caine, 1999; Mossey, 1997). Community studies show similarly poor outcomes (Broadhead, Blazer, George, & Tse, 1990; Howarth et al., 1992; Johnson, Weissman, & Klerman, 1992). This evidence suggests the importance of developing treatments applicable to the range of depressive syndromes seen in nursing homes.

Treatments for Depression in Late Life

For young adults, research shows clearly that depression is a disorder that can be effectively treated in the majority of cases, either through use of medication or psychotherapy. Much less is known about treatment responding among older adults, and even less is known about nursing home residents.

Psychopharmacological Interventions. Studies have shown that antidepressant medication can be effective for older adults (see Apfeldorf, Alexopoulos, Weill, & Weill, 1999; Lebowitz et al., 1997; Reynolds et al., 1998, for reviews). However, drug responses may be both delayed and more brittle than for young adults (Bump et al., 1997; Reynolds et al., 1996; Reynolds et al., 1998). Poor responses are most likely among elders who are older and not married (Little et al., 1998), or bereaved (Pasternak et al., 1997), characteristics that are typical of nursing home residents. The evidence concerning pharmacological treatment of depression among frail elders, including those in nursing homes, suggests that antidepressant medications can be effective, but has failed to improve functional disability or self-care (Katz, Simpson, Curlik, & Parmelee, 1990), mitigate bereavement (Reynolds, Miller et al., 1999), or eliminate hopelessness (Szanto, Reynolds, Conwell, Begley, & Houck, 1998). Both tricyclic antidepressants (TCAs) and serotonin reuptake inhibitors (SRIs) produce an increased risk of side effects in frail elders (Katz et al., 1989; Katz, Parmelee, Beaston-Wimmer, & Smith, 1994; Nebes et al., 1997; Thapa, Gideon, Cost, Milam, & Ray, 1998). These shortcomings suggest the need to develop psychosocial interventions that can either augment, or in cases where drugs cannot be tolerated, substitute for, pharmacotherapy (Reynolds, 1994; Reynolds, Miller et al., 1999). Among medical patients, research suggests that psychotherapy may be more successful than pharmacotherapy for depressive symptoms (Klerman et al., 1987; Mossey, Knott, Higgins, & Talerico, 1996; Paykel, Hollyman, Freeling, & Sedgewick, 1989).

Psychosocial Interventions. A number of psychotherapy approaches have been successfully adapted for use with older adults (Frank et al., 1993; Knight & Satre, 1999; Teri, 1991; Thompson, 1996). Studies have examined the efficacy of these interventions in comparison to control groups (e.g., Beutler et al., 1987; Sloane, Staples, & Schneider, 1985), and in comparison to one another (e.g., Gallagher & Thompson, 1982; Jarvik, Mintz, Steuer, & Gerner, 1983; Steuer et al., 1984; Thompson, Gallagher, & Breckenridge, 1987). Treatments were consistently superior to no-treatment controls, producing effect sizes comparable to effects shown in studies with younger adults (O'Rourke & Hadjistavropoulos, 1997; Scogin & McElreath, 1984; Zeiss & Breckenridge, 1997). The evidence slightly favors cognitive and behavioral treatments over psychodynamic approaches (McCusker, Cole, Keller, Bellavance, & Berard, 1998; Widner & Zeichner, 1993; Zeiss & Breckenridge, 1997), but there is substantial similarity in outcome among the treatments. Reynolds, Frank, and colleagues (1999) demonstrated benefits for interpersonal psychotherapy above those provided by antidepressant medication during maintenance treatment. It therefore appears that both cognitive-behavioral approaches and interpersonal therapy have promise for treating depression in older adults. However, both cognitive and interpersonal approaches require verbal and cognitive competence on the part of the patient, and frequently some form of active participation in the form of diary-keeping and other homework assignments. In a frail population with prevalent cognitive impairment, implementation of such treatments is often impractical.

A Successful Behavioral Therapy for Cognitively-Impaired Elders with Depression

Teri and her colleagues have developed a promising behavioral intervention for depression, specifically designed for patients with dementia

(Teri, 1994, 1997; Teri, Logsdon, & Uomoto, 1991). This therapy involves training caregivers to assess pleasant events in the lives of the elder with dementia, and then systematically increasing the frequency of those events. The treatment also involves teaching caregivers problem-solving strategies for handling behavioral problems of dementia that may interfere with pleasant events. The rationale for using a behavioral approach in the treatment of depression in dementia came from a combination of clinical wisdom, successful use of behavioral intervention strategies in management of other behavioral problems, and studies that have focused on caregiver behaviors in the successful management of dementia (Teri, 1997). Teri and her colleagues (Teri, Logsdon, Uomoto, & Curry, 1997) compared this intervention to two control conditions, a typical care (attention) condition, and a wait-list (no contact) control. Seventy-two patient-caregiver dyads were randomly assigned to treatment conditions; assessments were taken pre-, post-, and 6 months following intervention. The patients were all diagnosed with Alzheimer's dementia based on rigorous diagnostic procedures. The pleasant events condition was superior to the control conditions in terms of change in depression and response rates, but not superior to another active condition involving caregiver problem-solving. These differences held at 6 months as well.

The research by Teri and her colleagues demonstrates clear promise for a behavioral approach involving caregivers in treating elders who have significant cognitive impairment. Residents of nursing homes show a wide range of disability, both physical and cognitive. In part because of the diversity of the population, any intervention used in nursing homes will also need to be implemented on an individual level (Cohen-Mansfield & Werner, 1997). The success of the behavioral intervention described above with Alzheimer's dementia, and its applicability to other types of cognitive impairment (Teri, 1999, personal communication) suggests its appropriateness with nursing home residents.

A Conceptual Foundation for Behavioral Treatment of Depression in Nursing Homes

The Behavioral Model. The conceptual model that forms a basis for behavioral approaches to depression is one proposed by Lewinsohn (1975; Lewinsohn, Youngren, & Grosscup, 1979). As originally formulated, this model proposed that depression results from a low rate of response-contingent positive reinforcement. The theory suggested that due either to poor social skills or environmental deprivations, people who develop depression are unable to generate adequate levels of positive reinforcement from their social or physical environments, and that low rates of positive reinforcement would lead to dysphoria. Therapies developed from this model focused on social skills training and other techniques to increase clients' rates of pleasant events. As with many early psychological theories of depression, this theory was later reformulated by Lewinsohn, Hoberman, Teri, and Hautzinger (1985) to accommodate empirical evidence contradictory to the original hypothesis, and other evidence supporting multiple cognitive, behavioral, and biological contributors to depression. The newer model is an integrative one, positing that depression results from an interaction of predisposing factors, negative environmental events, disruption of regular behavioral patterns and emotional responses, and reduced availability of positive reinforcement. In vulnerable individuals, stressful events or circumstances disrupt behavioral regularity, leading to an increase in negative affect, accompanied by a reduced rate of positive reinforcement (reduced *positive affect*). Thus the balance between positive and negative affect is shifted to become more negative. An accompanying heightened state of negative self-awareness diminishes the person's ability to regulate positive affect, perpetuating dysphoria and inhibiting the person's ability to right the balance. Because the model includes several interconnections and feedback loops among its elements, it implies that interventions targeting one or more of these elements will have an impact on the entire system, resulting in decreased dysphoria and improved functioning. Thus, the model supports cognitive, behavioral, or medical interventions for depression. We propose that the choice of a behavioral intervention focused on increasing pleasant events is particularly compelling for long-term care environments, based on both theoretical and practical considerations.

The Importance of Regulating Positive Affect and Its Relationship to Negative Affect

One of the authors' expressed goals in proposing the reformulated behavioral model was to account for the primacy of dysphoria in depression (Lewinsohn et al., 1985). The term dysphoria is typically used to characterize the negative mood state that is clearly present in the majority of depressions. The model converges nicely with classical conceptions of depression that identify the primary impairment as anhedonia, or an inability to experience pleasure (e.g., Kraepelin, 1977/1921; Klein, 1974; Meehl, 1975). More recently, a number of researchers have focused on the relationship between positive and negative affect in characterizing general well-being (e.g., Diener, Suh, Lucas, & Smith, 1999), depression, and anxiety states (reviewed by Mineka, Watson, & Clark, 1998). As currently measured, positive and negative affect are conceptualized as separable dimensions of affective experience; high negative affect is a shared attribute of both anxiety and depression, and depression is differentiated from anxiety by low positive affect (Mineka et al., 1998). Collectively these perspectives suggest that increasing positive affect should be a goal of treatments for depression.

As they are typically measured in community populations, positive and negative affect are either independent, or moderately correlated (see, e.g., Diener, Smith, & Fujita, 1995) and have different relationships to life events. Positive events increase positive affect, but have little effect on negative affect. The impact of negative events is more pervasive, however, lowering positive affect as well as raising negative affect (Zautra & Reich, 1983). Schulz and Heckhausen (1997), articulating their life span theory of control, argue that the separation of affects makes sense from an evolutionary point of view. In positing primary control (control over behavior-event contingencies) as a fundamental goal of human development, Schulz and Heckhausen view positive and negative affect as essential parts of feedback loops in regulating human motivation and attainment of control. The fact that negative affect tends to be an enduring response to negative conditions, whereas positive affect is more transient, they argue, is necessary for the evolutionary success of the organism, related to the need for harm avoidance (see also Davidson, 2000). Affective asymmetry is supported by studies of emotional responding in the hemispheres of the prefrontal cortex of the brain (Davidson, 2000). As Schulz and Heckhausen put it, "From an evolutionary perspective, an asymmetric affective system that requires continuous change for maintaining positive affect and heightening responsiveness to adverse conditions is likely to promote survival by way of maximizing primary control" (p. 194). In other words, successful adaptation requires harm avoidance, combined with continuous regulation of positive affect. Recent theoretical work in the domains of emotion and neuroscience, then, suggests that regulation of positive affect is a critical adaptive function. In fact, Davidson (2000) defines *resilience* as "the maintenance of high levels of positive affect and well-being in the face of significant adversity" (p. 1198).

Zautra, Potter, and Reich (1997) have argued that the independence of positive and negative affects depends on context. Specifically, they argue that under conditions of stress, positive and negative affect become negatively correlated. Consistent with the Lewinsohn et al. (1985) model, Zautra et al. (1997) argue that stress is destabilizing, leading to increased uncertainty. That is, the person's expectations about "what comes next" are to some extent unreliable, and often accompanied by a diminished sense of control. Coping responses are commonly means of increasing control over this uncertainty. The pressures placed upon the information- and affect-processing systems under conditions of stress would make independent processing of affects inefficient, and thus Zautra et al. (1997) suggest that under stress the separate systems are unified to optimize level of functioning. To support this contention, they present evidence that the relationship between positive affect and pain becomes significant and inverse under stress, whereas under normal conditions negative affect is strongly correlated with pain, but positive affect is not (Zautra, Reich, & Guarnaccia, 1990). Conversely, elderly people with worsening disabling conditions reported that positive events had an impact on both positive and negative affect, whereas this relationship was not found for bereaved elders or those with no stressors.

Returning to the Lewinsohn et al. (1985) model, depression results from the combination of destabilizing negative events, increased negative affect, and unsuccessful regulation of positive affect through primary control efforts. Figure 1 roughly illustrates the model for elders living in nursing homes. The recent theoretical and empirical work cited above supports our belief that an effective intervention in this cycle is to increase the availability, frequency, and regularity of, and control over, positive events, thus facilitating the ongoing regulation of positive affect and restoring the balance of affects that will be optimal for adaptive functioning.

The Empirical Foundation for a Pleasant Events-Based Behavioral Intervention in Long-Term Care

The work of Lawton and his colleagues at the Philadelphia Geriatric Center extends our understanding of the relationships among positive and negative affect, and positive and negative events to frail, elderly populations. Lawton and his collaborators have conducted a systematic program of research examining affect states in elderly residents of long-term care that demonstrates a pattern of affect and relationships between affect and events consistent with our model (Lawton, 1997). They demonstrated different patterns of positive and negative affect between depressed and nondepressed nursing home residents (Lawton,

FIGURE 1. A Model of Depression in Nursing Homes

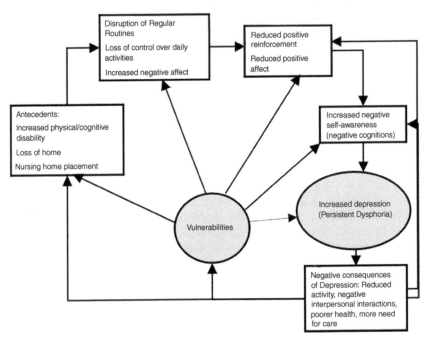

Adapted from Lewinsohn, P. M., Hoberman, H., Teri, L., & Hautzinger, M. (1985). An integrative theory of depression. In S. Reiss & R. R. Bootzin (Eds.) *Theoretical issues in behavior therapy.* New York: Academic Press.

Parmelee, Katz, & Nesselroade, 1996). For normals, negative affect was low and invariable, but positive affect was variable. For those people with major depression, positive affect was low and not very variable, but negative affect was highly variable. People with minor depression were variable on both negative and positive affect. These results, again, are consistent with findings and theoretical work on the structure of anxiety and depression in young samples (Mineka et al., 1998). Lawton and his colleagues have found greater variability in negative affect in the nursing home than in congregate housing, and lower positive affect. Nursing home residents with major depression reported more negative and fewer positive events than nondepressed residents. The affective tone of daily events was related to daily affect–if positive events occurred, positive affect was higher for that day. Similarly, the occurrence of negative health-related events was significantly related to higher negative affect (Lawton, 1997). Lawton, Van Haitsma, and Klapper (1994) demonstrated greater pleasure, contentment, and interest among residents with AD who participated in planned and informal activities. In summarizing a decade's work on positive and negative affect in relation to environmental contexts, Lawton (1997) stated, "Positive, diverting, environmentally engaging experiences heighten PA [positive affect] but do not ameliorate NA [negative affect]; negative, internal experiences, such as poor health and negative personal relationships that reflect on the self, contribute to negative affect but are less likely to impair PA" (p. 35). A pleasant events intervention should therefore have its primary impact on positive affect, and may not influence negative affect, which will be affected by the chronic health problems seen in this population, although the work of Zautra et al. (1997) suggests the possibility that those with chronic health problems may show changes in negative affect as well. To the extent that positive events interventions improve relationships between staff and residents, there may be a change in negative affect. A guiding assumption behind Lawton's research in long-term care has been that an excess of positive over negative affect defines positive mental health. A pleasant events intervention should increase positive affect, tipping the balance in the direction of mental health.

Surprising support for a behavioral, pleasant events emphasis comes from an elegant treatment dismantling study of cognitive-behavioral therapy (CBT) with young adults (Gortner, Gollan, Dobson, & Jacobson, 1998; Jacobson et al., 1996). These researchers found that the *behavioral activation* component of CBT was equally as effective alone as in the combination with the cognitive components. The behavioral activation component is very similar to behavioral treatments of depression based on Lewinsohn's model. Support also derives from the collective wisdom of a variety of clinical and empirical reports. Ethnographies of long-term care residents show prevalent concerns about depression, and that residents' personal prescriptions for maintaining mental health focus on remaining active in preferred pursuits (Luborsky & Riley, 1997). A number of interventions designed to treat behavioral problems in dementia incorporate pleasant events variations. These include pet therapy, recreational therapy, and art therapy (Beck, 1998). The use of audiotaped memories (Camberg et al., 1999), videos, music, conversation, and activity (Cohen-Mansfield & Werner, 1997) to increase positive affect and reduce agitation have received some empirical validation. Ryden et al. (1999) provide a set of practice recommendations for treating depression in nursing homes that recommend individualized care plans based on residents' strengths and previous preferences, emphasizing residents' comfort needs as well. There are preliminary reports of treatments for depression in nursing homes incorporating pleasant events from two different research groups (Lichtenberg, Kimbarow, Wall, Roth, & MacNeill, 1998; Ray et al., as cited in Thompson & Gallagher-Thompson, 1997; see also DeVries & Gallagher-Thompson, 1993; Marson, 1995) that suggest that such an approach may be effective, although no published efficacy studies are available.

Rosen and his colleagues (1997) reported a controlled evaluation of a nursing home intervention involving structuring leisure activities. A licensed recreational therapist was provided for the eight-week intervention who assessed participants' leisure interests, and facilitated their planning and implementation. Participants were residents of a large nursing facility without cognitive impairment or severe depression, randomly assigned to either the intervention or wait-list groups. Although there was a significant decrease in depression scores from pre- to post-intervention, there followed a significant *deterioration* over the follow-up period. Authors concluded that residents were unable to maintain socialization achieved during the intervention without the support of the outside staff, that is, residents returned to baseline following removal of the consultant. These results illustrate the potential of an activities-based intervention in nursing homes, but they also show that an intervention relying exclusively on outside consultation fails to produce lasting gains and points to the need for treatment that involves changing the ongoing nature of the nursing home experience through staff training.

Challenges of Adapting a Behavioral Treatment for the Nursing Home Setting

The research reviewed above provides a strong foundation for applying a behavioral intervention for depression in a nursing home setting. The groundbreaking work of Teri and her colleagues on behavioral intervention for depression in dementia provides the basic template for such an intervention. However, their intervention was used with family caregivers who had primary responsibility for the care of the depressed patients. The situation for nursing home residents is markedly different, in which the primary caregivers are nursing and other institutional staff members, and where there are numerous institutional constraints on activity availability and timing. Further, the experience of the Rosen et al.

(1997) study suggests that an intervention that relies on an outside consultant or mental health expert to implement changes in resident activities will ultimately fail when the expert is withdrawn. What is needed is an intervention that can be applied within the confines of institutional constraints and that will produce lasting change through ongoing institutional support of residents' positive activities.

Dementia and physical frailty, especially in combination, decrease the ability of an individual to engage in primary control activities. Their environments become fundamentally less accessible and pleasurable, and more filled with obstacles and frustrations. Environmental and interpersonal problems can be exacerbated by caregivers who interpret efforts at control as uncooperative or manipulative, and who unintentionally reinforce dependent behaviors (Baltes & Werner-Wahl, 1987). The behavioral intervention with family caregivers alters environmental contingencies and caregiver coping to allow more pleasant interactions between the patient and caregivers, and to increase the patient's access to other pleasurable events. Whereas orchestrating such changes within a dyadic or family system is relatively simple, within the institutional setting the challenges extend far beyond any individual caregiver-patient relationship, and require an approach that takes into consideration broader institutional goals and issues. We therefore advocate taking a public health approach to the development and testing of an intervention for depression in nursing homes.

Rationale for a Public Health Approach

The public health approach to mental health, as articulated in the 1999 Surgeon General's Report (Department of Health and Human Services, 1999), increases access by moving mental health services into community settings where vulnerable individuals may be found, and treatment research involves not only treating those who request services, but also deliberate and systematic case-identification and other efforts to overcome barriers to access (see also Katz & Coyne, 2000). Relevant research takes place in the clinical setting, includes the full range of comorbid problems typically seen in that setting, and involves adapted designs that combine features of randomized clinical trials and observational field studies (Niederehe, Street, & Lebowitz, 1999; Norquist, Lebowitz, & Hyman, 1999). The goal, as stated by Niederehe et al. (1999), is "to assure that research-based interventions are actually put to use in the settings and care systems where the patients who need them are typically seen and treated" (p. 3). Despite decades of evidence that nursing homes may have detrimental mental health consequences (e.g., Baltes & Werner-Wahl, 1987; Baltes, Kindermann, Reisenzein, & Schmid, 1987; Lindsley, 1964; Parmelee & Lawton, 1990; Szekias, 1985), and that there are a variety of promising behavioral techniques for addressing these consequences (Burgio & Stevens, 1998; Wisocki, 1991), generalization to nursing homes for routine use is limited (Schnelle, Cruise, Rahman, & Ouslander, 1998), and the majority of nursing home residents do not have access to, or do not receive, sufficient mental health care (e.g., Burns et al., 1993; Conn, Lee, Steingart, & Silberfeld, 1992; Meeks, Jones, Tikhtman, & La Tourette, 2000). Primary barriers to technology transfer appear to be the lack of professional expertise, or lack of reimbursement structures for professional expertise in nursing homes, and lack of staff training to implement interventions in the absence of such expertise. Even when expertise is available, as demonstrated by Rosen et al. (1997), intervention gains may not be maintained when the expert withdraws. It is imperative that nursing home treatment, and the research required to evaluate it, involve staff members (Burgio & Stevens, 1998).

The arguments presented above lead to the conclusion that intervention research in nursing homes must emphasize ecological validity. Because of their frailty, multiple comorbid medical conditions and accompanying polypharmacy, and high prevalence of cognitive impairment, nursing home residents as a group possess characteristics that would result in exclusion from most standard clinical trials. Interventions developed in the model of highly controlled clinical trials will fail when implemented in the typical nursing home. Because the same barriers exist for the practitioner implementing treatments, generalization of treatments from clinical trials conducted with community or inpatient elders is likely to be poor. The situation of depressed elders in long-term care is precisely the situation Norquist and his colleagues (1999) identify in arguing for research with a public health emphasis. Mental health treatments for nursing homes must be acceptable, and feasible, for both institutions and patients.

Recommendations for Treatment Development and Evaluation

Most clinicians working in long-term care will agree that, on an individual basis, traditional approaches to psychotherapy can be effective with depressed nursing home residents, particularly those who have a full range of cognitive abilities and who suffer from uncomplicated major depression. What we are advocating here, however, is a broader approach with the potential to affect patients with a range of cognitive/physical disabilities and a variety of depressive syndromes. The public health approach dictates that we not content ourselves with treating individual help-seekers on a case-by-case basis, but rather set as our goal change in institutions so that individuals in need of services get them in a timely fashion and that serious problems are prevented by establishing health-promoting environments. The conceptual and empirical review presented here demonstrates the potential of a behavioral intervention based on the successful manual developed by Teri and her colleagues (Teri, Logsdon, & Uomoto, 1991) to improve positive mental health and combat depression in nursing home residents with a variety of cognitive and physical disabilities. We make the following specific recommendations concerning the development, implementation, and evaluation of such a treatment in nursing home settings.

1. The intervention should be taught to, and implemented by, nursing home staff rather than a mental health professional or family members. The role of the mental health professional should be as assessor, teacher, and supervisory consultant. Family members and other significant people in the residents' lives may play an auxiliary role in providing access to pleasant social events.
2. The intervention should be implemented at the institutional level rather than at the level of individual residents. Case identification may be the shared responsibility of the mental health consultant, primary care physician, and staff members; systematic assessment by the mental health consultant is the ideal but often may be impractical. The broad goal is to change the way that nursing home staff respond to depressive symptoms on a routine basis, although the individual treatment plans are tailored to resident capacities, needs, and interests. Such a protocol-based response to symptoms fits well with the way nursing staff typically respond to physical symptoms, and therefore should increase adherence.
3. The ideal staff members for implementation are social service and activities staff. These are the staff who are primarily responsible for the leisure and social activities of nursing home residents. Further, high staff turnover among nurse aides, who are primary caregivers in long-term care, creates significant problems for intervention consistency and training (Burgio & Stevens, 1998; Schnelle et al., 1998). Turnover is less of a problem for the administrative-level staffs in social services and activities. Nevertheless, we also recommend that all nursing and administrative staff are made

aware of the intervention program, and receive training about depression, dementia, and the goals and approaches of the treatment (Burgio & Stevens, 1998).

4. Staff training should focus on three areas: understanding depression and dementia and problematic behaviors related to those disorders, understanding the nature and assessment of individualized pleasant events, and understanding the connection between pleasant events and positive mood states (see Teri et al., 1991).

5. Despite the public health focus, at the level of the individual patient, the intervention should be tailored to include preferred activities suitable to the individual patient's level of cognitive and physical ability. Assessment of pleasant events should be idiographic, and the identification of residents' previously enjoyed activities is the first objective of treatment. Adaptation of standardized assessment instruments such as the Pleasant-Events Schedule (Lodgson & Teri, 1997), as well as enlisting family members in selecting events that are agreeable to the patient, may assist in the process of individualizing the treatment. Evidence suggests that activity engagement is infrequent in the very frail elderly and particularly in long-term care settings (Horgas, Wilms, & Baltes, 1998), therefore, skill and creativity are needed on the part of clinicians and staff members to select events that are available, nondemeaning, and personally rewarding for a particular patient. Thereafter, frequency of pleasant events should be systematically increased, with an eye toward attaining early success experiences to gain momentum. In less cognitively impaired patients, visual charts of progress may be used for demonstrative purposes (Knight & Satre, 1999). The process of assessing and tracking individual residents' activity engagement should be easily incorporated in the individualized care plans that are standard practice in long-term care settings.

6. Evaluation should assess intra-individual as well as group change, to accommodate the wide heterogeneity in the nursing home population. Evaluation should also assess institutional and staff outcomes. Teri et al. (1997) found that their intervention improved not only patient depression, but also the depressed mood of family caregivers. It is possible that a successful intervention in the nursing home setting might have positive effects on staff morale and interpersonal interactions between staff and residents. If this is the case, long-term successful implementation should improve staff turnover as well.

REFERENCES

Ames, D. (1990). Depression among elderly residents of local-authority residential homes: Its nature and the efficacy of intervention. *British Journal of Psychiatry, 156*, 667-675.

Ames, D. (1992). Psychiatric diagnoses made by the AGECAT system in residents of local authority homes for the elderly; Outcome and diagnostic stability after four years. *International Journal of Geriatric Psychiatry, 7*, 83-87.

Apfeldorf, W., Alexopoulos, G., Weill, J., & Weill, S.I. (1999). Psychopharmacologic interventions in late-life major depression. *Annual Review of Gerontology and Geriatrics, 19*, 195-212.

Baltes, M.M., Kindermann, T., Reisenzein, R., & Schmid, U. (1987). Further observational data on the behavioral and social world of institutions for the aged. *Psychology and Aging, 2*, 390-403.

Baltes, M.M., & Werner-Wahl, H. (1987). Dependence in aging. In L.L. Carstensen, & B.A. Edelstein (Eds.), *Handbook of clinical gerontology* (pp. 204-221). New York: Pergamon.

Beck, C.K. (1998). Psychosocial and behavioral interventions for Alzheimer's disease patients and their families. *American Journal of Geriatric Psychiatry, 6*, S41-S48.

Beutler, L.E., Scogin, F., Kirkish, P., Schretlen, D., Corbishley, A., Hamblin, D., Meredith, K., Potter, R., Bamford, C., & Levenson, A. (1987). Group cognitive therapy and alprazolam in the treatment of depression in older adults. *Journal of Consulting and Clinical Psychology, 55*, 550-556.

Blazer, D., Hughes, D.C., & George, L.K. (1987). The epidemiology of depression in an elderly community population. *The Gerontologist, 27*, 281-287.

Blazer, D., & Williams, C.D. (1980). Epidemiology of dysphoria and depression in an elderly population. *American Journal of Psychiatry, 137*, 439-444.

Broadhead, W.E., Blazer, D.G., George, L.K., & Tse, C.K. (1990). Depression, disability days, and days lost from work in a prospective epidemiologic survey. *Journal of the American Medical Association, 264*, 2524-2528.

Bump, G., Reynolds, C., Smith, G., Pollock, B., Dew, M., Mazumdar, S., Geary, M., Houck, P., & Kupfer, D. (1997). Acceleration response in geriatric depression: A pilot study combining sleep deprivation and paroxetine. *Depression and Anxiety, 6*, 113-118.

Burgio, L.D., & Stevens, A.B. (1998). Behavioral interventions and motivational systems in the nursing home. *Annual Review of Gerontology and Geriatrics, 18*, 284-320.

Burns, B. J., Larson, D. B., Goldstrom, I. D., Johnson, W. E., Taube, C. A., Miller, N. E., & Mathis, E. S. (1988). Mental disorder among nursing home patients: Preliminary findings from the National Nursing Home Survey Pretest. *International Journal of Geriatric Psychiatry, 3*, 27-35.

Burns, B. J., Wagner, R., Taube, J. E., Magaziner, J., Permutt, T., & Landerman, R. (1993). Mental health service use by the elderly in nursing homes. *American Journal of Public Health, 83*, 331-337.

Camberg, L., Woods, P., Ooi, W., Hurley, A., Volicer, L., Ashley, J., Odenheimer, G., & McIntyre, K. (1999). Evaluation of simulated presence: A personalized approach to enhance well-being in persons with Alzheimer's disease. *Journal of the American Geriatrics Society, 47*, 446-452.

Cohen-Mansfield, J., & Werner, P. (1997). Management of verbally disruptive behaviors in nursing home residents. *Journal of Gerontology, 52A,* M169-M177.

Conn, D. K., Lee, V., Steingart, A., & Silberfeld, M. (1992). Psychiatric services: A survey of nursing homes and homes for the aged in Ontario. *Canadian Journal of Psychiatry, 37,* 525-530.

Davidson, R.J. (2000). Affective style, psychopathology, and resilience: Brain mechanisms and plasticity. *American Psychologist, 55,* 1196-1214.

Department of Health and Human Services (1999). *Mental health: A report of the Surgeon General.* Washington, DC: Author.

DeVries, H.M., & Gallagher-Thompson, D. (1993). Cognitive/behavioral therapy and the angry caregiver. *Clinical Gerontologist, 13,* 53-57.

Diener, E., Smith, H., & Fujita, F. (1995). The personality structure of affect. *Journal of Personality and Social Psychology, 69,* 130-141.

Diener, E., Suh, E.M., Lucas, R.E., & Smith, H.L. (1999). Subjective well-being: Three decades of progress. *Psychological Bulletin, 125,* 276-302.

Frank, E., Frank, N., Cornes, C., Imber, S.D., Miller, M.D., Morris, S.M., & Reynolds, C.F. (1993). Interpersonal psychotherapy in the treatment of late-life depression. In G.L. Klerman & M.M. Weissman (Eds.), *New applications of interpersonal psychotherapy* (pp. 167-198). Washington, DC: American Psychiatric Press, Inc.

Fries, B.E., Mehr, D.R., & Schneider, D. et al. (1993). Mental dysfunction and resource use in nursing homes. *Medical Care, 31,* 898-920.

Gallagher, D.E., & Thompson, L.W. (1982). Treatment of major depressive disorder in older adult outpatients with brief psychotherapies. *Psychotherapy: Theory, Research, and Practice, 19,* 482-490.

German, P.S., Shapiro, S., & Kramer, M. (1986). Nursing home study of the Eastern Baltimore Epidemiological Catchment Area Study. In M. Harper, & B. Lebowitz (Eds.), *Mental illness in nursing homes: Agenda for research* (DHHS Publication No. [ADM] 86-1459). Rockville, MD: DHHS.

Gortner, E.T., Gollan, J.K., Dobson, K.S., & Jacobson, N.S. (1998). Cognitive-behavioral treatment for depression: Relapse prevention. *Journal of Consulting and Clinical Psychology, 66,* 377-384.

Horgas, A.L., Wilms, H., & Baltes, M.M. (1998). Daily life in very old age: Everyday activities as expression of successful living. *The Gerontologist, 38,* 556-568.

Howarth, E., Johnson, A.J., Klerman, G., & Weissman, M.M. (1992). Depressive symptoms as relative and attributable risk factors for first-onset major depression. *Archives of General Psychiatry, 49,* 817-823.

Jacobson, N.S., Dobson, K.S., Truax, P.A., Addis, M.E., Koerner, K., Gollan, J.K., Gortner, E., & Prince, S.E. (1996). A component analysis of cognitive-behavioral treatment for depression. *Journal of Consulting and Clinical Psychology, 64,* 295-304.

Jarvik, L.F., Mintz, J., Steuer, J., & Gerner, R. (1982). Treating geriatric depression: A 26-week interim analysis. *Journal of the American Geriatrics Society, 30,* 713-717.

Johnson, J., Weissman, M.M., & Klerman, G.L. (1992). Service utilization and social morbidity associated with depressive symptoms in the community. *Journal of the American Medical Association, 267,* 1478-1483.

Kales, H., Blow, F., Copeland, L., Kammerer, E., & Mellow, A. (1999). Health care utilization by older patients with coexisting dementia and depression. *The American Journal of Psychiatry, 156,* 550-556.

Katz, I.R., & Coyne, J.C. (2000). The public health model for mental health care for the elderly. *Journal of the American Medical Association, 283,* 2844-2845.

Katz, I.R., Lesher, E., Kleban, M., Jethanandani, V., & Parmelee, P. (1989). Clinical features of depression in the nursing home. *International Psychogeriatrics, 1,* 5-15.

Katz, I.R., & Parmelee, P.A. (1997). Overview. In R.L. Rubinstein, & M.P. Lawton (Eds.), *Depression in long term and residential care* (pp. 1-25). New York, NY: Springer.

Katz, I.R., Parmelee, P.A., Beaston-Wimmer, P., & Smith, B.D. (1994). Association of antidepressants and other medications with mortality in the residential care elderly. *Journal of Geriatric Psychiatry and Neurology, 7,* 221-226.

Katz, I.R., Simpson, G.M., Curlik, S.M., & Parmelee, P.A. (1990). Pharmacologic treatment of major depression for elderly patients in residential care settings. *Journal of Clinical Psychiatry, 51,* 41-48.

Kennedy, G.J., Kelman, H.R., Thomas, C., Wisniewsky, W., Metz, H., & Bijur, P. (1989). Hierarchy of characteristics associated with depressive symptoms in an urban elderly sample. *American Journal of Psychiatry, 146,* 220-225.

Kim, E., & Rovner, B. (1995). Epidemiology of psychiatric disturbance in nursing homes. *Psychiatric Annals, 25,* 409-412.

Klein, D.F. (1974). Endogenomorphic depression: A conceptual and terminological revision. *Archives of General Psychiatry, 31,* 447-454.

Klerman, G.L., Budman, S., Berwick, D., Weissman, M.M., Damico-White, J., Demby, A., & Feldstein, M. (1987). Efficacy of a brief psychosocial intervention for symptoms of stress and distress among patients in primary care. *Medical Care, 25,* 1078-1088.

Knight, B.G., & Satre, D.D. (1999). Cognitive behavioral psychotherapy with older adults. *Clinical Psychology: Science and Practice, 6,* 188-203.

Kraepelin, E. (1977/1921). *Manic-depressive insanity and paranoia.* (R.M. Barclay, trans.). Manchester, NH: Ayer Company.

Lawton, M.P. (1997). Positive and negative affective states among older people in long-term care. In R.L. Rubinstein, & M.P. Lawton (Eds.), *Depression in long term and residential care* (pp. 29-54). New York, NY: Springer.

Lawton, M.P., Parmelee, P.A., Katz, I.R., & Nesselroade, J. (1996). Affective states in normal and depressed older people. *Journal of Gerontology: Psychological Sciences, 51B,* P309-P316.

Lawton, M.P., Van Haitsma, K., & Klapper, J. (1994). A balanced stimulation and retreat program for a special care dementia unit. *Alzheimer's Disease and Associated Disorders, 8* (Suppl. 1), S133-S138.

Lebowitz, B., Pearson, J., Schneider, L., Reynolds, C., Alexopoulos, G., Bruce, M., Conwell, Y., Katz, I., Meyers, B., Morrison, M., Mossey, J., Niederehe, G., & Parmelee, P. (1997). Diagnosis and treatment of depression in late life: Consensus statement update. *Journal of the American Medical Association, 278,* 1186-1190.

Lewinsohn, P.M. (1975). The behavioral study and treatment of depression. In M. Hersen, R.M. Eisler, & P.M. Miller (Eds.), *Progress in behavioral modification* (Vol. 1) (pp. 331-359). New York: Academic Press.

Lewinsohn, P.M., Hoberman, H., Teri, L., & Hautzinger, M. (1985). An integrative theory of depression. In S. Reiss, & R.R. Bootzin (Eds.), *Theoretical issues in behavior therapy.* New York: Academic Press.

Lewinsohn, P.M., Youngren, M.A., & Grosscup, S.J. (1979). Reinforcement and depression. In R.A. DePue (Ed.), *The psychobiology of depressive disorders: Implications for the effects of stress.* New York: Academic Press.

Lichtenberg, P.A., Kimbarow, M.L., Wall, J.R., Roth, R.E., & MacNeill, S.E. (1998). *Depression in geriatric medical and nursing home patients. A treatment manual.* Detroit: Wayne State University Press.

Lindsley, O.R. (1964). Geriatric behavioral prosthetics. In R. Kastenbaum (Ed.), *New thoughts on old age* (pp. 41-59). New York: Springer.

Little, J., Reynolds, C.F., Dew, M., Frank, E., Begley, A., Miller, M., Cornes, C., Mazumdar, S., Perel, J., & Kupfer, D. (1998). How common is resistance to treatment in recurrent, nonpsychotic geriatric depression? *The American Journal of Psychiatry, 155 (8),* 1035-1038.

Logsdon, R. G., & Teri, L. (1997). The Pleasant Events Schedule-AD: Psychometric properties and relationship to depression and cognition in Alzheimer's disease patients. *The Gerontologist, 37,* 40-45.

Luborsky, M.R., & Riley, E.M. (1997). Residents' understanding and experience of depression: Anthropological perspectives. In R.L. Rubinstein, & M.P. Lawton (Eds.), *Depression in long term and residential care* (pp. 75-117). New York, NY: Springer.

Lyketsos, C., Steel, C., Galik, E., Rosenblatt, A., Steinberg, M., Warren, A., & Sheppard, J. (1999). Physical aggression in dementia patients and its relationship to depression. *American Journal of Psychiatry, 156,* 66-71.

Lyness, J., King, D., Cox, C., Yeodiono, Z., & Caine, E. (1999). The importance of subsyndromal depression in older primary care patients: Prevalence and associated functional disability. *Journal of the American Geriatrics Society, 47,* 647-652.

Magaziner, J., Zimmerman, S.I., German, P.S., Kuhn, K., May, C., Hooper, F., Cox, D., Hebel, J.R., Kittner, S., Burton, L., Fishman, P., Kaup, B., Rosario, J., & Cody, M. (1996). Ascertaining dementia by expert panel in epidemiologic studies of nursing home residents. *Annals of Epidemiology, 6,* 431-437.

Marson, D.C. (1995). Modified self-management therapy for treatment of depression and anxiety in a nursing home resident. *Clinical Gerontologist, 16,* 63-65.

Masand, P. (1995). Depression in long-term care facilities. *Geriatrics, 50* (Suppl. 1), S16-24.

McCusker, J., Cole, M., Keller, E., Bellavance, F., & Berard, A. (1998). Effectiveness of treatments of depression in older ambulatory patients. *Archives of Internal Medicine, 168,* 705-712.

Meehl, P.E. (1975). Hedonic capacity: Some conjectures. *Bulletin of the Menninger Clinic, 39,* 295-307.

Meeks, S., Jones, M.W., Tikhtman, V., & La Tourette, T.R. (2000). Mental health services in Kentucky nursing homes: A survey of administrators. *Journal of Clinical Geropsychology.*

Meyers, B.S. (1998). Depression and dementia: Cormorbidities, identification, and treatment. *Journal of Geriatric Psychiatry and Neurology, 11,* 201-205.

Mineka, S., Watson, D., & Clark, L.A. (1998). Comorbidity of anxiety and unipolar mood disorders. *Annual Review of Psychology, 49,* 377-412.

Mossey, J.M. (1997). Subdysthymic depression and the medically ill elderly. In R.L. Rubinstein, & M.P. Lawton (Eds.), *Depression in long term and residential care* (pp. 55-74). New York, NY: Springer.

Mossey, J.M., Knott, K., Higgins, M., & Talerico, K. (1996). Effectiveness of a psychosocial intervention, interpersonal counseling, for subdysthymic depression in medically ill elderly. *Journal of Gerontology: Medical Sciences, 51A*, M172-M178.

Musselman, D.L., Evans, D.L., & Nemeroff, C.B. (1998). The relationship of depression to cardiovascular disease. Epidemiology, biology, and treatment. *Archives of General Psychiatry, 55*, 580-592.

National Center for Health Statistics (1997). Advance Data No. 89. Hyattsville, MD: Public Health Service. p. 3.

Nebes, R., Pollock, B., Mulsant, B., Kirshner, M., Halligan, E., Zmuda, M., & Reynolds, C.F. (1997). Low-level serum anticholingericity as a source of baseline cognitive heterogeneity in geriatric depressed patients. *Psychopharmacology Bulletin, 33*, 715-719.

Niederehe, G., Street, L.L., & Lebowitz, B.D. (1999). NIMH support for psychotherapy research: Opportunities and questions. *Prevention and Treatment, 2*, Article 0003a.

Norquist, G., Lebowitz, B., & Hyman, S. (1999). Expanding the frontier of treatment research. *Prevention and Treatment, 2*, Article 0001a.

O'Rourke, N., & Hadjistavropoulos, T. (1997). The relative efficacy of psychotherapy in the treatment of geriatric depression. *Aging and Mental Health, 1*, 305-310.

Parmelee, P.A., Katz, I.R., & Lawton, M.P. (1992). Incidence of depression in long-term care settings. *Journal of Gerontology, 47*, M189-M196.

Parmelee, P.A., & Lawton, M.P. (1990). The design of special environments for the aged. In J.E. Birren, & K.W. Schaie (Eds.), *Handbook of the psychology and aging* (3rd Ed., pp. 464-488). San Diego: Academic Press.

Pasternak, R.E., Prigerson, H., Hall, M., Miller, M.D., Fasiczka, A., Mazmdar, S., & Reynolds, C.F. III (1997). The posttreatment illness course of depression in bereaved elders. *American Journal of Geriatric Psychiatry, 5*, 54-59.

Paykel, E.S., Hollyman, J.A., Freeling, P., & Sedgewick, P. (1989). Predictors of therapeutic benefit from amitriptyline in mild depression: A general practice placebo-controlled trial. *Journal of Affective Disorders, 14*, 83-95.

Ray, W., Meador, K.G., Taylor, J.A., Gallagher-Thompson, D., & Thompson, L.W. Behavior therapy for major depression in nursing home residents: Model description and feasibility study. Unpublished Manuscript, cited in Thompson, L.W., & Thompson, D. (1997). Psychotherapeutic interventions with older adults in outpatient and extended care settings. In R.L. Rubinstein, & M.P. Lawton (Eds.), *Depression in long term and residential care* (pp. 169-184). New York, NY: Springer.

Regier, D.A., Boyd, J.H., Burke, J.D., Jr., Rae, D.S., Myers, J.K., Kramer, M., Robins, L.N., George, L.K., Karno, M., & Locke, B.Z. (1988). One-month prevalence of mental disorders in the United States. *Archives of General Psychiatry, 45*, 977-986.

Reynolds, C.F. (1994). Treatment of depression in late life. *The American Journal of Medicine, 97, suppl. 6A*, 39S-46S.

Reynolds, C., Frank, E., Kupfer, D., Thase, M., Perel, J., Mazumdar, S., & Houch, P. (1996). Treatment outcome in recurrent major depression: A post-hoc comparison of elderly ("young old") and midlife patients. *American Journal of Psychiatry, 153*, 1288-1292.

Reynolds, C.F., III, Frank, E., Mazumdar, S., Meltzer, C.C., Mulsant, B.H., Pilkonis, P., Pollock, B.G., Schulberg, C., Schulz, R., Shear, M.K., & Smith, G. (1998). Behavioral and pharmacologic interventions for depression in later life. *Annual Review of Gerontology and Geriatrics, 18,* 48-73.

Reynolds, C. F. III, Frank, E., Perel, J. M., Imber, S.D., Cornes, C., Miller, M.D., Mazumdar, S., Houck, P.R., Dew, M.A., Stack, J.A., Pollock, B.G., & Kupfer, D.J. (1999). Nortriptyline and interpersonal psychotherapy as maintenance therapies for recurrent major depression: A randomized controlled trial in patients older than 59 years. *Journal of the American Medical Association, 281,* 39-45.

Reynolds, C.F., Miller, M., Paternak, R., Frank, E., Perel, J., Cones, C., Houck, P., Mazumdar, S., Dew, M., & Kupfer, K. (1999). Treatment of bereavement related major depressive episodes in later life: A controlled study of acute and continuation treatment with nortriptyline and interpersonal psychotherapy. *American Journal of Psychiatry, 156,* 202-208.

Rosen, J., Rogers, J.C., Marin, R.S., Mulsant, B.H., Shabar, A., & Reynolds, C.F. III (1997). Control-relevant intervention in the treatment of minor and major depression in a long-term care facility. *American Journal of Geriatric Psychiatry, 5,* 247-257.

Rovner, B.W., German, P.S., Brant, L.J., Clark, R., Burton, L., & Folstein, M.F. (1991). Depression and mortality in nursing homes. *Journal of the American Medical Association, 265,* 993-996.

Rovner, B.W., German, P.S., Broadhead, J., Morriss, R.K., Brant, L.J., Blaustein, J., & Folstein, M.F. (1990). The prevalence and management of dementia and other psychiatric disorders in nursing homes. *International Psychogeriatrics, 2,* 13-24.

Ryden, M., Pearson, V., Kaas, M., Hanscom, J., Lee, H., Krichbaum, K., Wang, J., & Snyder, M. (1999). Nursing interventions for depression in newly admitted nursing home residents. *Journal of Gerontological Nursing, 25 (3),* 20-29.

Samuels, S.C., & Katz, I.B. (1995). Depression in the nursing home. *Psychiatric Annals, 25,* 419-424.

Schnelle, J., Cruise, P., Rahman, A., & Ouslander, J. (1998). Developing rehabilitative behavioral interventions for long-term care: Technology transfer, acceptance, and maintenance issues. *Journal of the American Geriatrics Society, 46,* 771-777.

Schulz, R., & Heckhausen, J. (1997). Emotions and control: A life span perspective. In M.P. Lawton, & K.W. Schaie (Eds.), *Annual Review of Gerontology and Geriatrics, Volume 17* (pp. 185-205). New York: Springer.

Scogin, F., & McElreath, L. (1994). Efficacy of psychosocial treatments for geriatric depression. A quantitative review. *Journal of Consulting and Clinical Psychology, 62,* 69-74.

Shah, A., Phongsathorn, V., & George, C. et al. (1993). Does psychiatric morbidity predict mortality in continuing care geriatric inpatients? *International Journal of Geriatric Psychiatry, 8,* 255-259.

Sloane, B.A., Staples, F.R., & Schneider, L.S. (1985). Interpersonal therapy versus nortriptyline for depression in the elderly. In G.D. Burrows, T.R. Norman, & L. Dennerstein (Eds.) *Clinical and pharmacological studies in psychiatric disorders.* London: John Libbey.

Steuer, J.L., Mintz, J., Hammen, C.L., Hill, M.A., Jarvik, L.F., McCarley, T., Motoike, P., & Rosen, R. (1984) Cognitive-behavioral and psychodynamic group psychotherapy in treatment of geriatric depression. *Journal of Consulting and Clinical Psychology, 52,* 180-189.

Strahan, G., & Burns, B.J. (1991). Mental health in nursing homes: United States, 1985. *National Health Survey: Vital and Health Statistics* (Series 13, No. 105, DHHS Publication No [PHS] 91-1766). Washington, DC: Department of Health and Human Services.

Szanto, K., Reynolds, C.F., Conwell, Y., Begley, A., & Houck, P. (1998). High levels of hopelessness persist in geriatric patients with remitted depression and a history of attempted suicide. *Journal of the American Geriatrics Society, 46*, 1401-1406.

Szekias, B. (1985). Using the milieu: Treatment-environment consistency. *Gerontologist, 25*, 15-18.

Teri, L. (1991). Behavioral assessment and treatment of depression in older adults. In P. Wisocki (Ed.), *Handbook of clinical behavior therapy with the elderly client* (pp. 225-243). New York: Plenum Publishing.

Teri, L. (1994). Behavioral treatment of depression in patients with dementia. *Alzheimer's Disease and Associated Disorders, 8*, 66-74.

Teri, L. (1997). The relation between research on depression and a treatment program: One model. In R.L. Rubinstein, & M.P. Lawton (Eds.), *Depression in long term and residential care* (pp. 129-153). New York, NY: Springer.

Teri, L., & Gallagher, D. (1991). Cognitive-behavioral interventions for treatment of depression in Alzheimer's patients. *The Gerontologist, 31*, 413-416.

Teri, L., Logsdon, R., & Uomoto, J. (1991). *Treatment of depression in patients with Alzheimer's disease. Therapist manual*. Seattle: University of Washington School of Medicine.

Teri, L., Logsdon, R.G., Uomoto, J., & McCurry, S.M. (1997). Behavioral treatment of depression in dementia patients: A controlled clinical trial. *Journal of Gerontology: Psychological Sciences, 52B*, P159-P166.

Teri, L., Truax, P., Logsdon, R., Uomoto, J., Zarit, S., & Vitaliano, P.P. (1992). Assessment of behavioral problems in dementia: The Revised Memory and Behavior Problems Checklist. *Psychology and Aging, 7*, 622-631.

Teri, L., & Uomoto, J. (1991). Reducing excess disability in dementia patients: Training caregivers to manage patient depression. *Clinical Gerontologist, 31*, 49-63.

Teri, L., & Wagner, A. (1992). Alzheimer's disease and depression. *Journal of Consulting and Clinical Psychology, 3*, 379-391.

Thapa, P., Gideon, P., Cost, T., Milam, A., & Ray, W. (1998). Antidepressants and the risk of falls among nursing home residents. *The New England Journal of Medicine, 339*, 875-882.

Thompson, L.W. (1996). Cognitive-behavioral therapy and treatment for late-life depression. *Journal of Clinical Psychiatry, 57* (Suppl.5), 29-37.

Thompson, L.W., & Gallagher-Thompson, D. (1997). Psychotherapeutic interventions with older adults in outpatient and extended care settings. In R.L. Rubinstein, & M.P. Lawton (Eds.), *Depression in long term and residential care* (pp. 169-184). New York, NY: Springer.

Thompson, L.W., Gallagher, D., & Breckenridge, J.S. (1987). Comparative effectiveness of psychotherapies for depressed elders. *Journal of Consulting and Clinical Psychology, 55*, 385-390.

Widner, S., & Zeichner, A. (1993). Psychologic interventions for the elderly chronic pain patients. *Clinical Gerontologist, 13*, 3-18.

Wisocki, P.A. (1991). Behavioral gerontology. In P.A. Wiscocki (Ed.), *Handbook of clinical behavior therapy with the elderly client* (pp. 3-51). New York: Plenum.

Wragg, R.E., & Jeste, D.V. (1989). Overview of depression and psychosis in Alzheimer's disease. *American Journal of Psychiatry, 146,* 577-587.

Wulsin, L.R., Valliant, G.E., & Wells, V.E. (1999). A systematic review of mortality of depression. *Psychosomatic Medicine, 61,* 6-17.

Zautra, A.J., Potter, P.T., & Reich, J.W. (1997). The independence of affects is context-dependent: An integrative model of the relationship between positive and negative affect. In M.P. Lawton, & K.W. Schaie (Eds.), *Annual Review of Gerontology and Geriatrics, 17,* 75-103.

Zautra, A.J., & Reich, J.W. (1983). Life events and perceptions of life quality: Developments in a two-factor approach. *Journal of Community Psychology, 11,* 121-132.

Zautra, A.J., Reich, J.W., & Guarnaccia, C.A. (1990). The everyday consequences of disability and bereavement in older adults. *Journal of Personality and Social Psychology, 59,* 550-561.

Zeiss, A.M., & Breckenridge, J.S. (1997). Treatment of late life depression: A response to the NIH Consensus Conference. *Behavior Therapy, 28,* 3-21.

Systemic Characteristics of Long-Term Care in Residential Environments: Clinical Importance of Differences in Staff and Resident Perceptions

Joyce Parr, PhD
Sara Green, PhD

SUMMARY. The perceptions of 276 residents and 94 staff of the systemic characteristics of a residential long-term care facility were examined. Factor analysis of resident and staff responses to questionnaire items yielded a five-factor, sixteen-item solution with a comparative fit index of .97. Comparison of resident and staff perceptions of the quality of these components, resident satisfaction, and resident control indicate that: (1) Staff members feel that residents are more involved and influential in the facility than residents themselves feel they are (p < .001); (2) Residents feel that their relationships with other residents are better than staff think they are (p < .05); and (3) Staff underestimate the degree of control residents feel they have over what is important in their lives

Joyce Parr is affiliated with the Foundation for Aging Research. Sara Green is affiliated with the Department of Sociology, University of South Florida.

Address correspondence to: Joyce Parr, 15350 Amberly Drive, Unit 1924, Tampa, FL 33647 (E-mail: christja@aol.com) or Sara Green, Department of Sociology, CPR 107, University of South Florida, 4202 East Fowler Avenue, Tampa, FL 33755 (E-mail: sagreen@luna.cas.usf.edu).

This article is based partially on a paper presented at the 102nd Annual Meeting of the American Psychological Association, Los Angeles, CA, August 15, 1994.

[Haworth co-indexing entry note]: "Systemic Characteristics of Long-Term Care in Residential Environments: Clinical Importance of Differences in Staff and Resident Perceptions." Parr, Joyce, and Sara Green. Co-published simultaneously in *Clinical Gerontologist* (The Haworth Press, Inc.) Vol. 25, No. 1/2, 2002, pp. 149-172; and: *Emerging Trends in Psychological Practice in Long-Term Care* (ed: Margaret P. Norris, Victor Molinari, and Suzann Ogland-Hand) The Haworth Press, Inc., 2002, pp. 149-172. Single or multiple copies of this article are available for a fee from The Haworth Document Delivery Service [1-800-HAWORTH, 9:00 a.m. - 5:00 p.m. (EST). E-mail address: getinfo@haworthpressinc.com].

149

(p < .001) and overestimate the contribution of facility components to such feelings (p < .05). *[Article copies available for a fee from The Haworth Document Delivery Service: 1-800-HAWORTH. E-mail address: <getinfo@haworthpressinc.com> Website: <http://www.HaworthPress.com> © 2002 by The Haworth Press, Inc. All rights reserved.]*

KEYWORDS. Systemic characteristics, long-term care, CCRC, staff perceptions, resident satisfaction, resident control

Clinical geropsychologists are increasingly providing services within long-term care (LTC) settings. Each setting presents as a complex system of variables and interrelationships intertwined with other systems including legislative and regulatory bodies, medical practitioners, families and community organizations. Within LTC settings, the system is hierarchically organized with residents having less decision-making authority than staff. Among staff, those who provide direct care to residents have less authority than administrative staff. Residents interact most frequently with direct support staff and the social climate of the facility is primarily determined by these interactions (Logsdon, 2000; Ogland-Hand and Zeiss, 2000; Qualls, 2000; Zarit, Dolan and Leitsch, 1998).

Like all organizational systems, LTC settings have open boundaries across which information, goods, services and social actors (e.g., residents, family members, visitors, staff, consulting geropsychologists) pass. Systems also have complex organizational plans and decision-making processes that coordinate and control information and activities toward the organization's official mission (Powers, 1988). In many ways, LTC systems are total institutions—that is, ". . . a social hybrid, part residential community, part formal organization . . ." (Goffman, 1961, p. 12). In total institutions, the day-to-day needs of a large group of residents are managed by a small number of staff. For residents, life within facility walls differs from life outside. Activities such as meals, recreation, transportation, etc., are desegregated. These activities occur at specified times, under supervision of staff and with a large number of other residents. Control over decisions about when, where and with whom these activities occur is limited. Thus, the individual agency accorded adults regarding these activities is limited. This contrasts with staff members who are able to maintain adult agency in the wider world outside of the facility. Further, the LTC setting constitutes multiple spheres of activity for residents yet it is relevant to only one sphere of life for staff. For staff, the facility is their place of work and the goal of that work is the provision of care. The training and licensing of LTC workers and the organization of work within facilities all act to create a clear dichotomy of social positions: staff as the givers of care vs. residents as the recipients of care (Diamond, 1992).

This distinction can lead staff members to view residents primarily as objects of their work rather than as complex individuals with rich personal histories (Goffman, 1961; Qualls, 2000). Such objectification may, in turn, affect the attitudes that staff members have about residents as human beings. Pietrukowicz and Johnson (1991), for example, gave nursing aides one of two versions of an anonymous resident's chart–one version included a life history of the resident while the other did not. Aides who read the chart without the life history rated the resident as less autonomous and personally acceptable than the aides who evaluated the chart with the life history. While staff tend to be very aware of the specific care needs of residents, they often are unaware of the familial and social contexts within which residents have previously lived (Qualls, 2000). Unless staff members come to know residents as whole people, rather than merely as the objects of their caregiving work, they are likely not only to underestimate residents' abilities but also to overestimate their degree of dependence.

Residents, on the other hand, may see staff through the lens of their former experiences with wait staff, housekeepers and other members of blue-collar service occupations. As one resident stated, "Sometimes they seem to forget that they work for us and not the other way around." Contrary to residents' previous encounters with service workers in the outside world, LTC staff members are generally more accountable to their supervisors than to the residents to whom they provide care (Diamond, 1992; Qualls, 2000). In fact, in many instances, the very fact of being a resident carries with it the assumption of incompetence. In front of residents, staff members frequently talk to each other or to family members about residents as if the resident were not present. This can be particularly offensive to people accustomed to being in control not only of their own lives but also of the workers who provide services to them. For example, Jim took his 97-year-old mother, Margaret, to the doctor after she stubbed her toe. The orthopedist examined the x-ray and began discussing the results with Jim. To the doctor's astonishment, Margaret interrupted: "Why are you talking to him? It's my toe that hurts." Failing to speak directly to the person involved, regardless of her or his infirmity or age, socially constructs an identity of incompetence. The organization of work within LTC settings encourages the view that the LTC system is merely a place in which passive, incompetent residents receive care rather than as a complex social system in which residents live their lives (Diamond, 1992). To residents, it is the character of this social system that is key to quality of life (Logsdon, 2000). Of particular importance to residents is a ". . . friendly, cheerful and compassionate staff . . ." (Logsdon, 2000, p. 133). Training programs for direct support staff tend not to address these key components of quality of life. Rather, they focus on the incompetence and dependency of LTC residents and their need for care (Diamond, 1992).

Negative staff attitudes about the value and competence of residents can have negative consequences for residents. It is well known that long-term treatment as an incompetent social actor leads to reduced feelings of self-efficacy and personal control (Goffman, 1961) and that feeling that one is not in control of one's life can be detrimental to well-being (Mirowsky, 1995; Mirowsky and Ross, 1990; Timko and Rodin, 1992). Margaret Baltes and colleagues (Baltes, Neumann and Zank, 1994; Baltes and Wahl, 1992) have proposed, however, that the social construction of residents as dependent recipients of care can sometimes be used as a mechanism of control by residents. Staff members expect resident dependence and reinforce it and residents use this expectation to control the course of social contacts with staff. Thus, a dependency-support script develops for resident-staff interactions in which residents give up some control in order to get the social support they desire. This exchange may have benefits for successful aging (Baltes and Wahl, 1992). These authors caution, however, that this script may be detrimental to maintenance of functional capacity in the long run because residents do not use the skills they have.

In summary, staff and residents of LTC facilities are likely to hold divergent views of the reality of life within the facility, themselves and each other. "Each point of view has as a crucial element an image of the other grouping. Although . . . it is seldom of the kind that leads to sympathetic identification" (Goffman, 1961, p. 93). As the objects of the caregiving work, residents are likely to be seen by staff as more dependent than they really are. Residents may, however, see staff members in terms of their former relationships with blue-collar service workers and may be more critical and competent judges of the quality of the care provided in the facility than staff believe them to be. Residents may also use the dependency role expected and rewarded by staff in order to garner the social and emotional attention they desire from staff members.

Continuing Care Retirement Communities (CCRC) are particularly interesting LTC facilities in which to investigate resident-staff discrepant views of system reality. These facilities share with total institutions and other long-term care settings the basic system characteristics and organization of work that can lead to discrepancies between resident and staff perceptions of resident competence. Unlike other total institutions, however, residents of CCRCs choose to move in and retain the option of moving out if the facility or the attitudes and actions of staff members prove unacceptable. Thus, residents have exercised control in voluntarily giving up control over some details of life but retain the option to leave the system at any time. Administration is well aware that residents have and can exercise this option. Resident satisfaction, thus, becomes a major goal and part of the definition of reality within the CCRC. Resident and staff perceptions of resident satisfaction and control, as well as resident competence, therefore, become important issues in these settings.

Discrepancies between CCRC residents and staff members in terms of the components of the facility's system and the contribution of these components to resident satisfaction and feelings of control over the important events and things in life are examined in the sections that follow. Specifically, the following research questions are addressed:

1. From the resident's perspective, what are the qualities of the system components in these continuing care retirement centers?
2. How do staff members' perceptions of the qualities of these system components compare to those of residents?
3. How do staff members' perceptions of the degree to which residents are satisfied with life within the facility compare to the residents' own assessments of their degree of overall satisfaction?
4. How do staff members' perceptions of the degree to which residents are in control of their lives compare to residents' own assessments of their degree of control?
5. How do residents' perceptions of individual system components relate to their satisfaction with life within the facility?
6. How do staff members' perceptions of individual system components relate to their assessments of residents' satisfaction with life within the facility?
7. How do residents' perceptions of system components relate to their feelings of control over the important things and events of their lives?

8. How do staff members' perceptions of system components relate to their assessments of the degree of control residents have over their lives?

METHODOLOGY

Data used for this study are drawn from a longitudinal data set collected from 1978 through December of 1991 by the Foundation for Aging Research (FAR)–a public, not-for-profit research organization in Florida that was incorporated from 1977 through 1999. The data set contains information on residents of two CCRCs located on the west coast of Florida. The older of these facilities opened in 1975, the newer in 1978. Although the facilities experienced several changes in ownership and management over the years during which the data were collected, they remained "sister" facilities (owned and managed by the same firms). The facilities' sale to new corporate owners in 1989 caused disruptive changes. Thus, new cases were not added to the file after this date. Both facilities offered life care contracts and lease arrangements.

Data Collection Procedures

Basic demographics at entry, status changes (moving out, death, death of a spouse, permanent transfer to the skilled nursing facility [SNF], etc.) and the total number of days spent each year in the SNF were recorded for all residents who moved in prior to 1989. Information was updated annually through December of 1991. In addition, a "Resident and Staff Satisfaction Instrument" (RASSI) was created and administered to residents and staff members in 1987 (Time 1) and again in 1989 (Time 2). A meeting with the executive committee of the residents' council resulted in agreement that the survey was appropriate and could be a useful medium for resident expression. Prior to each administration of RASSI, the executive directors of each facility made an announcement of the upcoming survey. A copy of the questionnaire was placed in the mailbox of each "Independent Living" and "Assisted Living" resident. Residents were assured that facility personnel would not see their individual answers, but would be provided with a facility-wide summary of results. Residents were supplied with business reply envelopes addressed to the researchers and asked to put the completed surveys in the mail. At Time 1, these procedures yielded a return of 276 questionnaires (59% of residents). The Time 2 replication of the RASSI survey yielded 199 returns (53% of residents).

At both the Time 1 and Time 2 administrations of RASSI, staff members were asked to complete parallel questionnaires. Like residents, staff members were also promised that their individual answers would be shown to no one other than members of the research team. Their questionnaires included no identifying information. A total of 94 staff members completed questionnaires at Time 1 (approximately 67%) and a similar percentage participated at Time 2.

Measures

System Variables. The RASSI is a 26-item questionnaire designed to evaluate social, physical, programmatic, policy and service characteristics of life within the CCRC. The items were created specifically for RASSI and were designed for the CCRC environment. The general domains covered by the items are quite similar to those included in measures of quality of acute care facilities (see Cleary and McNeil, 1988; Cryns, Nichols, Katz and Calkins, 1989; Maciejewski, Kawiecki and Rockwood, 1997), home care (see Edebalk, Samuelsson and Ingvad, 1995; Forbes, 1997) and skilled nursing facilities (see Davis, Sebastian and Tschetter, 1997; Kane et al., 1982; Kruzich, Clinton and Kelber, 1992; Simmons et al., 1997; Zinn, Lavizzo-Mourey and Taylor, 1993). Of the 26 original items, 21 are included in the analyses reported here. Five were eliminated because of missing data or lack of sufficient variance in response. Items included in the analyses are listed as worded in the resident version of the RASSI questionnaire in Table 1. Parallel questions are included in the staff version by substituting "resident(s)" for "you" and/or "your" in items 3 through 8, 10 through 13, 15, 17, 20 and 21. Response categories for both residents and staff are (3) "Most of the Time," (2) "Some of the Time," and (1) "Rarely."

Resident Satisfaction with Life Within the Facility was measured in the resident version of the RASSI questionnaire by the question: "How do you rate your overall satisfaction with your present housing situation?" Response categories are: (5) "Excellent" (15% of residents), (4) "Very Good" (38% of residents), (3) "Good" (38% of residents), (2) "Poor " (9% of residents) and (1) "Very Poor" (0.4% of residents). In the staff version, perception of resident satisfaction with the facility overall is measured by the question: "How do you feel residents rate their overall satisfaction with their housing situation?" Response categories are the same as those in the resident version and the distribution of staff responses is as follows: "Excellent" = 8%, "Very Good" = 36%, "Good" = 49% and "Poor" = 8%. No member of the staff rated resident satisfaction as "Very Poor."

Degree to Which Residents Have Control Over Their Lives is measured in the questionnaire administered to residents by the question: "Do you feel pretty much in control of the important things and events in your life?" Response categories are: (3) "Most of the Time " (87% of residents), (2) "Some of the Time" (12% of residents) and (1) "Rarely" (2% of residents). In the staff version of the questionnaire, the parallel question is: "Do you feel residents are pretty much in control of the important things and events in their lives?" Again, the response categories used in the staff version are identical to those of the resident version. The staff distribution on this item is: "Most of the Time" = 60%, "Some of the Time" = 34% and "Rarely" = 6%.

FINDINGS

Question One: From the resident's perspective, what are the qualities of the system components in these continuing care retirement centers?

The first step in the analysis related to question one was an exploratory principle components factor analysis using the resident data from Time 1. The second step was to determine the degree of fit using a confirmatory factor analysis of the previously identified factor structure. All the factor analyses were conducted using EQS for Windows (Bentler, 1995; Bentler and Wu, 1995; Byrne, 1994). The goal was to determine whether clear and separate clusters of system characteristics could be identified. The third step was a replication of the best-fit model identified from Time 1 with the data from Time 2.

As can be seen from Table 1, a six-factor structure was identified. Five of the six factors had clear patterns of factor loadings. Factor 1 contains six items related to caring, supportive relationships with members of the staff. Three items related to relationships with other residents loaded on Factor 2. The third factor is comprised of three items related to food and maintenance. The four items that load on Factor 4 are related to the physical plant of the facility and its basic programs and Factor 5 is comprised of three items related to the degree to which residents are actively involved and have influence in the facility's system. Factor 6 contains only one item (#20) that does not also load on another factor. Item #21 has loadings of between .30 and .40 on three factors (#1, #4

TABLE 1. Five Components of the Retirement Center System: Results of Exploratory Factor Analysis with Orthogonal Rotation

Factor names and item descriptions	Factor loadings					
	# 1	# 2	# 3	# 4	# 5	# 6
Factor one: Supportive relationships with staff.						
1. Do staff care about residents as people?	.58	.13	.07	.41	.21	.38
2. Are staff members helpful and friendly?	.54	.05	.11	.33	.28	.40
3. Do you feel comfortable with the security of the building?	.46	−.14	.25	.30	−.01	.12
4. Do you feel that staff respect your dignity and individual rights?*	.41	.08	.16	.24	.14	.63
5. Do the residents care about staff members as people?*	.50	.19	−.09	.02	.30	.14
6. Do you feel free to invite your friends or family to visit you at the facility?*	.65	.19	.12	.07	−.03	.10
Eigen value = 6.466, Alpha = .75 (Items 1 - 3 only)*						
Factor two: Relationships among residents.						
7. Are you able to achieve the level of interaction that you want with other people?	.14	.60	−.01	.16	.08	.06
8. Do you feel comfortable with most of the other residents?	.10	.59	−.01	−.14	.17	.11
9. Do you feel that residents help each other and give each other support?	.11	.54	.21	.17	.21	.11
Eigen value = 1.953, Alpha = .59						
Factor three: Personal services.						
10. Are you satisfied with the quality of the food served?	.02	.08	.65	.16	.03	.32
11. Are you satisfied with the quality of the service at meal time?	.11	.17	.64	.12	.05	.06
12. Are your maintenance requests handled in an effective manner?	.21	−.21	.56	.11	.16	.05
Eigen value = 1.511, Alpha = .64						
Factor four: Physical and programmatic environment.						
13. Do you feel that health care and assistance is available when you need it?	.16	.02	−.01	.64	.18	.11

TABLE 1 (continued)

Factor names and item descriptions	Factor loadings					
	#1	#2	#3	#4	#5	#6
14. Do you feel that management is concerned about maintaining the physical condition of the property?	−.00	.12	.33	.55	−.04	.10
15. Are the common areas suited to your needs?	.34	.02	.18	.53	.16	.13
16. Do you feel that, on the whole, staff members are doing their jobs well?	.21	.06	.22	.49	.26	.38
Eigen value = 1.259, Alpha = .71						
Factor five: Resident involvement and influence in the facility.						
17. Do you feel that you know pretty much what's happening in the building?	.09	.09	.10	.07	.67	.15
18. Does the residents' association function effectively on behalf of residents' needs and concerns?	.11	.26	.01	.22	.55	.15
19. Are there interesting activities in the building?	.03	.32	−.01	.28	.40	.09
Eigen value = 1.135, Alpha = .63						
Factor six**						
20. Are staff members informed and able to secure answers to your questions?	.09	.12	.12	.08	.15	.67
Eigen Value 1.010						
Items not clearly associated with any single factor.						
21. Are common areas suited to your needs?	.34	.14	.15	.39	.10	.35

*Because confirmatory analysis indicated that deletion would improve the fit of the model (see Table 2), Items 4, 5 and 6 were not used in the composite measure of Supportive Relationships with Staff.

**Factor 6 was neither named nor used in further analyses because of its very low Eigen Value, the fact that it contains only one item not already included in another factor, and because its correlation with four out of five of the other factors exceeds .30.

and #6) and thus does not clearly belong to any one component. These two items and Factor 6 were eliminated from further analyses.

The results of the confirmatory factor analysis of the nineteen-item, five-factor model as presented in the first column of Table 2 indicate a fit that is borderline and could be improved by modifications. Lagrange

Multiplier Test results suggested that the fit could be improved by eliminating three items from Factor 1 (#4, #5 and #6) and one item from Factor 2 (#8). Since dropping Item #8 left only two items in Factor 2, however, it was retained. The results for this sixteen-item, five-factor model are presented in the second column of Table 2 and show that the fit is quite good with a Comparative Fit Index (CFI) of .97. Thus, from the point of view of residents, the quality of the system within the facility has five distinct components: Supportive Relationships with Staff; Relationships Among Residents; Personal Services; Physical and Programmatic Environment; and Resident Involvement and Influence in the Facility. Composite measures were created by averaging resident responses to the items included within each component. Each composite measure has a minimum possible score of 1 and a maximum possible score of 3.

Results presented in the third column of Table 2 suggest that while the fit of the model for the Time 2 data is not as good as for the Time 1 data on which it was based, it is adequate (Marsh and Hocevar, 1985). Alphas for the items included in Factors 1 through 4 at Time 2 (Factor 1 = .80, Factor 2 = .58, Factor 3 = .65, Factor 4 = .61) are quite comparable to those presented in Table 1 for Time 1 (Factor 1 = .75, Factor 2 = .59, Factor 3 = .64, Factor 4 = .71). The alpha for the items included in Factor 5 is much higher at Time 2 (.93) than at Time 1 (.63). Thus, the structure of the five-component model is fairly stable–indicating reasonable reliability. Paired samples t-tests of differences between means on the composite measures for the two administrations also indicate good pre-

TABLE 2. Indices of Fit for the Nineteen-Item, Five-Factor Model and the Final Sixteen-Item,[a] Five-Factor Model.

	Nineteen-item model	Sixteen-item model[a]
Chi square	237.11***	112.21
Degrees of freedom	142	94
Relative likelihood ratio	1.67	1.19
Comparative fit index (CFI)	.88	.97

[a] Lagrange Multiplier Tests indicated that fit could be improved by dropping Items 4, 5, 6 and 8. Confirmatory Factor Analysis with the remaining fifteen items yielded a CFI of .97. Because dropping Item 8 left the measure of Relationships Among Residents with only two items, Item 8 was introduced in the sixteen-item model reported here.

* p < .05, ** p < .01, *** p < .001

dictive validity. As noted in the methodology section, the facilities were in the midst of considerable turmoil in 1989. They were in some financial difficulty and were in the process of being sold. It is reasonable to expect that the uncertainty of these circumstances would affect resident perceptions of at least some aspects of the facility's system. Relationships with staff and the personal services of food and maintenance might be expected to be particularly amenable to the impact of short-term budget shortages and the turmoil of an impending sale. Paired samples t-tests were conducted with the 97 residents for whom data were available for both years. Results indicate that while Time 1 and Time 2 means for Relationships Among Residents $t(96) = -0.53$, $p > .05$), Physical and Programmatic Environment $t(96) = -1.49$, $p > .05$) and Resident Involvement and Influence in the Facility $t(96) = 1.70$, $p > .05$) did not differ significantly from one another, the Time 2 means were significantly lower than those at Time 1 for Supportive Relationships with Staff $t(96) = -2.84$, $p < .01$) and Personal Services $t(96) = -3.52$, $p < .001$). These findings, therefore, suggest that the composite measures of the five aspects of the facility's system are sensitive to changes in the environment in ways that affirm their predictive validity.

Question Two: How do staff members' perceptions of the qualities of these system components compare to those of residents?

For the purposes of addressing questions 2 through 8, the responses of the 276 residents and 94 staff members included in the Time 1 administration of RASSI were compared. Time 1 was selected over Time 2 because of the larger number of residents included and because of the possibility that the special circumstances present at the Time 2 administration might affect results in relation to these questions. Question 2 is addressed by means of discriminant analysis in which residents and staff members are the groups, and composite measures of the five system components identified above are the independent variables. Results are presented in Table 3.

As can be seen from the table, 77 percent of the cases were correctly classified as to resident/staff status on the basis of the multivariate discriminant equation. The table also shows that when the two groups are compared on each component individually, residents' scores are significantly higher than those of staff members on Relationships Among Residents. Residents' scores are significantly lower than those of staff, however, on Resident Involvement and Influence in the Facility. Thus, staff members feel that residents get along with each other

TABLE 3. Difference Between Resident and Staff Ratings of Components of the Facility's System: Results of Discriminant Analysis

System components	Residents (n = 259) mean (s.d.)	Staff (n = 90) mean (s.d.)	F	Standardized discriminant function coefficient
Supportive relationships with staff	2.85 (.34)	2.79 (.32)	2.87	.27
(min. = 1, max. = 3)				
Relationships among residents	2.77 (.36)	2.67 (.39)	4.33*	.58
(min. = 1, max. = 3)				
Personal services	2.55 (.48)	2.44 (.53)	3.34	.30
(min. = 1, max. = 3)				
Physical and programmatic environment	2.78 (.33)	2.75 (.30)	0.74	.02
(min. = 1, max. = 3)				
Resident involvement in the facility	2.43 (.49)	2.73 (.32)	28.35***	−1.12
(min. = 1, max. = 3)				

Group centroids: residents = .26, staff = −.74

Percent of cases correctly classified: 77%

Canonical correlation: .40

* $p < .05$, ** $p < .01$, *** $p < .001$

less well and have more influence over the system of the facility than residents themselves feel they do.

> *Questions Three and Four: How do staff members' perceptions of the degree to which residents are satisfied with life within the facility compare to the residents' own assessments of their degree of overall satisfaction? How do staff members' perceptions of the degree to which residents are in control of their lives compare to residents' own assessments of their degree of control?*

Questions three and four are addressed by means of independent samples t-tests of the difference between scores of residents and staff members on the measures of resident satisfaction with life within the facility and degree to which residents have control over their lives. Results are presented in Table 4 and show that the mean on the resident satisfaction variable for staff members does not differ significantly from satisfaction reported by residents themselves. In terms of resident control over life, however, the two groups do differ significantly. The mean for residents' scores is significantly higher than that for members of the staff. Thus, while staff members are fairly accurate in their estimation of the degree to which residents are satisfied with life within the facility, they underestimate the degree of control residents feel they have over their lives.

> *Questions Five and Six: How do residents' perceptions of individual system components relate to their satisfaction with life within the facility? How do staff members' perceptions of individual system components relate to their assessments of residents' satisfaction with life within the facility?*

In order to address questions five and six, the individual relationship of each system component to resident satisfaction is assessed separately for residents and staff members by means of correlation analysis (Pearson Product Moment). The difference between the resident and staff correlation coefficients is then tested by means of t-tests for difference between correlation coefficients from independent samples (McNemar, 1955). The multivariate relationship of the group of system components to satisfaction is then evaluated separately for residents and staff members by means of stepwise multiple regression analyses with resident satisfaction dependent. Stepwise entry was used because the amount of variance shared among the components caused underestimation of their

TABLE 4. Resident/Staff Differences in Perceptions of Resident Satisfaction and Control: Results of Independent Samples t-tests

	Residents Mean (S.D.)	Staff Mean (S.D.)	Mean Difference	t
Satisfaction (min. = 1, max. = 5)	3.58 (.86)	3.44 (.75)	0.14	1.52
Control (min. = 1, max. = 3)	2.85 (.41)	2.55 (.60)	0.30	4.41***

* p < .05, ** p < .01, *** p < .001

individual effects on satisfaction when all variables were entered simultaneously.

As can be seen from the t-test results presented in Table 5, staff members do not differ significantly from residents in terms of the magnitude of the correlation between any of the individual system components and perceived resident satisfaction. They do differ from residents, however, in terms of the single component that best predicts resident satisfaction. To residents, perceived quality of the personal services of food and maintenance is clearly the best predictor of overall satisfaction with life within the facility. The correlation between Personal Services and satisfaction for residents is considerably higher than that of any of the other components. This component enters the stepwise equation first and once it is controlled, none of the other variables makes a significant additional contribution to the equation. This component alone explains 28 percent of variance in residents' satisfaction with life within the facility (R squared = .28).

The table shows that staff estimates of resident satisfaction, on the other hand, are related to a wider variety of components. Correlations between staff members' assessments of resident satisfaction and staff perception of the degree to which resident relationships with staff are supportive, the quality of the personal services of food and maintenance, the quality of the physical and programmatic environment and resident involvement are all significant and of similar magnitude. The Physical and Programmatic Environment enters the stepwise equation first and other system components fail to add significantly to the predictive power of the equation once it is controlled. The equation containing this single component, however, explains only 13 percent of variance in staff perception of resident satisfaction (R squared = .13). It is, therefore, a much less powerful predictor of staff estimation of resident satisfaction than is the component of Personal Services of satisfaction among residents themselves (R squared = .28).

Questions Seven and Eight: How do residents' perceptions of system components relate to their feelings of control over the important things and events of their lives? How do staff members' perceptions of system components relate to their assessments of the degree of control residents have over their lives?

The final research questions are addressed by replicating the analyses related to questions five and six with resident control rather than satisfaction as the dependent variable. Results are presented in Table 6 and

TABLE 5. Resident/Staff Differences in Contributions of Facility System Components to Perceptions of Resident Satisfaction: Results of Pearson's Correlation and Step-Wise Regression Analyses

System component	Residents (N = 247)				Staff (N = 89)				t-test of difference in r values
	Pearson r	B	(S.E.)	Entry at step	Pearson r	B	(S.E.)	Entry at step	
Supportive relationships with staff	.30***	—	—	—	.29**	—	—	—	0.08
Relationships among residents	.13*	—	—	—	.15	—	—	—	0.16
Personal services	.53***	0.96***	(.10)	1	.36***	—	—	—	1.36
Physical and programmatic environment	.35***	—	—	—	.36***	.90***	(.25)	1	−0.08
Resident involvement and influence in the facility	.26***	—	—	—	.30**	—	—	—	−0.32
R squared:		.28***				.13***			

* p < .05, ** p < .01, *** p < .001

show that the differences between residents and staff with respect to relationship of the system components to resident control are more dramatic than differences in their relationship to satisfaction. The magnitude of the correlation between staff perception of the quality of the personal services of food and maintenance and the degree to which residents feel in control of the important things and events in their lives is significantly larger than the correlation between residents' feelings about the quality of these services and their actual feelings of control over their lives. Similarly, the correlation between staff perceptions of resident involvement in the facility and resident control over life is significantly larger than the correlation between this system component and actual feelings of control over life among residents themselves. Stepwise regression results for residents show that of the five system components, Supportive Relationships with Staff has the strongest relationship to feelings of control and once it has entered the equation, Relationships Among Residents also makes a significant contribution to the multivariate equation predicting control. This two variable equation, however, explains only 7 percent of variance in the degree to which residents feel in control of the important things and events in their lives (R squared = .07). Staff perception of degree of resident control, on the other hand, is best predicted by Personal Services. Once this variable is in the equation, Resident Involvement and Influence in the Facility also contributes significantly to prediction of staff assessment of resident control over life. The two variables together explain 27 percent of variance in staff perception of resident control (R squared = .27).

Summary of Findings

It is clear that residents and staff members of these CCRCs have different views of the reality of the system within the facility in which they live and work. From the point of view of residents, there are five distinct components of system quality measured by the RASSI instrument: Supportive Relationships with Staff; Relationships Among Residents; Per-

TABLE 6. Resident/Staff Differences in Contributions of Facility System Components to Perceptions of Resident Control: Results of Pearson's Correlation and Step-Wise Regression Analyses

System component	Residents (N = 255)				Staff (N = 89)				
	Pearson r	B	(S.E.)	Entry at step	Pearson r	B	(S.E.)	Entry at step	t-test of difference in r values
Supportive relationships with staff	.20***	0.22**	(.08)	1	.26**	—	—	—	−0.24
Relationships among residents	.20**	0.16*	(.08)	2	.38***	—	—	—	−1.44
Personal services	.18**	—	—	—	.44***	0.36**	(.11)	1	−2.08*
Physical and programmatic environment	.22***	—	—	—	.26**	—	—	—	−0.32
Resident involvement and influence in the facility	.17**	—	—	—	.43***	0.59**	(.19)	2	−2.08*
R squared:			.07*					.27***	

* p < .05, ** p < .01, *** p < .001

sonal Services; the Physical and Programmatic Environment; and Resident Involvement and Influence in the Facility. Residents and staff members differ considerably with respect to their perceptions of these five components. Staff members believe that residents are more involved and influential in the facility than residents think they are while residents think that their own relationships with other residents are better than staff members believe them to be. While staff members are reasonably accurate in predicting resident satisfaction with the facility, they underestimate the degree to which residents feel in control of the important things and events of life. This is particularly interesting in light of the previous finding that staff believe that residents have greater influence over life within the context of the facility system than residents themselves feel they have. Thus, staff members see residents as more in control of the facility in which staff work but less in control of what is important in their own lives. This suggests that staff may lack real understanding of what is important in the personal lives of residents.

Staff members also differ from residents with respect to which components predict their estimation of resident satisfaction and control. Among residents, satisfaction is primarily related to perceived quality of personal services while among staff, estimation of overall resident satisfaction is related to a wider variety of system components. Differences between staff and residents in terms of components that predict resident control are even more dramatic. Among residents, the small amount of variance in sense of control explained by facility components is related to the social components–Supportive Relationships with Staff and Relationships Among Residents. Among staff members, a greater amount of variance in perception of resident control is related to facility components–primarily Personal Services and Degree of Resident Involvement and Influence in the Facility. Again, findings related to resident and staff differences in perceptions of control are particularly interesting. Staff members seem to both overestimate the degree of control residents feel they have within the specific context of the CCRC and to overestimate the importance of this limited type of control to resident feelings of control over what is important in life. For residents, feeling that they as a group have influence over the system within the CCRC has little impact on feelings of control over the important things and events in their lives which is primarily related to factors other than the system components measured here.

DISCUSSION

The findings reported here demonstrate that the overall systemic characteristics of a long-term care facility can be identified. Knowing these characteristics provides an understanding of the context within which resident and staff function and should suggest ways in which plans for systemic changes could benefit both groups.

Staff members see residents only in the context of the residential environment. It is not surprising that they perceive that the quality of the physical environment and resident involvement in the facility contribute most to resident satisfaction. These are the variables that staff members see on a day-to-day basis. More importantly, however, in terms of resident feelings regarding the important things and events in their lives, staff members overestimate the importance of facility characteristics to residents' feelings of control. Results of previous studies would suggest that this could be because staff members do not see the whole of the residents' life but only the portion related to their current living environment. Many factors that affect general feelings of control are simply outside of the realm of the facility. While the concept of locus of control was originally proposed as a fairly stable trait (Rotter, 1966), there is ample evidence that it can be affected by a variety of life circumstances including aging, poor health and disability (Baltes, Wahl and Schmid-Furtoss, 1990; Mirowsky, 1995; Mirowsky and Ross, 1990; Rodin and Timko, 1992; Lachman, 1986; Schieman and Turner, 1998). If staff were able to develop more personal relationships with residents they might come to better understand what factors other than those specific to the facility itself affect residents' feelings of control.

Another possibility is that general feelings of control and situation-specific control operate in different ways for elderly individuals. It is generally recognized that locus of control can be multidimensional and domain specific. It has been suggested, for example, that elderly individuals may be better able than the general public to maintain a sense of personal efficacy with regard to health while also acknowledging that medical practitioners and chance can also affect health outcomes (Lachman, 1986; Robinson-Whelen and Storandt, 1992). Similarly, CCRC residents may be able to maintain a general sense of control over the important things in life while simultaneously relinquishing control over specific staff functions. Residents may, in fact, decide to move to a CCRC in order to give up control over some day-to-day activities while maintaining control over things that are important to them. In such cases, individuals have prioritized what is most important to them and have decided to use their energies in ways other than maintaining a house, car, or the necessity of preparing meals. From the vantage point of younger age, staff may be unable to distinguish between control over the details of life within the facility and control over what is important to residents.

This distinction between situation-specific and general control may be comfortable for most residents. For others, a condition of unresolved conflict over lifetime expectations and the situation-specific variables in a congregate living community may be a source of anger and/or depression. Such persons may well be some of those referred to clinicians for evaluation and treatment. In either case, it is clear from these findings that staff do not understand the relationship between these two types of control among residents.

One of the serious potential outcomes of poor resident-staff mutual understanding is abuse. Tarbox (1983) reports that the most common form of abuse to residents is benign neglect. He suggests that this process may occur in a totally unconscious and nonmalicious fashion, but that symptoms of staff burnout are likely to increase the frequency of neglect. Lichtenberg (1994) describes a situation in which ". . . lonely and neglected patients were served by a staff that was equally lonely and neglected" (p. 4). In these studies, situational variables that directly affect the quality of staff-patient interactions have been found to be the best predictors of patient abuse (Pillemer and Finkelhor, 1988; Pillemer and Moore, 1989). Significant predictors of abuse were staff who: frequently think of quitting, believe that residents are like children who need occasional disciplining, scored high on Mashlach's Burnout Inventory, had frequent arguments or conflicts with patients or were experiencing stress in their own lives. LTC staff are not villains but are engaged in highly stressful, physically and emotionally demanding work with little monetary reward or public recognition (Burgio and Burgio, 1990; Diamond, 1992; Kramer and Smith, 2000; Feldman, 1994; Foner, 1994a, 1994b; Oberer, 1995). "Steps to reduce this stress and to improve the ability of staff to resolve conflicts in more constructive ways have the potential to bring about substantial improvements in nursing home care" (Pillemer and Bachman-Prehn, 1991, p. 91).

One step toward reducing stress for direct support staff might be to include them in an interdisciplinary team approach to treatment. The data presented here indicate that the variables of most importance to residents' sense of control (and perhaps well-being within the residence) are meaningful personal relationships. The organization of work within LTC facilities makes it difficult for staff to provide these relationships (Diamond, 1992). In contrast, ". . . mental health practitioners seek a partnership with their patients and spend time creating a trusting relationship" (Lichtenberg, 1998, p. 172). The problems which clinicians are most likely to be asked to address are those most difficult for the staff to handle–i.e., depression, anxiety, and anger. Involving staff in the development and implementation of treatment plans should have benefits for staff members, residents and clinicians. Such interdisciplinary work may also affect relationships among staff (Lichtenberg, 1998) and help to relieve all too frequently occurring problems of staff morale and turnover (Baltes, Neumann and Zank, 1994; Lichtenberg, 1994).

Some of the discrepancies between resident and staff perceptions might also be addressed through training opportunities in which residents and direct care staff jointly participate. In contrast to the common assumption of resident incompetence encouraged by the organization of work in LTC facilities, evidence exists that even frail and seriously ill nursing home residents recognize constructive and destructive aspects of their surroundings (Burgio and Sinnott, 1990; Diamond, 1992; Heiselman and Noelker, 1991; Stein, Linn and Stein, 1986). Studies such as that conducted by Fisher and Carstensen (1990) suggest, further, that, with clinical assistance, residents can learn to modify undesirable staff behaviors in positive ways. Diamond (1992), in fact, suggests that LTC residents have caregiving expertise of their own and should be directly involved in the training of the staff members who provide care. These findings are worth further pursuit and may provide guidelines for joint resident/staff training encounters. Involving direct care staff and residents in joint discussions about how care could be improved might have the potential of changing the dichotomized organization of work within LTC settings. Such change could improve empathy and understanding between residents and staff and decrease discrepancies in the ways in which the two groups view each other and the LTC setting in which they live and work.

REFERENCES

Baltes, M., Neuman, E. & Zank, S. (1994). Maintenance and rehabilitation of independence in old age: An intervention program for staff. *Psychology and Aging, 9,* 179-188.

Baltes, M. & Wahl, H. (1992). The behavior system of dependency in the elderly: Interaction with the social environment. In M. Ory, R. Abeles & P. Lipman (Ed.), *Aging, health and behavior* (pp. 83-106). Newbury Park, CA: Sage.

Baltes, M., Wahl, H., & Schmid-Furtoss, V. (1990). The daily life of elderly Germans: Activity patterns, personal control and functional health. *Journals of Gerontology, 45,* 173-179.

Bentler, P. (1995). *EQS: Structural equation program manual.* Encino, CA: Multivariate Software, Inc.

Bentler, P. & Wu, E. (1995). *EQS for windows: User's guide.* Thousand Oaks, CA: Sage.

Burgio, L. & Burgio, K. (1990). Institutional staff training and management: A review of the literature and a model for geriatric, long-term care facilities. *International Journal of Aging and Human Development, 30,* 287-302.

Burgio, L. & Sinnott, J. (1990). Behavioral treatments and pharmacotherapy acceptability ratings by elderly individuals in residential settings. *The Gerontologist, 30,* 811-816.

Byrne, B. (1994). *Structural equation modeling with EQS and EQS/Windows.* Thousand Oaks, CA: Sage.

Cleary, P. D. & McNeil, B. J. (1988). Patient satisfaction as a indicator of quality care. *Inquiry, 25,* 24-36.

Cryns, A. G., Nichols, R. C., Katz, L. A. & Calkins, E. (1989). The hierarchical structure of geriatric patient satisfaction: An older patient satisfaction scale designed for HMOs. *Medical Care, 27,* 802-816.

Davis, M. A., Sebastian, J. G. & Tschetter, J. (1997). Measuring quality of nursing homeservice: Residents' perspective. *Psychological Reports, 81,* 531-542.

Diamond, T. (1992). *Making grey old: Narratives of nursing home care.* Chicago, IL: University of Chicago Press.

Edebalk, P. G., Samuelsson, G. & Ingvad, B. (1995). How elderly people rank-order the quality characteristics of home services. *Aging and Society, 15,* 83-102.

Feldman, P. (1994). "Dead end" work or motivating job?: Prospects for frontline paraprofessional workers in LTC. *Generations, 18,* 5-11.

Fisher, J. & Carstensen, L. (1990). Generalized effects of skills training among older adults. *Clinical Gerontologist, 9,* 91-107.

Foner, N. (1994a). *The caregiving dilemma: Work in an American nursing home.* Berkeley, CA: University of California Press.

Foner, N. (1994b). Nursing home aides: Saints or monsters? *The Gerontologist, 34,* 245-250.

Forbes, D. A. (1997). Clarification of the constructs of satisfaction and dissatisfaction with home care. *Public Health Nursing, 13,* 377-385.

Goffman, E. (1961). *Asylums: Essays on the social situation of mental patients and other inmates.* New York: Anchor Books.

Heiselman, T. & Noelker, L. (1991). Enhancing mutual respect among nursing assistants, residents and residents' families. *The Gerontologist, 31,* 552-555.

Jenkins, H. & Allen, C. (1998). The relationship between staff burnout/distress and interactions with residents in two residential homes for older people. *International Journal of Geriatric Psychiatry, 13,* 466-472.

Kane, R., Riegler, S., Bell, R., Potter, R. & Koshland, G. (1982). *Predicting the course of nursing home patients: A progress manual.* Santa Monica, CA: RAND.

Kramer, N. & Smith, M. (2000). Training nursing assistants to care for nursing home residents with dementia. In V. Molinari (Ed.), *Professional psychology in long term care* (pp. 227-256). New York: Hatherleigh Press.

Kruzich, J. M., Clinton, J. F. & Kelber, S. T. (1992). Personal and environmental influences on nursing home satisfaction. *The Gerontologist, 32,* 342-350.

Lachman, M. (1986). Locus of control in aging research: A case for multidimensional and domain-specific assessment. *Psychology and Aging, 1*, 34-40.

Lichtenberg, P. (1994). *A guide to psychological practice in geriatric long-term care.* New York: The Haworth Press.

Lichtenberg, P. (1998). *Mental health practice in geriatric health care settings.* New York: The Haworth Press.

Logsdon, R. (2000). Enhancing quality of life in long-term care. In V. Molinari (Ed.), *Professional psychology in long term care* (pp. 133-159). New York: Hatherleigh Press.

Maciejewski, M., Kawiecki, J. & Rockwood, T. (1997). Satisfaction. In R. L. Kane (Ed), *Understanding health care outcomes research* (pp. 67-90). Gaithersburg, MD: Aspen Publishers.

Marsh, H. & Hocevar, D. (1985). Application of confirmatory factor analysis to the study of self-concept: First and higher order factor models and their invariance across groups. *Psychological Bulletin, 97*, 562-582.

McNemar, Q. (1955). *Psychological statistics (2nd Edition).* New York: John Wiley and Sons, Inc.

Mirowsky, J. (1995). Age and the sense of control. *Social Psychology Quarterly, 58*, 31-43.

Mirowsky, J. & Ross, C. (1990). The consolation prize theory of alienation. *American Journal of Sociology, 95*, 1505-1535.

Oberer, D. (1995). *Independence and dependence in activities of daily living: People with dementia and their caregivers.* Unpublished doctoral dissertation, Teachers College, Columbia University, New York.

Ogland-Hand, S. & Zeiss, A. (2000). Interprofessional health care teams. In V. Molinari (Ed.), *Professional psychology in long term care* (pp. 257-277). New York: Hatherleigh Press.

Pietrukowicz, M. & Johnson, M. (1991). Using life histories to individualize nursing home staff attitudes toward residents. *The Gerontologist, 31*, 102-106.

Pillemer, K. & Bachman-Prehn, R. (1991). Helping and hurting: Predictors of maltreatment of patients in nursing homes. *Research on Aging, 13*, 74-95.

Pillemer, K. & Finkelhor, D. (1988). The prevalence of elder abuse: A random sample survey. *The Gerontologist, 28*, 51-57.

Pillemer, K. & Moore, D. (1989). Abuse of patients in nursing homes: Findings from a survey of staff. *The Gerontologist, 29*, 314-320.

Powers, M. (1988). *Expanding systems of service delivery for persons with developmental disabilities.* Baltimore, MD: Paul H. Brookes.

Qualls, S. (2000). Working with families in nursing homes. In V. Molinari (Ed.), *Professional psychology in long term care* (pp. 91-112). New York: Hatherleigh Press.

Robinson-Whelen, S. & Storandt, M. (1992). Factorial structure of two health belief measures among older adults. *Psychology and Aging, 7*, 209-213.

Rodin, J. & Langer, E. (1980). Aging labels: The decline and fall of self-esteem. *Journal of Social Issues, 36*, 12-29.

Rodin, J. & Timko, C. (1992) Sense of control, aging, and health. In M. Ory, R. Abeles & P. Lipman (Eds.), *Aging, health and behavior* (pp. 174-236). Newbury Park, CA: Sage.

Rotter, J. (1966). Generalized expectancies for internal versus external control of reinforcements. *Psychological Monographs, 80* (whole no. 609).

Schieman, S. & Turner, H. (1998). Age, disability and the sense of mastery. *Journal of Health and Social Behavior, 39*, 169-186.

Simmons, S. F., Schnelle, J. F., Uman, G. C., Kulvicki, A. D., Lee K. O. H. & Ouslander, J. G. (1997). Selecting nursing home residents for satisfaction surveys. *The Gerontologist, 37*, 543-550.

Small, N. (1991). Impact of attitudes on the quality of nursing care: Patient and staff perceptions. In M. Harper (Ed.), *Management and care of the elderly* (pp. 207-217). Newbury Park, CA: Sage.

Stein, N., Linn, M. & Stein, E. (1986). The relationship between nursing home residents' perceptions of nursing home staff and quality of nursing home care. *Activities, Adaptation & Aging, 8*, 143-156.

Tarbox, A. (1983). The elderly in nursing homes: Psychological aspects of neglect. *Clinical Gerontologist, 1*, 39-52.

Timko, C. & Rodin, J. (1985). Staff-patient relationships in nursing homes: Sources of conflict and rehabilitation potential. *Rehabilitation Psychology, 30*, 93-108.

Zarit, S., Dolan, M. & Leitsch, S. (1998). Interventions in nursing homes and other alternative living settings. In I. Nordus, G. VandenBos, S. Berg & P. Fromholt (Eds.), *Clinical geropsychology* (pp. 329-343). Washington, DC: American Psychological Association.

Zinn, S., Lavizzo-Mourey, R. & Taylor, L. (1993). Measuring satisfaction with care in the nursing home setting: The nursing home resident satisfaction scale. *The Journal of Applied Gerontology, 12*, 452-465.

A Team Effort
for Treating Depression in Dementia

Donald G. Slone, PhD

SUMMARY. Managing depression or other challenging behaviors in people with dementia requires a team effort for optimal treatment outcomes. Developing a team approach in a dementia unit requires planning and coordination. Teamwork concepts and practical guidelines are described including: (a) Why a team approach is necessary, (b) Deciding who should be involved in a team effort, (c) When to involve the team in developing behavior management programs, (d) Using formal versus informal mechanisms to coordinate teamwork, (e) Focusing team based behavior management planning by using basic categories of intervention strategies, and (f) Different team dynamics to consider when developing or troubleshooting team functioning. *[Article copies available for a fee from The Haworth Document Delivery Service: 1-800-HAWORTH. E-mail address: <getinfo@haworthpressinc.com> Website: <http://www.HaworthPress.com> © 2002 by The Haworth Press, Inc. All rights reserved.]*

KEYWORDS. Team, depression, dementia, behavior management

Caring for people with dementia, by its very nature, requires a team effort. The need for teamwork is even further emphasized when dementia is complicated by issues such as depression or behavior problems (Lichtenberg, 1994). When consultants are called upon to intervene

---

Donald G. Slone is affiliated with Western State Hospital, Tacoma, WA.

[Haworth co-indexing entry note]: "A Team Effort for Treating Depression in Dementia." Slone, Donald G. Co-published simultaneously in *Clinical Gerontologist* (The Haworth Press, Inc.) Vol. 25, No. 3/4, 2002, pp. 173-196; and: *Emerging Trends in Psyhological Practice in Long-Term Care* (ed: Margaret P. Norris, Victor Molinari, and Suzann Ogland-Hand) The Haworth Press, Inc., 2002, pp. 173-196. Single or multiple copies of this article are available for a fee from The Haworth Document Delivery Service [1-800-HAWORTH, 9:00 a.m. - 5:00 p.m. (EST). E-mail address: getinfo@haworthpressinc.com].

with depression or other behavioral difficulties, the process is team focused from start to finish, beginning with assessment based on input from caregivers, followed by intervention strategies formulated from this input, and finishing with intervention efforts which are carried out largely by caregivers (Zarit & Zarit, 1998).

Slone and Gleason (1999) describe the critical role that the dynamics of the caregiving team have on the success or failure of intervention efforts. Despite the impact team dynamics can have on treatment outcomes for people with dementia, teamwork issues often seem to be overlooked. This article is designed to emphasize, first, that a coordinated team effort is critical to optimal treatment outcomes. Second, once the nature of teamwork is understood, the very nature of clinical practice must change to provide optimal treatment for behavioral complications of dementia. Lichtenberg (1994), in his review of efforts to create interdisciplinary teams in nursing homes, points out that an effective team requires a combination of elements. The lack of one component may render other components ineffective.

The topic of teamwork is complex in both theory and practice. For purposes of discussion, two approaches will be used to simplify this topic. First, the issue of depression in nursing home residents with dementia will be used as a focal point to illustrate teamwork concepts. The teamwork concepts and processes apply equally well to other behavioral challenges of dementia.

Next, the teamwork concepts and practical guidelines will be organized according to issues of why, who, when, how, and what.

a. Why? The reasons teamwork is necessary will be discussed.
b. Who? Some key team members in a nursing home and their unique contributions to the overall team effort will be considered.
c. When? Time frames for engaging a team effort will be described.
d. How? Formal versus informal mechanisms for coordinating teamwork will be contrasted.
e. What? A practical method for breaking down different aspects of dementia behavior to consider when developing intervention strategies will be offered.
f. What? Eight components of effective teams will be distinguished as a framework improving or troubleshooting dementia caregiving teams.

WHY? THE NEED FOR A TEAM EFFORT

Mary was a persistent complainer with drawn out, whining speech. She was overweight and had weakness in her arms and legs, making personal care difficult. Staff tended to avoid her except when absolutely necessary. A psychologist, new to the team, realized that Mary was depressed. The diagnosis of depression, along with pharmacological treatment for depression, had somehow been dropped during her prolonged hospitalization. During efforts to discuss her depression it became apparent that her somatic complaints were used to divert attention from her more painful issue of depression. Treatment involved psychotherapy with patient efforts to refocus conversation from somatic complaints to depressive topics. Mary was taught more appropriate ways to ask that her needs be met. Staff were educated and encouraged not to avoid her persistent demands as she learned more appropriate ways to ask that her needs be met. Efforts to re-institute antidepressant medication were pursued. Recreation staff helped her write letters to her husband, who she desperately missed. Upon her successful discharge she was happier, more functional, and much more pleasant to be around.

An understanding of teamwork begins with the question of "why?," or "Do we really have to?" The case of Mary demonstrates that a coordinated team effort is sometimes needed for effective treatment outcomes. However, attempts to coordinate a team effort are not always successful. Experience shows that working with a dysfunctional team can result in a state of "team purgatory," where the team dysfunction ". . . may cause the entire team to feel like they are spending time in purgatory, a place or state of temporary suffering or misery where people wait with uncertainty and a restricted sense of control over their final destiny" (Drinka & Streim, 1994, p. 541). Efforts to improve teamwork may not meet with success. Teamwork can become a struggle for influence, where team meetings are boycotted and the focus on patient care is lost in the struggle (Lichtenberg, 1994). Team members may become discouraged and develop a sense of helplessness regarding any ability to influence the team process in a constructive direction. It becomes easy to understand the temptation to just focus on one's specific duties and avoid issues that involve a team process.

Unfortunately, effective teamwork is inextricably linked to such issues as quality of care, staff satisfaction, productivity, and staff turnover (Lichtenberg, 1994). It is important to understand why working together with other team members becomes so critical when caring for a depressed, demented nursing home resident. Both the complexity of the illness and the dynamics of the caregiving situation demand a team approach for optimal care.

The complex nature of depression in dementia and the relationship of this to teamwork can be illustrated by four basic principles of dementia care. First, there is no simple formula for treatment. A behavioral problem in dementia can have multiple potential causes (Robinson, Spencer, & White, 1989). Intervention efforts begin with a catalog of potential causes to consider. The same behavior problem, when manifested by 10 different dementia residents, may easily require different solutions for each resident. Treatment solutions for depression or other problems in this population must be unique and individualized. Finding solutions becomes an exercise in creativity. The implication for teamwork is that this problem solving process is accomplished much more effectively as a team, rather than having each team member working in relative isolation.

A second principle is that there is no single cure. Geriatric issues tend to be complicated. Treatment is no longer regarded as a search for a single cause, but as a combination of multiple contributing variables (Blazer, 1995). These multiple variables are likely to fall within the purview of several different team members. Given that multiple team members are involved, it becomes unavoidable that treatment planning is best accomplished as a coordinated team effort.

A third principle involves the diversity of approaches by different staff members. In a nursing home environment, a given resident will be approached by a number of different caregivers, each with their own personality, caregiving style, expertise, training, and experience. It is typical that one staff member will be the first to discover an intervention strategy that a given resident responds positively to. It is also common that this staff member tends to enjoy problem-free interactions with this resident, while other team members remain frustrated and unaware that an effective intervention strategy has been discovered. With multiple caregivers attempting multiple caregiving strategies, the result may be a more efficient discovery of effective intervention strategies. However, more effective and efficient overall treatment will result only to the extent that these discoveries are shared with other team members. Otherwise, having an effective overall treatment program must wait until team members discover effective interventions on their own.

The fourth principle is that managing behavioral complications in dementia residents typically requires more observation, expertise, and time than any one caregiver has to offer (Tsukuda, 1990). Again, the implication is that a team effort is required. Considering the implications that these four principles have for teamwork, working together well becomes more than a workplace pleasantry. An integrated team intervention is necessary for effective treatment.

The second set of issues that illustrate why teamwork is necessary might best be described as the dynamics of the caregiving situation. These dynamic issues might be grouped according to team dynamics, resident dynamics, and the dynamics of the illness. First, of course, is the issue of team dynamics. As discussed previously, team dynamics can either help or hinder efforts to provide optimal dementia care.

The second dynamic factor involves the resident. In general, nursing home residents have distinct personalities. This may involve clear preferences for working with one staff member rather than another. This, in turn, may facilitate or hinder caregiving efforts. Different staff may be faced with very different caregiving scenarios depending on these resident preferences. A resident dynamic which is more specific to depression in dementia is manifested by responses such as, "Of course I'm depressed. I'm old." Overcoming strongly held beliefs that depression is an inevitable consequence of aging is often a critical first step in treating depression in this population. Instilling hope and the belief that depression is a treatable illness can be a challenge. Similarly, other resident variables such as personality, belief systems, or preferences can impact efforts to provide treatment.

The third dynamic is that of the illness itself. Depression in general has a more subdued presentation in older adults. When depression exists in addition to dementia, the characteristics of the dementia such as poor insight, poor memory, and expressive deficits result in an even more poorly defined presentation of depression (Bungener, Jouvent, & Derouesne, 1996; Jenkins et al., 1996). In addition, mood fluctuations in dementia mean that depression in dementia may not be as apparent at some times as others. This is especially troublesome when the depression is not apparent when the psychiatrist visits. As a result of these characteristics of depression in dementia, depression is often overlooked in this population. Whether or not observations that may indicate the presence of depression are reported to team members who might play a role in assessment and intervention is a matter of teamwork. Hughes and Medina-Walpole (2000), for example, found that one clear outcome of better teamwork on a dementia specialty unit was more effective detection and treatment of depression.

If we can accept that treating depression in residents with dementia is a complicated and dynamic task which is best accomplished by caregivers who work effectively as a team, how does this affect our practice? The critical next step is to realize that effective teamwork is a complex and challenging task and is unlikely to happen by accident. A program for working with dementia residents must be redesigned to include the teamwork component. The remainder of this article will focus on the issues of how to incorporate teamwork into a dementia program. This will include who to include, when to involve the team, how to structure this, and what factors need to be considered when developing intervention strategies. Finally, key elements of effective teams will be described as a guide to developing and troubleshooting dementia caregiving teams.

WHO? KEY TEAM MEMBERS
AND THEIR UNIQUE CONTRIBUTIONS

Every afternoon at about 3:00 Elizabeth would stand by the entrance to the Alzheimer's Special Care Unit, crying and desperately pleading with anyone entering or leaving the unit. She insisted on going home to care for her children, because they were due home from school. Staff knew that, in reality, her children were long since grown. The unit social worker and the nurse manager were at their wits' end due to both the mournful pleas and the time consuming task of passing through the door where Elizabeth waited. A consultant was called in. During the course of the evaluation, the consultant happened to ask a nurse's aide, Larry, about Elizabeth. Larry was somewhat surprised by this question, but patiently explained. "That's no problem. She likes to help. I ask her to come help me in the kitchen. We have a cup of coffee, chat for a few minutes, and she forgets all about it." Larry's solution was easily implemented by all concerned, and needed only to be shared with other team members.

Deciding who to include as a part of the team when working with depressed dementia residents in a nursing home setting requires some consideration. This may involve core team members or extended team members. Extended team members may include those not normally involved as everyday team members, such as psychologists and psychiatrists. Ultimately, teams should be formed on the basis of who is needed to solve the problem at hand (Tsukuda, 1990). The list of potential team members and their roles could become lengthy. However, as Lichtenberg (1994) points out, a poor understanding of the roles of other disciplines on the team becomes a major barrier to effective team functioning. Knowing who to involve in a given issue depends upon a familiarity with the roles and potential contributions of other team members. Also, being familiar with roles is important because working with a dementia population usually requires that professional staff redefine their roles somewhat. Working in an institutional setting means some degree of role overlap with other disciplines, which requires that roles and tasks must be negotiated at times (Tsukuda, 1990). Although deciding which team members to involve depends upon the situation, it may be helpful to highlight the roles of a few key team members in a nursing home setting. This is not intended to be a comprehensive list or to exclude any potential team members. The roles of a few common nursing home team members were chosen as examples in order to highlight some of the unique contributions that different team members can have.

Nursing Assistants (NAs) are often overlooked as key team members. Lichtenberg (1994) points out how NAs are often discouraged from verbalizing ideas about patient care and are not regarded as a part of the team. Yet, quality of care is improved when the NAs are included in decision making processes. The NAs are the team members who spend the most time with residents. They have the greatest observational baseline for resident behaviors, including signs of depression that may become evident. Also, they have the most experience with trying different ways of working with residents and, ultimately, will be the ones to implement many intervention strategies. Involvement of the NAs is essential to assessment and to developing intervention strategies. Programs must be designed to include input from these team members.

Activities staff often spend considerable time with residents and offer a unique perspective. Engaging residents in activities is a major component of a program for treating depression in dementia residents (Teri & Logsdon, 1991). Activities staff tend to have the most experience with exploring the upper limits of what residents are able to do and with attempting to engage residents in activities. Activities programming for dementia is a specialized field. Dementia residents are unable to participate in many standard nursing home activities. Yet, when activities are based upon an assessment of a resident's abilities and are designed so that dementia residents are able to engage in activities, the payoff includes happier and less anxious residents (Orsulic-Jeras, Judge, & Camp, 2000). Ultimately, the expertise and efforts of activities staff are critical to designing and implementing intervention programs for depression in dementia residents.

A third group who deserves special mention as team members is family members. Family members are often not considered as part of the team. They may be seen as intrusive or contentious. Yet, family members can be invaluable assets to nursing home programs. Their knowledge of premorbid personality, history of depression, and intervention strategies used before admission can be invaluable, and their willingness to help can be incorporated into the overall treatment program. Gladstone and Wexler (2000) offer guidelines as to how families and nursing home staff can work together to form a collaborative working relationship.

A fourth person who deserves special consideration is the team coordinator. In order to have a coordinated team intervention, someone must have the coordinator role (Tsukuda, 1990). In general, the team coordinator should be capable of working with others in a collaborative way where each member is regarded equally with consideration given to their particular knowledge, experience, expertise, and observational opportunity (Lichtenberg, 1994; Tsukuda, 1990). A caution should be given to nurse supervisors, who are in an authority role. It is important that an authoritarian style does not dominate the team coordinator role, as this may quash the input from subordinates that the team coordinator role is designed to facilitate. Otherwise, the team coordinator can be any team member who has the talent and inclination to perform this role.

Many other team members have unique contributions to make and could be considered in this discussion. It becomes clear that many people may be involved in the care of a depressed dementia resident. The task of coordinating an overall treatment effort may seem to be daunting and time consuming. It may help to weigh this against the costs of not performing this task, which may include excess disability for the resident, increased stress and effort for the caregivers, and increased overall costs from a resident who requires more staff time than is necessary. Overall, the time spent in this effort is a good investment.

WHEN? TIME FRAMES FOR ENGAGING A TEAM EFFORT

Norma was being evaluated for depression subsequent to a stroke which left her with mild cognitive impairment. During the course of the evaluation, the medication nurse reported that Norma's mood brightened every day when the nurse asked for stories about the farm Norma was raised on. The consultant included a recommendation that this strategy be continued. The Director of

Nursing, upon receiving a copy of the report, looked askance at this recommendation, wondering why this would be expected of her staff. The consultant explained that one of her staff was already using this approach effectively, and that the intent was to encourage others to try it also. Obviously, this is not an intervention that was within the abilities or conceptual models of all of the staff. Further implementation of this strategy would probably depend on how well it fit the model of the Director of Nursing.

As described by Zarit and Zarit (1998), the time frames for engaging a team in the process of treating depression in dementia residents involves three points. First, input from key team members must be sought when assessing the resident and when formulating possible treatment approaches. As described earlier, different team members may have unique perspectives to offer. Second, the team needs to be considered when making recommendations for a treatment program. Third, the team needs to be consulted to monitor implementation of treatment recommendations and the resident's response to these. These three points are important to observe. However, the greater challenge for effective teamwork is in the second step: recommendations. It is easy to make recommendations that are consistent with one's own discipline and training. To coordinate a team effort, treatment interventions must target the entire team. Three points may be helpful to consider when formulating an overall treatment program.

First, it is important to include all good strategies, regardless of the source. The expert model and the authoritarian model of leadership both suggest that the team leader should be the source of ideas. In a team oriented model, it does not matter whose idea it was. If all the team coordinator does is share a working solution so that others may use it, this coordinator has been successful. Oftentimes an NA may know how to manage a problem behavior, or may have a critical observation, but the solution is never implemented because the information is not shared.

Second, intervention strategies should be phrased in a brief, concise format that is useable by line staff as much as possible. Basic interventions for depression in dementia include activities, medication, and some adaptation of psychotherapy. As a psychologist, this author has struggled with the idea of translating psychotherapeutic interventions into a form useable by NAs. Some situations are complex and require a trained psychotherapist. However, assessment sometimes reveals strategies that may be implemented by NAs. For example, one resident could be consistently redirected from a depressive mood simply by changing the topic to one that cheered her up. This strategy worked and could easily be used by caregivers. Of course, different team members have varying levels of talent as lay psychotherapists, so some knowledge of staff abilities is essential. After due cautions are considered, it is important to attempt to tailor basic "talking cure" interventions for use by NAs and other team members (Zarit & Zarit, 1998). The best interventions for dementia are often those that can be utilized consistently by multiple caregivers throughout the day (Feil, 1992; Feil, 1993).

Third, it is important to consider the potential roles of different disciplines and to develop intervention strategies for those who may help in a given situation. For example, activities, or pleasant events, are a key component of treatment for depression in dementia (Teri & Logsdon, 1991). Yet, depressed residents can be irritable and withdrawn, giving the distinct impression that they are not interested in activities. It is important to be sure that activities staff understand this. A resident's right to choose should be respected, but irritability, withdrawal, and poor initiative to become involved in activities are part of depression. Some consistent encouragement may play a critical role in treating this resident. Likewise, it is important to consider other disciplines that might help and to convey information necessary to engage them in the treatment effort.

Developing intervention programs that are based on input from all staff, that have concise strategies that are useable by all, and that are targeted to all potential disciplines will help build intervention programs that harness the potential of the entire team.

HOW? MECHANISMS FOR TEAMWORK COORDINATION

Unit nursing staff were reluctant to attend a meeting to discuss ways to manage behavior problems. Staff reported that they had worked together on the unit for a long time, they socialized together, and they had active discussions about behavior management strategies. At the first meeting, they discussed a resident named Richard. Richard would grab staff firmly by the arm and attempt to pull them along with him. If staff resisted, he would strengthen his grip so it became painful, and would become assaultive if staff continued to pull away. Staff were uniformly frustrated, concerned, and at a loss as to how to manage this behavior. Debbie, a nurse's aide, came late to the meeting. When asked for her input, she was somewhat shy and reluctant to offer input. However, she reported no difficulty in managing this behavior. She would let Richard take her arm, would walk with him a short distance, and talk conversationally. She could then easily redirect his attention to another activity of interest, such as the television. He would release his grip and she could be on her way. Debbie's colleagues were surprised to hear that she was able to manage this behavior so easily.

Developing team based intervention programs for depression or other behavioral issues in dementia depends on team members sharing observations and ideas. Typically, staff do this on an informal basis, sharing ideas as conversational opportunities present themselves. This informal process has the advantage of requiring no planning. However, both clinical experience and research suggest that ideas are often not shared and that communication in nursing home settings tends to be very limited (Lichtenberg, 1994).

Team based interventions are likely to be better developed if a more formal process for team coordination is utilized. The standard process of treatment planning conferences is, theoretically, the appropriate process for gathering and consolidating input from different team members about treatment related issues. This has advantages over an informal process for developing a team based intervention program, and has the major advantage of being a familiar component of all facilities. In practice, however, two limitations often emerge in treatment planning conferences. First, NAs and other hands-on caregivers are often not included among the team members present at these conferences. Second, the focus may be more on producing a good document than on encouraging a sharing of ideas. For these reasons, it may be preferable to set up a separate meeting, sometimes referred to as behavior rounds, as a mechanism for collecting team input. This information, once gathered, can easily be transcribed into treatment plans.

Conducting a behavior rounds meeting is not difficult. In general, behavior rounds are scheduled at a time that will allow NAs and other nursing staff to attend. They are scheduled through the nursing supervisors to assure that nursing staff can fit this meeting into their schedule, and to assure that staff know attendance is authorized. Schedules of other key team members can usually be accommodated to fit this schedule. Basic guidelines for behavior rounds are straightforward. First, they are kept short, typically 30 to 45 minutes once per week, to assure that staff have time to attend. Second, it is essential that key team members can attend, especially NAs who tend to spend the most time observing and working with residents.

The process of a behavior rounds meeting involves first describing any symptoms or behavioral issues of concern for the resident under discussion. Then participants describe any observations, ideas, or intervention strategies that may help with either understanding problems or developing intervention strategies. One person typically takes notes from the meeting, so that others may focus on the discussion, and ideas are then written up for each resident who is discussed. It helps if this write-up is then put in the form of minutes to be circulated so that team members who are not present may read them. The more team members present, the more effective the sharing of ideas can be. The minutes can be reviewed at future meetings to track any changes or progress. Key team members who may not be present, for example, primary care physicians, should be informed of observations that may affect them, such as the possibility of previously undetected pain.

The behavior rounds process in clinical practice has been an effective means of encouraging and consolidating input from various team members, and tends to have a more active participation and a much more enthusiastic tone than traditional treatment conferences. Also, the emphasis on the behavior management aspect of staff-resident interactions not only supports treatment efforts, but it highlights an aspect of team members' duties about which they tend to have much pride and work satisfaction. In any case, having a mechanism for gathering, documenting, and disseminating intervention strategies is essential for a team treatment effort.

WHAT? BASIC COMPONENTS
OF INTERVENTION STRATEGIES

Ralph presented a complex and challenging behavior management scenario. He was known for sudden outbursts with accusations toward certain staff, demands for immediate attention, physical pursuits of targeted staff, and assaultive behavior. In confidence, he offered that his mood was "down," but this was not something he shared with his treatment team, seeming to prefer angry outbursts. He had a surprising amount of insight about his cognitive deficits and his need for assistance. He seemed willing to accept assistance, suggesting that a working relationship with him could be built and that he could learn to trust and rely on staff for help. However, his very brief tolerance for waiting for assistance made this difficult to implement. Despite his gruff manner, his history as a boxer, and his history of verbal and physical abuse of his wife, he seemed genuinely surprised when asked about becoming angry and assaultive, insisting that this was not like him. He said he would want to know if he became angry. When he did become over-whelmed during an interview and suddenly glared with anger, he easily accepted a plan to handle this by continuing the interview later. He made ambiguous reports of pain, possibly related to a prior hip injury, but it was unclear how effective his pain medica-tion was in managing this. Obviously, developing an overall man-agement plan for Ralph was a complicated matter which would require consideration of multiple facets of his situation.

Whether an informal style, a traditional treatment planning confer-ence, or a behavior rounds type meeting is used to structure team input about depression or other behavioral issues, the next consideration is the content. What types of interventions should be considered? Lichtenberg (1994) emphasizes that simply assembling staff together is not enough. "The focus of teams should be on the services to be delivered" (p. 60).

A classic compilation of the types of interventions that have been found to be useful for dementia residents has been prepared by Robin-son, Spencer, and White (1989). This is a comprehensive reference list, but may be too much to consider in a brief meeting. On the other hand, psychologists tend to recommend the antecedent-behavior-conse-quence (ABC) model (Zarit & Zarit, 1998). While this model is cer-tainly concise, it tends to put diverse categories such as hunger, boredom, and interactions with caregivers all in one category as antecedents.

A more beneficial format for focusing a discussion about behavioral issues might have several features. The list should be moderate in size, with a manageable number of items. It should be developed from every-day conceptualizations of behavior problems so that it has a familiar, common sense quality for line staff. It should have categories that stim-ulate caregivers to think about a diverse array of potential causes and solutions of behavior problems. One example of such a list, which has been described in detail elsewhere (Slone & Gleason, 1999), will be re-viewed briefly with reference to applications to depression in dementia. Each of these categories has potential causes of behavior problems as well as corresponding intervention strategies.

Comfort Needs. Comfort needs includes issues such as hunger, feel-ing cold, pain, and medical conditions. Providing physical comfort, rec-ognizing and treating medical conditions, and treating pain are important components of a treatment program for depression in dementia. Morrison (1997), for example, offers a checklist with 42 common medical conditions that are associated with depression. Also, remember that depressed older adults tend to emphasize somatic complaints more than psychological symptoms as a manifestation of depression (Jenkins et al., 1996), so that the physical and psychiatric issues are closely related in depression.

Mood. Assessing for the presence of depression is, obviously, a critical step in the treatment of depression in dementia. This is not a simple task, however, given that the manifestation of depression tends to be less distinct in older adults and even less distinct in dementia (Bungener, Jouvent, & Derouesne, 1996; Jenkins et al., 1996). Also, consider that depression in the elderly may present as dementia. This is referred to as pseudodementia, and differentiating dementia from depression may be difficult or impossible (Jenkins et al., 1996; Peskind & Raskind, 1996). Both the recognition of depression and treatment are best accomplished as a team effort. Remember that team input should include a consideration of whether symptoms of depression have been observed. If so, a referral for assessment may be necessary. Possible intervention strategies should be considered, including medications, activities, and an appropriately adapted form of psychotherapy.

Anger. The general issue here is, if the resident makes anger based responses such as assaultiveness, threats, or verbal abuse, do they see this as appropriate? If so, helping them learn more appropriate responses is indicated. In relation to depression, it is important to realize that the current generation of elderly was raised at a time when depression was not seen as a biochemical imbalance for which treatment is indicated. Many viewed depression as a character flaw for which the solution was to "pull yourself up by your bootstraps." Being depressed, therefore, may be personally unacceptable. Depressed feelings may be channeled into angry feelings and responses, which, though not laudable, may be more fitting with a strong self image. If this appears to be occurring, strategies for both managing anger and identifying symptoms of depression may be necessary. Also, working with the resident for a more acceptable definition of depression, which includes identified symptoms, may be helpful.

Resident's Perception of the Problem. This general strategy refers to efforts to understand the resident's explanation of the problem behavior in question. Depressed dementia residents may believe that being depressed is how an older person in a nursing home is supposed to feel. Challenging this belief, if present, is a critical first step in an overall treatment program. It is important to instill a sense of hope and the idea that depression is a very treatable illness.

Activities. Decreased interest or pleasure in activities and decreased energy for activities are both key symptoms of depression. Also, increasing involvement in activities is a basic intervention strategy for depression in dementia (Teri & Logsdon, 1991). Therefore, assessing current activities, both potential for activities and actual involvement in activities, is a critical component of developing intervention programs for depressed dementia residents.

Triggers and Pattern of Escalation. These two general intervention strategies often work together. Triggers refers to events that may precede an episode of a behavioral problem, and represents a lay person's understanding of antecedents. Pattern of escalation refers to the observation that behavioral episodes in dementia often escalate over time, rather than being instantaneous. Implications for treatment programs are to eliminate or minimize triggers, and to learn to recognize the escalation pattern and intervene as early as possible for better results. These strategies may apply to depression, depending on the specific behavioral manifestations.

Relevant Personal History. Understanding a dementia resident's past history, activities, and premorbid personality is often useful in both understanding and developing intervention strategies for behavioral issues. With depressed residents who have a milder dementia, helping them to identify something in their life that they are proud of may be the first positive turning point in psychotherapy. For more impaired residents, discovering topics from their past that are associated with a positive emotional state may be helpful. Caregiving staff can then refer to these topics when working with the residents in an attempt to redirect residents toward a more positive mood and to enhance their cooperation with caregiving procedures.

Staff Intervention Style. Asking "Who works best with the resident?" and "What do they do?" is probably the single best method for identifying the individualized approaches that are effective for particular residents. Intervention programs are developed by identifying effective approaches and sharing them with other team members. Sometimes other team members can use these strategies directly. However, often it is necessary to modify these strategies to fit either different personal styles or different caregiving situations of other team members. Of course, simply calling upon the team member who has discovered a successful strategy and asking them to intervene with the resident is acceptable as a short-term strategy. However, having an overall treatment program demands that other caregivers ultimately learn how to intervene effectively in their own interactions.

Level of Cognitive Functioning. This general strategy refers to determining what the resident's cognitive abilities are, then comparing this to the level of performance that is being expected of the resident to determine whether these two are consistent. Often, caregivers become frustrated because they are expecting the resident to perform activities that exceed the resident's abilities. It becomes necessary to design approaches to match abilities so the caregiving experience is positive and successful for all. Depression changes this equation because depression superimposed upon dementia may cause excess disability (Pearson, Teri, Reifler, & Raskind, 1989). The extent to which a resident's disability is exacerbated by the presence of depression must be considered so that an optimal functional level can be targeted.

These ten categories of intervention strategies can be used within the context of team problem solving efforts to facilitate consideration of a broader range of intervention strategies.

WHAT? BASIC ELEMENTS OF EFFECTIVE TEAMWORK

Karen had been an RN for many years, but she was relatively new to the Alzheimer's unit. She was very conscientious about her nursing duties and made sure that her patients received good medical care. She tended to stay to herself, as she had plenty to do. She was somewhat impatient with the amount of time other nursing staff spent socializing with the residents or with other staff. When the team started having behavior rounds she was skeptical and was usually too busy to attend. After all, what these residents needed was good, basic nursing care. After hearing some of the ideas that came out of these meetings, she eventually began to attend. Other team members noticed that Karen became more open to their input. She reluctantly started sharing her input during behavior rounds, which often was quite valuable to her team members. Her interactions with residents became noticeably more therapeutic, and she was overall much more pleasant to work with.

The final aspect of teamwork to consider when formulating a team approach to the treatment of depression in dementia is the issue of how to build or maintain an effective team process. A number of authors have addressed the issue of how to diagnose and intervene with team dynamics in a geriatric treatment team (Drinka & Streim, 1994; Heinemann, Farrell, & Schmitt, 1994; Lichtenberg, 1994; Tsukuda, 1990). All agree that (a) treatment in geriatrics should be a collaborative team effort, and (b) teamwork can be effective or ineffective depending on how it is conducted. Exactly what constitutes an effective team process in geriatrics is an emerging concept that is difficult to define precisely at this time. Given the importance of this issue, it seems prudent to outline some general aspects of a functional team.

Eight key elements of effective teamwork will be presented here. These elements were synthesized from both the geriatric teamwork literature and clinical experience with teamwork. They are intended as a guide for diagnosing team functioning and for developing strategies to improve teamwork. The eight elements to be considered are a specialist mentality, foundational themes, basic training, understanding team roles, barriers to teamwork, team coordination, conflict resolution, and maintaining morale. Examples of symptoms of team dysfunction and types of corrective strategies will be offered for each.

A Specialist Mentality. A pervasive belief about dementia is that nothing can be done about it, so why bother trying? A day of caregiving with dementia residents presents many opportunities to wonder whether anything can be done about the challenges that present themselves to the caregiver. The first and most important indicator of team health is the extent to which the team members believe that something can be done. A specialist mentality involves distinguishing what can be treated, such as medical complications, behavior problems, and depression, from what cannot be changed, such as loss of brain functions from dementia.

Signs of a poor specialist mentality include pointing the finger at other team members to intervene when problems occur, expressing a sense of helplessness about intervention possibilities, or simply failing to consider how to intervene when challenging behaviors occur. A healthy team has a positive sense of its ability to solve challenging behaviors and has an open and active stance toward understanding and developing interventions when challenging behaviors occur. A healthy team should build and develop a repertoire of success stories to remind team members of past successes in managing challenging situations.

Foundational Themes. A number of underlying assumptions form the foundation for effective teamwork. Four basic assumptions will illustrate this aspect of teamwork. First, of course, is whether or not the team members believe teamwork is an essential component of dementia care. Many talented team members believe that just focusing on their specific role constitutes effective dementia care, and that collaborating with team members is not important.

A second underlying theme is the realization that caring for dementia residents requires a special talent. Many people find a true purpose for themselves in their work with dementia, and others abhor this role. Working effectively with dementia residents means focusing on and utilizing remaining abilities. However, this requires caregivers, ". . . to value what is still there and not dwell on functions the person has lost" (Raia, 1999). This shift in focus from deficits to abilities is not always easily done. Lichtenberg (1994) points out how this task can raise personal issues that may cause some to avoid working with elderly populations.

The difference in those who are and are not able to make this shift in focus is easily observed in practice. Teams who fail to appreciate team members or family members who have this talent may not be honoring this specialist talent. Likewise, team members who fail to thrive in this work should be free to transfer elsewhere, and family members who find it difficult to interact with these residents should not receive excessive pressure to do so.

A third underlying theme is evidenced by an atmosphere of creative experimentation. A caregiver who believes that a truly competent caregiver should know how to manage a challenging behavior, or who believes that they should have known sooner, is showing signs of weakness in this theme. There is no clear guideline for intervening with a given resident. Finding the solution is a creative effort, and a healthy team should appreciate and support the process. Finding an intervention that works should be regarded as an important discovery, something to be appreciated and shared with others.

A fourth underlying theme is expectations for change. For example, some challenging behaviors change slowly, and change in small increments. Recognizing and appreciating the changes as they occur, however slowly, is important for effective teams.

A shared understanding of these underlying beliefs in teamwork, a specialist mentality, an atmosphere of creative experimentation, and realistic expectations for change forms the foundation for effective teamwork.

Basic Training. Perhaps the simplest component of effective teamwork to remedy is whether or not the team shares a common knowledge of dementia and commonly accepted intervention strategies. Having a team member express exasperation that a resident is being "manipulative" is, for example, typical evidence that the cognitive deficits of the residents are not well understood or accommodated. Failure to report sudden changes in the resident's level of alertness or functioning may be a sign that the impact of medical illness is not appreciated. Assuring that the team members have a basic knowledge of dementia, and refreshing this from time to time, may be the best starting point for improving team functioning.

However, Lichtenberg (1994), in his review of nursing home training efforts, cautions that, ". . . training for nursing home staff is a necessary, but not sufficient, condition for improving psychological care" (p. 52). Other teamwork components must be present, such as ongoing contacts to guide the creation of practical interventions, communication mechanisms, and team conflict management. An absence of other teamwork components can, ". . . overwhelm any training effort and make the knowledge to nursing assistants seem remote and unimportant" (pp. 51-52).

Understanding Team Roles. The previous discussion of who to include in team problem solving processes emphasized the different roles that various dementia team members have. Team members are trained primarily in the roles of their own discipline. Learning the roles of other team members is essential to becoming an effective team (Lichtenberg, 1994). In addition, roles overlap somewhat in an institutional setting where many team members work together. Team members must learn to flex, adapt, and negotiate their respective boundaries and roles (Tsukuda, 1990).

Team symptoms of poor role recognition may appear in several forms. First, team members must learn where they can complement and support each other's roles. As in the case of depression in dementia, the team members who observe signs of depression must know to report these signs to team members whose role it is to act on these observations. Another classic example of this is with pain in dementia. The staff who provide direct care are most likely to observe signs of pain, and may not realize the importance of reporting these signs to medical staff whose role it is to diagnose and treat the pain.

A second symptom of poor role recognition is disrespect for other's roles. Recreation staff, for example, may be the least respected members of the dementia team. Yet, experience shows that engaging residents in well suited recreational activities enhances their quality of life and can decrease the frequency of behavior problems. This, in turn, makes everyone else's job easier. Other team members can do much to support the efforts of activities staff, such as escorting residents to activities or scheduling personal care prior to activities.

Finally, a symptom of poor role recognition is failing to find time to collaborate with other team members. Time is at a premium on a dementia team, but team members who appreciate the value of collaboration are more likely to find time.

Barriers to Teamwork, or "One Way–My Way!" There are many potential barriers to effective teamwork on a dementia team. The impact of these barriers can be illustrated by focusing on a few which warrant special mention. Consider the following case scenario of teamwork gone astray. The nursing staff are annoyed by the seemingly perpetual disruptive vocalizations of one resident who has hearty vocal assets. One day they decide enough is enough and they take action. They place this resident right outside the nurses' station, only a few feet from where the physician normally sits. They know that once he becomes annoyed by her yelling he will finally take action and prescribe something for it. Aside from the fact that the nursing staff seem unaware that there is no specific anti-yelling medication, this case scenario helps illustrate several common barriers.

First, the classic medical model is accompanied by an authoritarian model, which dictates that communication occurs primarily in one direction, from the top down. This expectation is in place for these staff so much that they do not even consider more direct communication with the physician, as a collaborative model would suggest. It would be surprising if the physician would manage to deduce their intended message.

Second, this is a classic example of finger-pointing. Rather than consider what role they might play in managing the disruptive vocalizations, they assume that it is the task of another team member and delegate the entire task of developing an intervention program to the physician.

A third classic teamwork barrier, which is not apparent in this example, is the "One way–My way!" scenario. Team members who are untrained in behavioral interventions may make a classic error. Once they discover one way to intervene with a behavior problem, they may assume that it is the only way. If they are forced to admit that someone else's intervention strategy is effective, they secretly assume that their method is actually more effective. In fact, there may be many ways to manage a given behavior problem. Different methods may work better for different caregivers or at different times. It is especially important to consider what others do because someone must be the first to discover a successful strategy. When this occurs, the remainder of the team should consider how they might use this strategy, or how to adapt the lessons learned to their style or task. The value of having many caregivers with different styles is that someone is likely to discover the answer sooner, but this only helps the resident's program if other team members know, appreciate, and implement this solution.

These are just a few classic examples of barriers to teamwork. It is clear, however, that barriers such as these have a direct impact on the quality of resident care. It is important to teach team members to recognize such barriers, and to build an expectation of how teams should function, so that teams are better prepared to intervene as barriers occur.

Team Coordination. The mechanism for team coordination has already been discussed in some detail. This is a critical aspect of effective teamwork, but it is necessary here only to reemphasize that some type of mechanism for coordinating team input, intervention efforts, and overall treatment program is essential.

Conflict Resolution. The point has also been made that a good dementia team will generate a diversity of perspectives and ideas, so that learning how to manage the inevitable conflicts and to maintain a constructive direction in the face of these differences must become a routine task of the team (Lichtenberg, 1994). While overt conflict is not difficult to recognize, it is also important to recognize indirect conflict. Less obvious but equally destructive processes include a consistent lack of support of certain team members, intolerance of dissenting opinions, or acceptance of ideas without due consideration of potential drawbacks (Heinemann, Farrell, & Schmitt, 1994). A few conflict management strategies to consider include the following:

a. Remember that some degree of conflict is necessary and healthy.
b. Team members may express ideas in a way that is offensive, vague, or awkward. Restating these ideas in a manner that is more diplomatic, clear, or task focused may facilitate the team process. Offering such diplomatic assistance should become a routine expectation of team members.
c. Seek out opinions from key team members on important issues.
d. When disagreement is voiced, ask whether other team members share similar concerns before weighing pros and cons.
e. If tensions are high, consider whether an immediate decision is necessary. It may take time to formulate the best solution. Keeping minutes of meetings helps assure that issues are not simply forgotten.
f. When in doubt, err on the side of trying new ideas. Incorporate precautions and reevaluate the effectiveness of ideas as soon as possible.

g. If a team becomes stagnant, start by acting on small ideas to build momentum and develop teamwork.

h. Make a special effort to help new team members adjust. Offer support, education, guidance, and patience.

Maintaining Morale. A final element in the effectiveness of a team process is morale. Dementia work can be slow, difficult, and frustrating. Indications of poor morale may include statements indicating that dementia caregiving is an impossible and pointless task, or statements indicating a lack of pride in one's work. Finding ways to improve and maintain morale is important for the long-term maintenance of dementia teams.

Morale maintenance methods can be creative. The starting point is to realize that the best source of emotional support is usually fellow dementia caregivers. Fellow caregivers understand the nature, frustrations, and value of the work. Simply sharing frustrations with a colleague may help. Staff get-togethers, such as potlucks, or attending conferences about dementia, provide opportunities for supportive connections with colleagues.

Another strategy goes back to the question of "Why bother?" When friends, family, colleagues, visitors, or others ask this question, it helps to have a good response. The team can develop a sales pitch. The sales pitch might include the nature of dementia, the challenge of managing related problems, and the special talent the team has that enables them to accomplish this. Once this sales pitch is developed and practiced, having an opportunity to deliver it can be uplifting to team members.

A third strategy to consider is developing hospitality guidelines. It does well for the team to remember that the impression that others have of their work may depend largely upon how the team members treat visitors or callers. Basic telephone courtesy, greeting visitors, and being hospitable all convey a positive impression. Having others appreciate the talents of the team, in turn, helps support team morale.

Together, these eight elements of teamwork provide a basis for diagnosing the effectiveness of team processes and for formulating strategies to address specific team issues.

CONCLUSIONS

Teamwork is, in the best of circumstances, a complicated proposition. Whether working with depression or other behavioral issues in dementia residents, teamwork becomes necessary for effective treatment. This overview of teamwork in the treatment of dementia residents has included a description of the complex and dynamic nature of dementia that makes teamwork a necessity, a discussion of who should be included in the team effort, different times in the process to engage a team effort, how to coordinate a team effort, an outline of what aspects of intervention to consider in the overall treatment program, and a description of a model for diagnosing a dementia team along with some suggestions for improving teamwork.

In closing, it may help to consider that working effectively as a team allows us to accomplish what others may have thought impossible. Our teamwork allows even those with the most distressing experience of dementia to come to a comfortable and caring existence. Most of all, being part of an effective team, and sharing in the remarkable accomplishments of that team, is perhaps the most personally fulfilling aspect of dementia caregiving.

REFERENCES

Blazer, D. G. (1995). Geriatric syndromes: An introduction. *Psychiatric Services, 46*, 31.
Bungener, C., Jouvent, R., & Derouesne, C. (1996). Affective disturbances in Alzheimer's disease. *Journal of the American Geriatrics Society, 44*, 1066-1071.
Drinka, T. J. K., & Streim, J. E. (1994). Case studies from purgatory: Maladaptive behavior within geriatrics health care teams. *The Gerontologist, 34*, 541-547.
Feil, N. (1992). *V/F validation: The Feil method: How to help disoriented old-old.* Cleveland, Ohio: Edward Feil Productions.
Feil, N. (1993). *The validation breakthrough: Simple techniques for communicating with people with "Alzheimer's type dementia."* Baltimore: Health Professionals Press.
Gladstone, J., & Wexler, E. (2000). A family perspective of family/staff interaction in long term care facilities. *Geriatric Nursing, 21*, 16-19.
Heinemann, G. D., Farrell, M. P., & Schmitt, M. H. (1994). Groupthink theory and research: Implications for decision making in geriatric health care teams. *Educational Gerontology, 20*, 71-85.
Hughes, T. L., & Medina-Walpole, A. M. (2000). Implementation of an interdisciplinary behavior management program. *Journal of the American Geriatrics Society, 48*, 581-587.
Jenkins, M. A., Westlake, R., & Salloway, S. (1996). The diagnosis and treatment of geriatric depression. *Journal of Practical Psychiatry and Behavioral Health, 6*, 336-349.
Lichtenberg, P. A. (1994). *A guide to psychological practice in geriatric long term care.* New York: Haworth Press.
Morrison, J. (1997). *When psychological problems mask medical disorders.* New York: The Guilford Press.
Orsulic-Jeras, S., Judge, B. A., & Camp, C. J. (2000). Montessori-based activities for long-term care residents with advanced dementia: Effects on engagement and affect. *The Gerontologist, 40*, 107-111.

Pearson, J. L., Teri, L., Reifler, B. V., & Raskind, M. A. (1989). Functional status and cognitive impairment in Alzheimer's disease with and without depression. *Journal of the American Geriatrics Society, 37,* 1117-1121.

Peskind, E. R., & Raskind, M. A. (1996). Cognitive disorders. In E. W. Busse, & D. G. Blazer (Eds.), *The American Psychiatric Press textbook of geriatric psychiatry* (2nd ed., pp. 213-234). Washington, D.C.: American Psychiatric Press.

Raia, P. (1999). Habilitation therapy. A new starscape. In L. Volicer & L. Bloom-Charette (Eds.), *Enhancing the quality of life in advanced dementia* (pp. 21-37). Massachusetts: Alzheimer's Association of Eastern Massachusetts.

Robinson, A., Spencer, B., & White, L. (1989). *Understanding difficult behaviors: Some practical suggestions for coping with Alzheimer's disease and related illnesses.* Ypsilanti, Michigan: Eastern Michigan University, Geriatric Education Center of Michigan.

Slone, D. G., & Gleason, C. E. (1999). Behavior management planning for problem behaviors in dementia: A practical model. *Professional Psychology: Research and Practice, 30,* 27-36.

Teri, L., & Logsdon, R. (1991). Identifying pleasant activities for Alzheimer's disease patients: The pleasant events schedule. *The Gerontologist, 31,* 124-127.

Tsukuda, R. A. (1990). Interdisciplinary collaboration: Teamwork in geriatrics. In C. K. Cassel, D. E. Reisenberg, L. B. Sorensen, & J. R. Walsh (Eds.), *Geriatric medicine* (pp. 668-675). New York: Springer-Verlag.

Zarit, S. A., & Zarit, J. M. (1998). *Mental disorders in older adults: Fundamentals of assessment and treatment.* New York: The Guilford Press.

Training in Long-Term Care Facilities: Critical Issues

Lee A. Hyer, EdD, ABPP
Amie M. Ragan, PhD

SUMMARY. Caregivers can make a difference in the quality of life of residents in long-term care facilities (LTC) through the application of behavioral management techniques. This is widely accepted, but has little supporting data. In reality, a clear definition of the practice of caregiving in these facilities does not yet exist. Here, we present an overview of extant training in an LTC facility, identify problems, and point to core modules for such training. We also discuss quality of care in these settings. We discuss studies that support these ideas. We then discuss what we call the necessary ingredients of care. These involve the caregiver, the resident, and the system. Importantly, all must be committed for quality indicators to change. *[Article copies available for a fee from The Haworth Document Delivery Service: 1-800-HAWORTH. E-mail address: <getinfo@haworthpressinc.com> Website: <http://www.HaworthPress.com> © 2002 by The Haworth Press, Inc. All rights reserved.]*

KEYWORDS. Nursing homes, long-term care facilities, training, elderly, caregiving

Caregivers make the difference in the quality of life of residents of long-term care (LTC) facilities in positive and negative ways. Caregivers

---

Lee A. Hyer and Amie M. Ragan are affiliated with the University of Medicine & Dentistry, New Jersey, Piscataway, NJ.

[Haworth co-indexing entry note]: "Training in Long-Term Care Facilities: Critical Issues." Hyer, Lee A. and Amie M. Ragan. Co-published simultaneously in *Clinical Gerontologist* (The Haworth Press, Inc.) Vol. 25, No. 3/4, 2002, pp. 197-237; and: *Emerging Trends in Psychological Practice in Long-Term Care* (ed: Margaret P. Norris, Victor Molinari, and Suzann Ogland-Hand) The Haworth Press, Inc., 2002, pp. 197-237. Single or multiple copies of this article are available for a fee from The Haworth Document Delivery Service [1-800-HAWORTH, 9:00 a.m. - 5:00 p.m. (EST). E-mail address: getinfo@haworthpressinc.com].

can have the most positive effect by utilizing appropriate knowledge and application of behavioral management techniques (Dupree & Schonfield, 1998; Molinari, 2000). Good care, however, is a nebulous concept that defies clear definition. Despite this fact, there has amassed an entire industry and federal and state regulatory commissions to monitor the application of what is perceived to be good care (Colenda et al., 1999). And, there is no shortage of training models applied to caregivers in LTC facilities, most with common elements and virtually none with efficacy.

Here, we address the issue of good care in LTC facilities and provide what we consider the necessary methods of care based on behavioral principles and a basic medical understanding of the patient. First, we address an overview of LTC facilities since the Omnibus Budget Reconciliation Act of 1987 (OBRA, 1992). We then consider the realities of LTC facilities and the problems that will occur. Toward this end, we consider training in these facilities: the history, the current status, efficacy, and the necessary conditions for training to be meaningful. Next, we address the problem of the medical model in LTC facilities and consider newer models of care. We then consider the issue of QL (quality of life) as the new and necessary way for care. In this effort we summarize data on our own work and present the core ingredients of caretaking, labeled transformation of care. We provide practical advice and discuss the training as we applied it.

Our argument is that training is the key to important change. Importantly, whatever the exact model of training used, it should highlight the elements discussed here.

OVERVIEW OF LTC FACILITIES

A recent report to Congress by the Department of Health and Human Services, based on eight years of research, states that most nursing homes are understaffed to the point where residents are endangered (Pear, 2000). The 1987 OBRA law asserts that nursing homes must have enough staff to provide services enabling each resident to achieve "the highest practical, physical, mental and psychosocial well-being" (OBRA, 1992). You might say that this is the macro-goal for LTC facilities in this nation. One sizable obstacle toward achieving this goal is the lack of basic understanding for managing disruptive behavior.

Borson et al. (2000) surveyed just under 900 directors of nursing (DONs) on the issue of handling of disruptive behavior in LTC facilities. They found that there are substantial deficits in the skill of staff members at all levels in the management of disturbed behaviors and a need for a broad-based improvement in skills. Only 15% of the DONs were satisfied with the current level of expertise. This study closely followed a study that showed that DONs highly valued nonpharmacologic interventions.

Borson et al. (2000) emphasize:

> A nursing home interdisciplinary team training program should generate a common, evidence-based understanding of the causes and consequences of disruptive behavior; train members of each staff discipline to identify opportunities for prevention and treatment and teach validated, specific, and practical interventions tailored to the unique roles in patient care. Appropriate content includes techniques for modifying antecedent and environmental contingencies that promote disturbed behavior, interpersonal strategies that minimize the risk of disrupted consequences, design and implement programs that engage residents in activities incompatible with disrupted behavior, and safe and effective psychopharmacologic treatments for ameliorating the varied forms of disrupted behavior commonly associated with agitated states, psychosis, anxiety, and depression. (p. 251)

Research indicates that usual care in LTC facilities does not seriously address mental health problems (Frazer, 1995). State mandates under the direction of HFCA are typically interested in the necessary basic care and the prevention of poor care. Even psychological assessment assesses for weaknesses and often gives no information regarding an individual's potential for optimal functioning (Camp, Koss, & Judge, 1999). For example, what does a Mini-Mental State Exam (MMSE) score truly say about the rehabilitative potential of the person? The typical psychiatric evaluation seeks to type dementia and evaluate for psychopharmacologic intervention for problem behaviors. These interventions are "resident limiting" and "system comforting." "Quality management" then often only applies to meet the minimal needs of state and federal agencies. There is typically only consideration for the risk of adverse application of care. More cynically, it can be argued that the canons of care are profit or maintenance and sanction avoidance. They have a human cost. Erving Goffman's (1959) "total institution" seems to apply.

In Defense of LTC Facilities

To the defense of the LTC facility, its "industry" is experiencing a revolution of ideas in design, programming and care. The following information is offered:

- The 1.6 million residents in LTC facilities will double by 2030, triple by 2050.
- There is a decrease in the increase of cost in these facilities (25% in three years 1993-1996).
- Residents are sicker than ever before.
- Upwards of 80% have behavior problems.

LTC facilities are used for many reasons these days, including housing people with mental health needs as well as an acute way station for hospital patients. In addition, LTC facilities are the target of just about every evaluation possible. They are "attacked" by issues of financing, reimbursements, quality management, service delivery, as well as treatment and practice. As Costa and McCrae (1988) noted about adult development in general, we may be having a hard time now trying to actually define what is the best area to be critical of. Given that the history of LTC facilities has been poorly administered and has undergone such a radical change in recent years, the ready critic can initiate action anywhere.

REALITIES OF LTC CAREGIVERS

Healing is not forcing the sun to shine, but letting go of that which blocks the light.

–Steven and Ondrea Levine

In LTC facilities it is the nursing assistant (NA) that applies the day-to-day care. Licensed practical nurses and nursing assistants hold the majority (88%) of full-time positions in hospitals and over half of all positions in geriatric long-term care (Kasteler, Ford, White, & Carruth, 1979; Smyer, Cohn, & Brannon, 1988). Nursing assistants outnumber licensed practical nurses 4 to 1 and licensed practical nurses outnumber registered nurses 3 to 2 (Kasteler et al., 1979). Turnover among the nursing assistants is high, is costly to the institution and has considerable effect on quality (Kasteler et al., 1979; Schwartz, 1984; Smyer et al., 1988; Waxman, Carner, & Berkenstock, 1984). Turnover rates have been identified as high as 75% per year (Kasteler et al., 1979; Schwartz, 1984). Waxman et al. (1984) found it to vary from 5% to 76% per year among seven long-term care facilities.

There is evidence too that the average NA is frustrated. As a group they suffer from low morale, burnout, and stress (Baillon, Scothern, Neville, & Boyle, 1996; Karuza & Feather, 1989). A majority are disenchanted with the understaffing and overwork, along with the organizational problems such as poor supervision and communication (Kasteler et al., 1979). Waxman et al. (1984) concluded that a rigid organizational structure, one that did not allow the NAs to communicate with professional staff, was a major contributor to turnover. Smith, Discenza, and Saxberg (1978) found that 71% of the NAs and licensed practical nurses had contact with the director of nursing only through their charge nurses. NAs are discouraged from verbalizing their ideas about patient care and are not routinely considered as part of the treating health care team (Faulkner, 1985; Kasteler et al., 1979; Sbordone & Sterman, 1983; Schwartz, 1984; Smith, Discenza, & Saxberg, 1978; Stein, Linn, & Elliot, 1986). Thus, although nursing assistants are heavily involved in difficult patient care, they often feel isolated, ignored, and neglected. Finally, we note that these conditions can cause their own problems. Baltes, Neumann and Zank (1994) showed that carers can increase dependence. They have also been shown to be inefficient on the job (Baillon et al., 1996).

Given their level of involvement in day-to-day care, it should be no surprise that innovations to improve the quality of geriatric long-term care can occur only by involving NAs and licensed practical nurses. NAs must be part of the interdisciplinary team. It is logical that they need better support and training for working with older adults. Assertiveness training may be helpful because it gives the nursing assistants a tool for communicating their resident concerns. This was made evident by time sampling methodology on nursing assistants and licensed practical nurses (Burgio et al., 1990; Kahana & Kiyak, 1984) which revealed that resident care and interacting with patients were the predominant activities in LTC facilities. Training is also key (see below). Finally, administrative support also is crucial (Lichtenberg, 1994).

Training in LTC Facilities

We believe that there is a robust record that the actions of the nursing staff can make a difference in the quality of care for residents, but an anemic one that there is efficacy in the application of its efforts. Historically, training has been a secondary concern in LTC facilities. In 1964, Lindsley discussed the possibility that the physical environment and reinforcement schedules could optimize resident care. "Prosthetic environments" could be developed and make a difference. In the 1980s, Baltes and colleagues (Baltes, Kindermann, Reisenzein, & Schmid, 1987) conducted a series of studies that described an environment that is overresponsive and overprotective, thereby fostering dependent behavior at the cost of independent behaviors (Baltes & Wahl, 1991). It appeared that most of the NAs were learning "on the job" and what they were learning was fostering a negative environment (Baltes & Wahl, 1991).

It was really not until OBRA in 1987 that training became a serious issue. Currently, there are two forms of training in an LTC facility, in-service and in vivo. Most models involve some variation of the two methods. In-service training involves classroom didactics. Often efforts are not successful, as pre-post tests show no changes (Feldt & Ryden, 1992). In fact, it is the usual case that an LTC facility will provide training through its DON or contract for this service (especially if the site is part of a corporation). Pre- and post-measures are rarely taken in this case.

In vivo training is also used with NAs in LTC facilities. Rather than viewing this as strictly negative, consider that on-the-job training provides NAs with immediate performance-based training and feedback. This has been done, for example, with some success on prompted voiding (Schnelle, Newman, & Fogarty, 1990). Unfortunately, after training stopped, so did the skill learned. Using a coding form designed to monitor in-service training after the fact, the Burgio group (Burgio et al., 1990; Stevens et al., 1996) followed up three weeks of behavior management skills training with success. Immediate feedback was provided on correct and incorrect tasks.

Several studies have provided positive findings for other techniques in training NAs. Several formal programs have been applied to the training of CNAs with success, using memory books (Bourgeois, Beach, Schultz, & Burgio, 1996; Bourgeois, Burgio, Schultz, Beach, & Palmer, 1997; Bourgeois, Burgio, & Schultz, 1992), didactic training (Burgio & Stevens, 1999), and family groups (Pruchno, 1995). A recent study by the Burgio group (Burgio et al., 2001) examined the effects of a communication skills training and the use of memory books by CNAs on verbal interactions with residents. This study was important because it applied several methods that are related to treatment enactment and treatment receipt–didactic training, behavioral supervision, staff motivational system, and computer-assisted observations. There were over 60 residents and CNAs. Residents had moderate levels of cognitive impairment. CNAs were taught to use communication skills and memory books. Also, a staff motivational system was included. Results were compared to a no treatment control group on a matched unit. The trained group used more positive statements and used more specific instructions without increases in total time for the resident. Results held up to two months after the research staff exited the facility.

In a train-the-trainer model Smith et al. (1994) used a two-day intensive training session. They used modules focusing on the behavioral principles that address problem behaviors, using the ABCs (antecedent-behavior-consequence) model. Cohn, Horgas, and Marsiske (1990) applied a behavioral model and the result was positive. Mathews and Altman (1997) used a similar model but included more in-service practice to good effect. In post-testing both the trainers and trainees improved. Of course, knowledge acquisition in no way guarantees skill performance.

Typically, studies have applied intense training and assessed outcomes directly after. For six weeks Vaccaro (1998), for example, had staff lavishly reward residents with tangible rewards after no aggressive behavior and punish aggressive behavior with reprimands and time outs. Aggressiveness was reduced markedly. In other venues, Pillemer et al. (1998) developed a *Partners in Caregiving* program for the training of caregivers and family members. They trained caregivers on areas related to communication and conflict resolution. Satisfaction was high. Brodaty and Gresham (1989) employed a 10-day intensive training program and applied booster sessions over a year on caregivers. Gains were substantial and were maintained over the year period. In parsing apart the results, they noted that caregivers are all different. They also noted that it is best not to intervene when there is stress but that the situation is solvable. Mittelman (1996, 2000) and Hinchliffe et al. (1992, 1995) also had similar programs and found similar results, one with spousal caregivers and the other in an LTC facility.

Finally, rehabilitation is a more controversial notion applied here. Regarding these efforts on older people, West, Welch and Yassuda (2000) describe the results of seminal studies on cognitive rehabilitation as regards older people: memory strategies, even the complex techniques, can be learned by older adults; training can lead to improvement that can last for long periods; training tends to be task-specific with little or no transfer of tasks not incorporated into the training regimen. In a much cited meta-analysis of this area, Verhaegen et al. (1992) endorse training and its effects. This group noted that four factors enhance training; pretraining, group sessions, shorter sessions, and younger participants. They also note modest effect sizes due to training.

Often two approaches are used to discuss training, restorative and compensatory approaches. The restorative approach applies cognitive retraining to facilitate recovery of functioning. The goal is to improve the person. The compensatory approach, on the other hand, accepts that the cognitive functioning will be impaired and attempts to train the resident to function by use of compensating strategies. Typically the former is used in a nonprogressive brain disorder and the latter for the progressive dementias.

We should note too that the mix of training and behavioral management principles has also been applied with limited success in the rehabilitation of the person. As one example, Royall (1994) highlighted the use of this mix with a dementing patient. The environmental stimuli serve as cues for overlearned subroutines and evoke compensatory behavior. Both employ two areas of focus, external and internal. He suggests that the resident can be managed by:

• Establishing a daily ritual
• Using new routines to break old habits
• Building good habits through repetition
• Listening to what the environment is saying to the resident
• Using social and environment cues to your advantage
• Removing or altering cues that seem to trigger problem behaviors

In sum, training is mandatory: it is going to happen. In general, it can be said that, when the primary focus is on the training of the caregiver, data are equivocal. Education is helpful but does not lead to immediate effects, generalized results, or utility for the resident. Sustained education, however, seems to positively affect morale and staff attitudes, caregiver-resident communication (Kihlgren et al., 1992; Post, Ripich, & Whitehouse, 1994), as well as reduced psychotropic medication and restraint (Rovner, 1994). There have also been reductions in behavior problems and depressed mood (Hagen & Sayers, 1995; Rovner, Steele, & Folstein, 1996). Regarding training packages (courses for caregivers), Edberg, Hallberg and Gustafson (1996) sum up these efforts by noting: Caregivers deliver more informal and human care and have a rehabilitative effect on residents, even those with a dementing illness. But, whatever is happening in the LTC facility to the nurse or CAN, more is required.

System Support

The administration must also be involved in active ways. Motivational systems also have targeted the skills of the supervisory staff. Performance Based Training (Snyder-Halpern & Buczkowski, 1990), Competency Based Training (del Bueno, Barker, & Christmyer, 1981), and Mastery Learning (Pickney-Atkinson, 1980), as well as TQM (Total Quality Management) (Deming, 1986) are popular ones. TQM (Deming, 1986) and Performance Management (Daniels, 1994) especially have been proposed as methods to assist in this area. TQM emphasizes the inter-relatedness of individuals and systems that make up the care setting, as well as the satisfaction of the customers. Zinn, Brannon, and Weech (1997) note that TQM involves five factors: a written statement of philosophy, a structured problem solving approach including measurement, use of employee teams for the analysis and improvement of processes, assessment of resident satisfaction, and empowerment of employees to identify and respond to quality improvement opportunities. It is also a system that emphasizes feedback for the group and not the individual. As a whole, a central problem seems to be the hierarchy of the system: DONs, RNs, LPNs, and CNAs. The Burgio group (Burgio & Burgio, 1986; Burgio et al., 2001) have addressed this area of concern as a major one.

Hallberg (in press) and Austrom (1996) independently conducted staff training according to TQM principles. Hallberg supplemented routine meetings with regular bi-weekly clinical supervision. A key component of the Austrom group (Austrom, Class & Unverzagt, 1997) was to conduct ongoing staff meetings in which staff and administration discuss care options for residents and exchange ideas. Results for both efforts were positive.

Performance Management has less success. This is a method of analyzing and implementing a management system based on antecedents (instruction), consequences (feedback), and multi-component staff management systems. Burgio and Burgio (1986) attempted this with limited success. The use of the multi-component system especially needed work.

In addition, more formalized and measured methods have been applied, including the Statistical Process Control (SPC) (Zinn et al., 1997) which looks for outliers along selected dimensions, as in the percentage of incontinence. Feedback is given to the entire unit, never an individual. Schnelle and colleagues (Schnelle, Newman, Fogarty, Wallston, & Ory, 1991; Schnelle, Ouslander, & Cruise, 1997) examined the SPC at improving incontinence and reducing physical restraints. It worked but only while in progress. A subsequent study (Schnelle, McNees, Crooks, & Ouslander, 1995) also found this to be the case.

Teams

The necessity of team care is often underrated. This starts with the organizational climate in an LTC facility. In an early study Sbordone and

Sterman (1983) reported that increased communication among hierarchies of staff led to reduced turnover and improved staff morale. Chartock, Nevins, Rzetelny, and Gilberto (1988) were able to increase staff time for bathing so that emotional as well as physical needs could be attended to, and they were able to get nursing assistants included in the treatment team meetings.

Clearly the interaction of the system and the individual teams on the unit is critical. Team care is then most relevant. In fact, the healthcare team is one of the key elements of care (see Finkel, 1998). Teams have long been hailed in health care as the best way to deliver care, despite the fact that few methodologically sound studies have been performed on team care. Residents receiving LTC services tend to have multiple, interrelated problems that require the skills and expertise of an interdisciplinary staff. Frequently, the staff operates in an inter-professional team structure to facilitate the development and implementation of a coordinated and comprehensive care plan (Zeiss & Steffen, 1996). Psychologists in LTC facilities frequently spend as much of their time working with staff as they do with the patients (Lichtenberg, 1994).

In addition, the experiences of some clinicians and teams are quite sobering (Bates-Smith & Tsukudo, 1984; de Santis, 1983). de Santis found that team members from a long-term care facility spent their time vying for influence rather than focusing on patient goals, and that team meetings were routinely boycotted. Bates-Smith and Tsukudo found that value differences and role confusions too often deter team functioning. These studies are useful in that they illustrate the necessity to plan team interactions and to build team cohesiveness.

Summary

In an effort to accommodate the many elements discussed here, a study was conducted at this facility (Hyer & Sohnle, 2001). Two LTC facilities were targeted for training, one an assisted living facility and one an NH. Three staff members provided the training. They followed a manual that addressed the issues in Table 1. The core modules were based on the ABC model (Teri et al., 2000). This model has been used in several training curricula of care (e.g., Wertheimer et al., 1992). It is based on learning theory. This model was also supplemented with core areas of memory problems, depression, and agitation. The trainee was also given training in the use of the autobiographical memory and ethical thinking, as well as stress reduction. These were given to bolster confidence and broaden perspectives.

Each setting provided 10 members for the training. Trainees committed to the program and attendance was required. No one dropped out. The participants consisted of CNAs (8), SW (3), nurses (3), rehabilitation medicine (4), and administrators (2). The class was made up of people from differing units and a "train the trainer" framework was used. After each session the trainee was asked to do homework and check in with staff. Trainees worked as teams. In the first and last sessions the DON and administrator were present and confirmed the support over time. Rewards were built in and applied over time. The administration was involved and afforded support and were in attendance at the end. A booster session was also applied at 6 months.

Table 2 consists of the core issues in the training. Several are noteworthy. Caregivers were "convinced" that they made a difference in the

TABLE 1. Training Modules

Session 1. Pre-test and expectancies exercise
            Model
            ABCs

Session 2. ABC film material and cases
            Use guidelines for care

Session 3. ABCs
            Dementia
            Memory (external ways of help)

Session 4. ABCs #1 problem → Memory
            External techniques
            Spaced retrieval

Session 5. ABCs #2 problem → Depression or not
            Thriving

Session 6. Special problems
            ABCs plus medication
            Agitation
            Severe depression
            CMI
            Pain
            Extreme frailty

Session 7. Autobiographical memory

Session 8. Ethics

Session 9. Overview of stress in LTC
            Simple techniques that work

Session 10. Administration support
            Post-test

Booster Sessions

On-call

QL of residents through the application of behavioral management techniques. They were empowered. While the content of the course consisted of behavioral and humane principles as well as the basics of decline in an LTC facility, the emphasis was on the caregivers. They were made the center part of the treatment team. Others were instructed to listen to them regarding day-to-day activities. It was noted that caregivers all differ, that caregiver distress causes problems, that it is important especially to control the situation when stressful, and that caregivers could work as teams and request assistance. It was emphasized that the system would support and encourage this program. In fact, caregivers were incentivized. Finally, an evaluation of the caregiver too was essential for success.

Measures were conducted before and after the training. Results showed that trainees' skills changed for the better. Staff rated themselves as more confident in the modules on the A-B-Cs, Depression, Memory, Agitation, and Overall confidence in "me." They also showed that they had learned the skills, by testing and by observation. These results were maintained at six months.

Caregivers can make a difference with residents when trained. As we have been discussing, the situation can be altered, at the person level and the level of training, as well as at the level of the system. At the person level, staff characteristics have been found to affect quality of care (Edberg, Nordmark Sandgreen, & Hallberg, 1995; Hallberg, Holst, Nordmark, & Edberg, 1995). At the level of training, improvements have been seen in any number of areas, including the usual outcomes of hygiene as well as behavioral management. At a system level (and as we noted above), the FSM (Formal Management System) for one has added measurably to the myriad forms of skills training. This includes clear descriptions of tasks, self-monitoring by nursing assistants, supervisory monitoring, supervisory performance feedback and praise and incentives.

MODELS OF CARE

Medical Model

The medical model still presides over care. Becker and Kaufman (1988) discuss two common assumptions that have prevented a paradigm shift to the therapeutic model of care in LTC facilities: aging is considered a physiological event foremost, and aging is considered a

TABLE 2. Key Training Perspectives

1. Caregivers can make a difference in the quality of life (QL) of residents of long-term care facilities (LTC) through the application of behavioral management techniques.

2. Like other professionals, caregivers must be incentivized (to make a difference). Like mothers, some are intuitive and naturally good; others not.

3. Residents can be understood, "read," and addressed according to behavioral and humane principles.

4. Residents have more insight into their condition than originally appreciated.

5. The person and the context of behaviors needs to be appreciated; otherwise a collection of symptoms is treated.

6. Caregivers (NAs) should be a center part of the treatment team. Others listen to them regarding day-to-day activities.

7. An evaluation of the caregiver is essential for success, especially after training. No one caregiver is like another.

8. Caregiver distress causes problems. As residents show problems, caregivers get worse, more stress and more depression.

9. It is important to control the situation when stressful and leave alone when not. The emotional relationship (between resident and caregiver) in particular is relevant to QL.

10. The system must support and encourage this program beyond the need for training.

time of illness and withdrawal from social life. As such, "medical care" is doled out by "nurses" and custodial care by NAs. Unfortunately, the philosophy of OBRA emphasizing psychosocial care has yet to meaningfully trickle down to the level of quality of care in most LTC facilities. At base, the medical model versus autonomy model clash.

At one level, it appears that the gross overmedication has been reduced. Regulations state that each resident's drug regimen be free of medically unnecessary drugs, defined as drugs of excessive doses and for excessive duration without adequate indicators, or in the face of adverse consequences that indicate that dose should be reduced or discontinued. In a recent study of five nations Hughes et al. (2000) found this to be the case. The policy has had an impact on the prescription of psychotropic medications in U.S. nursing homes compared with other countries, but it is unclear whether this has resulted in better outcomes.

At another level, it is unclear how the "medical" of the medical model alters care. Brown and Zinberg (1982) and Qualls (1988) focused on the differences between the medical and psychosocial model. In the diagnostic process, for instance, the medical model uses a "ruling out" or determining one etiology approach, whereas the psychosocial model uses a "ruling in" approach, acknowledging the effects of a variety of factors (i.e., loss, health, stress, depression). Medical practitioners are usually more paternalistic with patients and more concerned with immediate results, versus psychosocial practitioners, who view the patient more as a partner and use slower methods of assessment. The differences in these models may lead to conflicts among practitioners on a team. It is important both to understand the models of functioning brought by other team members and to make oneself understood.

At a molecular level, medication presents its own problems. For starters, the rate of success is not good. In a meta-analysis of 33 controlled studies of patients who had dementing problems, Schneider (1996) revealed that the response rate was 59% for the drug treatment and 41% for the placebo. This study consisted of over 252 patients studied up to eight weeks. In another metaanalysis of 16 controlled studies Lanctot et al. (2000) found these rates to be 64% and 38% respectively. Sunderland (2000) notes: Neuroleptics are more beneficial than placebo; however, only 20% of patients derived significant benefit. The same applies to depression. They take awhile and the necessity to titrate to symptom remission is unending in an aging decline process. There is always the need to monitor and adjust. Medication also causes side effects–"bad" ones that interfere with rehabilitation and "real bad" ones that cause side effects, like dyskinesias.

And, no medication does the complete job. Also there is no FDA medication approved for psychotic level problems in cognitive decline, for example. A partial list of behaviors that medication does not alter includes wandering, repetitions, shadowing, hoarding, lack of insight, perseveration, and poor social judgement. Unfortunately, pharmacologic interventions work from the model-cure to the disease (give a medication and see the result). This thinking is excessively utilitarian and begs the question of science in the area of the patient: Do anything until it works even if it causes many other effects. "Works" in this case can mean that the caregiver is no longer having to put up with annoying behavior.

As noted above, mental health is a problem in LTC facilities. Smyer, Shea and Streit (1994) reported that fewer than 20% of residents with mental illness received services at any point during their stay; fewer than 5% of these residents received services from psychologists. Standards of practice for psychologists in LTC settings, for example, have been published that delineate state-of-the-art psychological practice (Lichtenberg et al., 2000). They do not include the routine use of medications. But the political forces in Congress are encouraging the continued integrity of the Medicare system with proposed increases in spending in one large area: medications. Even the most recent White House Conference on

Mental Health emphasized biological treatments of mental disorders as the first line of treatment (Saeman, 1992). And, in a recent editorial for the American Association of Geriatric Psychiatrists, the supplication was made that increased medication should be applied to more residents to improve care (Reichman, 2001a). Behavioral health services such as psychotherapy continue to be the stepchild of mental health interventions (Bonder, 1994; Molinari, 2000).

There is one other important cost here: To the extent that the caregiver relies on the medication, to that extent they are out of the equation. This may occur in many ways; being less active with the resident as on a "doctor watch." Under such a watch, behavior is seen as a function of the medication. The person is behaving well because the medication is working; not well, if the medication is not working. The caregiver becomes a handmaiden of the pill bottle. By dint of this they give up the role of active caregiver and settle. If, as we imply, the caregiver is the key environment of the resident, there will be a reduction in care.

Medication is of course necessary for many, perhaps even most, declining residents. Regarding the data on those behaviors where medications show some efficacy, there is an axiom: Behavior management must co-occur. Medication works then in many areas but they always require a caregiver. Jacobo Mintzer (1997) and colleagues note that after a thorough review of the medicaments that subserve dementia, non-pharmacologic interventions constitute the basis for care of this disease.

Newer LTC Models

In recent days something has changed. It has become more apparent that the decline in residents is not inevitable. The environment can make a difference. OBRA (1987) clearly endorsed this idea. The days of custodial care should no longer be present. In fact, OBRA recommended that NAs be trained in behavior principles (American Health Care Association, 1990). In fact, OBRA '87 established a comprehensive training regimen for staff. It also noted that better care involved a lessened emphasis on medications. Conversely, the lack of training in these facilities has been linked to a number of negative characteristics, including overdependence on staff for daily care and poor QL.

Residents had to be better managed, behaviorally and environmentally (Coons & Mace, 1996). It did not mandate specific skill development that would assist in the care of resident problems. Thus, there is more training, not necessarily better training. Frazer (1995) notes that the need for specialized training, especially behavioral skills, is enormous. It may be unclear what direction to take. As Kelly said about psychotherapy, even bad theory may be helpful.

We have more than bad theory for models of care in LTC facilities. Covering all bases, Cohen-Mansfield (2000) noted that behavior can be altered through better medical care, staff training, increased socialization, and decreased stress. In general, however, there are two psychosocial theories that apply to the care of residents. They are the environmental competence press or control framework. Most theories are a combination of both. The former seeks to control the environment; the latter seeks to control the person. In fact, the latter entails the universal imperative achieved by the use of primary mechanisms of change of the immediate environment or secondary one, involving the change of emotions or cognitions.

Many models of care in these settings exist: Beck (1998), Hall and Buckwalter (1987), Lawton (1999), and Ryden (1989), to name a few. In addition, the work of Cameron Camp (2000), Cohen-Mansfield (2000), and Michelle Bourgeois (1991), again among others, have attacked the heart of the problem–the cognitive decline of dementia. They involve the endless and creative pursuit of a heuristic and practical intervention that works. In addition to providing structure, these models do something valuable: They parse apart the environment for the "right" person/environment fit for change using sound, videos, light, touch, social interaction, to name the more assessed ones.

There is also the behavioral model (Teri & Logsdon, 1991). These authors have given us the one technique that has been evaluated and matches mainstream psychological skills, the applied behavioral analysis program. This method applied in a validating environment with a motivated staff seems to have merit.

Quality of Life

> Once you have seen one person with dementia, you have seen one person with dementia.

A major focus of both the academic community and the government in recent years has been quality of life (QL). This issue has over 500 publications in two years. Prior to this period, QL has meant the absence of a bad or undesired outcome. Under such a definition, chemical restraints could be viewed as acceptable. Under such a definition, a risk averse environment was in vogue.

Well-being or QL is an umbrella term of psychological health consti-
tuting an amalgam of various affective, experiential, and cognitive
components that act and interact with one another in complex ways.
They interact with health, social support, positive outlook, and social
and emotional resources. The term is associated with affect, mood,
self-esteem, and autonomy. In the depression literature, for example,
Kennedy (2000) pointed out the importance of QL when there is a remission of depression without a restoration of independence. The disability that is attached to depression is also a central part of change, one
related to QL. Quality of life then applies to all psychiatric maladies and
settings.

The Agency for Health Care Policy assesses heath care services
(Bierman et al., 1998). This agency seeks out what works, for which patients, and at what cost. It also seeks when this happens and from whose
perspective. In short, they look at outcomes. They have made an aggressive effort to link the changing political and market environment for
LTC facilities to the quality of care necessary for well-being. As a
by-product of their efforts, several messages about LTC facilities have
resulted: that the cure model is not apt, that patients do best when involved in decision making, that there are many forms of positive outcomes, and that we need to broaden the definition of outcomes in this
variance-laden population (see Logsdon, 2000). Perhaps most of all, we
know that mental health needs are modal in these settings, that this issue
requires attention for the overall care of residents, that the (mental
health) needs are special, and that good care is grossly wanting
(Lombardo et al., 1995). It is clear too that LTC facilities require different outcomes than drug trials. In fact, this tests both the researcher and
health care provider to be both scientific and curative.

Unfortunately, we do not yet know with any certainty what constitutes the best care at what cost for what residents. We do not yet know
how to match residents with good care. When there is much variation,
simplicity ascends, often masking real issues. And in LTC facilities,
there is variance: people who seek rehabilitation or active recuperation,
people with chronic disabilities (those who will decline), those with primarily cognitive impairment, those in vegetative states, and those who
are terminal. Quality of life differs among these groups.

In fairness, this whole evaluation/monitoring process is a burden for
all. The surveyor of the LTC facility has the burden of recognizing and
documenting clear infractions based on the "regulations." The result is
that criteria emphasize concrete aspects of care, such as dirt, safety haz-
ards, and documentation in the medical record. To avoid the horror of

sanction, the LTC facility must meet these standards. They are encouraged for little else beyond the minimum (Lawton, 1999). Eloquently, Penrod, Kane, and Kane (2000) note the state is unforgiving, creating a risk-averse environment: the desire for the perfect is driving out the good. It may even be that innovations do not correspond to the surveyors criteria and penalties are given.

In defense of HFCA, QL is now a priority (Lawton, 1999). Aspects of QL have been extended to include psychological and social aspects of care. The relevance of these features in the environment is now on the radar screen. But criteria are not ready, any review is not standardized, and the methods of evaluation far from fair.

From the macro-perspective of the Resident Assessment Instrument and Minimum Data Set (MDS), Hawes, Phillips and colleagues (Fries, Hawes, Morris, & Phillips, 1997; Phillips & Hawes, 1992; Phillips, Chu, Morris, & Hawes, 1993; Phillips, Morris, Hawes, & Fries, 1997; Phillips & Sloane et al., 1997) investigated the relationship between the degree and type of regulation and QL. In a series of articles they concluded that something positive seems to be happening in LTC facilities. It involves an increased attentiveness on the part of the LTC facility to resident care. In general, these authors suggest that improvements have been found in the completeness and comprehensiveness of care plans, dehydration and stasis ulcers have a significantly lower prevalence rate, and hospital rates have declined. At some risk of simplification they suggest that comprehensiveness and accuracy of the MDS are associated with a wide array of outcomes that reflect better quality of care. This involves "direct problems" (e.g., bedsores) and "indirect problems" (e.g., family involvement). In addition, the accuracy of the data is better and there is some evidence that staff is increasingly accepting and appreciating this instrument. To date, however, the MDS has not been integrated well into care.

This group also found that regulation was indeed associated with better QL in a number of areas. Licensure alone was found to be effective at ensuring that LTC facilities provided care at or above the threshold of minimum performance. These areas included social aids, safety, and supportive features. Unfortunately, regulation was found to have no effect on other aspects of QL. These included staff training, staff knowledge in any number of areas, availability of licensed nurses, and cleanliness and attractiveness of homes. Faulk (1988) also assessed this issue. He evaluated 124 residents in Pennsylvania on QL. Results showed that, if only minimum QL was met, there were no gains in QL. Better QL occurs when social integration needs were fostered. The bottom line appears to be that autonomy and control are highly valued by residents.

There is also the problem of a "dilemma of dependency," excess disability as applied to an LTC facility. Despite the value of autonomy, many residents have basic needs that require assistance and these are compounded with excess help. Agich (1993) noted that lack of control results because of the need for assistance from others. Dowd (1975) also pointed out that power is lost relative to those who provide the service. Baldwin and colleagues (1993) noted that most LTC facilities have policies for the fostering of autonomy AND have policies that restrict the implementation of this value, such as limits on staff time.

From a research perspective, efforts are made to parse apart the construct QL. It is considered a multidimensional concept encompassing social, psychological, and physical domains. Perkins, Morton, and Ball (1997) found the QL encompassed 14 domains. Brod, Stewart, Sands, and Walton (1999) have also offered several areas for measurement of QL. These include self-esteem (thoughts and feelings about themselves), positive affect/humor (frequency of being cheerful, hopeful), negative affect (frequency felt afraid, lonely), feelings of belonging (frequency felt useful), and sense of aesthetics (extent pleasure obtained from sensory awareness, appreciation of beauty). Stewart and King (1994) even indicated that the central features of QL are agreed to: physical functioning, self-maintenance and self-care, usual activities, social functioning, sexual functioning, psychological well-being and distress, cognitive functioning, pain and discomfort, energy and fatigue, sleep, self-esteem, sense of mastery and control, perceived health, and satisfaction. It is important too that the ultimate test of QL comes from the persons most involved, the residents. And, it appears that increasingly there is an effort to assess QL from the perspective of the resident (Logsdon, 2000).

To assist in this debate Lawton (1999) identified six caveats in the measurement of QL. They include:

1. Documentation indicators of quality: If QL is limited to what is measurable, then we are impoverished.
2. Incorrect citations have a cost: Surveyors must be trained in new concepts if QL is to be represented in a broader fashion.
3. The absence of an obvious ultimate validity criterion: Typically we are rating "hard stuff"–death rates, morbidity rate, etc. Many of the criteria for QL are process criteria.

4. By whose perspective is QL to be judged?: If the emphases are on the consumer (the resident), there will be problems, as only a few will rate the condition; if only the environment is evaluated, we also miss something.
5. Representing both positive and negative QL: Most survey is centered around identifying the negative–deficits, risks. The opposite is the essence of QL.
6. Does QL vary by user group? Residents in LTC facilities are not all alike. The existence of a special unit in an LTC facility is evidence of this.

They appear to capture many of the problems of this debate at the research level. To this, Kane (1998) suggested the need for a taxonomy and a clearer identification of the key components (of QL). He suggests to:

1. Identify the basic taxonomy of patient groups in LTC facilities in order to develop outcomes for each group.
2. Identify multiple outcome clusters including physiological, functional, affect, cognitive, and psychosocial factors.
3. Identify appropriate institutional activities to achieve these outcomes.
4. Implement a CQM plan to identify meaningful problems at the level of the individual nursing home beyond that noted by the MDS. (This plan would incentivize local facilities to identify important problems and not just address those that are easiest to fix.)

Quality of life also depends on the goodness of fit between a person's unique needs and the ability of the facility to meet these. In this way, QL is interactive. Post (2000) says that the QL of a dementing person is entirely conditioned by that of his or her caregivers. It makes little sense (the argument goes) to focus on the concept without a caregiver. Zgola (1999) too notes that caregivers can perform the task much better by the relationship. In fact, this is the centerpiece, without it there is no good environment: QL is dialogical and reasonably fulfilling for the caregiver. Logsdon (2000) also has discussed these issues and provides a measure of care.

People are treated at the micro-level. Behavior in decline is not random. A person reacts because there is something awry in the physiology, safety, love or belonging, or self-actualization. In an LTC facility, Camp (2000) notes that QL is most driven by activity. This can be determined by the focus on the resident, the interests of the resident. Vygotsky (1997) noted that people have a "zone of proximal development." It is here that the work of change can occur. The more windows that are open to the resident, the better the QL. In this regard, positive behaviors are not shadows of the negative behavior. Good can occur then, just when bad things are not present.

Perhaps we need two forms for QL, one for the cognitively intact and one for those who do not have this. If so, it would include the input of the person. But the axioms of care that apply to normals apply also to one who is dementing. All people, dementing or not, are afraid of rejection, want acceptance, want their self-esteem nurtured, want to talk about themselves, can be petty, wear a social mask, and have unique values, beliefs, learnings, and lives. Zarit, Dolan, and Leitsch (1998) remind us that the real task in the care of a resident in an LTC facility is one that builds on the competencies of the resident with a supportive, yet challenging, environment that maximizes the potential for prolonged functioning. In fact, the effort to affect change in a dementing person can be as important as altering the course of the illness. Again, Camp (2000) notes that the LTC facility has the person for the rest of their life.

NECESSARY INGREDIENTS OF CARE

We now discuss necessary conditions for a transformation of care in LTC facilities. We break these down according to the resident, the caregiver, and the system.

Resident

> Deprivation of sight or hearing, partial paralysis of muscles, loss of limbs, even the conceptual blindness that is agnosia–all misfortunes, however disabling, still allow us to live on the distinctly human plane . . . but deprived of our intellectual minds, we are deprived of our humanity.

–Mortimer Adler

There are two issues addressed. First, we discuss a model of care, the stage model provided by Williams, Wood, Moorleghen, and Chittuluru (1995). It provides a way to see the problem from its simplest purview. Second concerns a psycho-philosophy, a necessary understanding for change. This second issue also involves the issue of insight as applied to a declining person.

Stage Model of Care

What must the caregiver do when there is a problem? Williams et al. (1995) identified a practical decision-making model for care to reduce chemical and physical restraints. It includes optimal stimulation, problem ownership, stimulus control, and applied analysis of behaviors. The caregiver assesses whether there is proper stimulation, whose problem is involved, and what stimulus control is necessary for alteration. If these choice points fail the situation, the ABC model is applied (see below). This model has been widely promulgated and is used here because it allows the caregiver to simply and realistically appreciate the condition of the resident. One can proceed with clarity.

Psycho-philosophy

The caregiver who knows that the person with whom they are working is still a person does better on all care indices. Several positions have been helpful. These are given in Table 3. In essence, the caregiver is taught that there is a real person that is being cared for. The "unbecoming" of the person is not random and can be altered and assisted.

It is recommended that a psycho-philosophy of dementia be developed. In a recent book on dementia Castleman, Gallagher-Thompson, and Naythons (1999) argue that *There Is Still a Person in There.* Duffy (1999) and Feil (1999) also advocate for the importance of affective-oriented strategies as these apply to a debilitated population where cognitive strategies do not. It is most unlikely that in the course of dementia there is someone in there locked in with lots of thoughts and feelings. It is much more likely that things are vacant and barren. The world has a sequence of meaningless sights and smells, partly experienced consciously and partly unknown. As the person disintegrates, there is probably little coherence in the feeling and no understanding. The person will feel the humiliation of their lost position; the lost something or other, then it goes. It is jumbled, only to return in an unconnected way during the next frustration. That is never far.

Insight and Personality

Insight and personality are key indicators of the new psycho-philosophy. For starters, we know that estimates of dementia in an LTC facility reach 80% (Sunderland & Silver, 1988). We know further that psychiatric symptoms increase across the dementing disorder (Finkel & McGue, 1998; Mega, Cummings, Fiorello, & Gornbein, 1996), causing more prob-

TABLE 3. Caregiver Philosophy and Perspectives

1. Very little is known about the experience of a dementing person. Some seem fully aware, some are partially aware, some are aware in moments, and some are not aware at all.

2. The dementing person needs ANOTHER to have personhood continue. The dementing person requires an environment for being a person. The further the dementia process, the more the need for person work. The environmental docility hypothesis.

3. The belief that a caregiver takes is most relevant. As the person "unbecomes," each is the pure victim of the medical disease. The medical view is that one can do nothing. OR, a position can be accepted that the medical condition is part of the process. The former holds that "there is nothing one can do." The latter says that many problems are the result of reactions to the disease process. Problems are the direct result of feeling lost; problems exist because others cannot enter into their world. People they do not know call them names, expect things from them, and otherwise exceed their capacities.

4. There may be ways of rediscovering identity and even enjoying the decline. The latter position may be an act of faith; the idea that the person can be sustained only by having an "us" makes a difference.

5. People are individuals and lumping is not good. Dementia just establishes the disease. Perhaps a hospice model of 5 or so people caring and being responsible for the person makes the most sense.

6. Communication with a dementia patient can be considered like a tennis match where the goal is to keep the ball going. What is the person actually saying at any given time? Fostering empowerment involves being a good observer, waiting for the right path to open up, and for the right response.

7. "Violence is the voice of the unheard." Behavior problems are adaptive attempts of the person to avoid a confrontation with the reality of the condition and its limits. What does the behavior mean? It may be a valid response to the phenomenological world. It comes from fear or frustration.

8. Value of the life story–The photo album of the person. This is the narrative, the who-they-are of the person. The process alone is important; so is the information. Do not be concerned about narrative truth.

9. Zen of the non-response–When are the caregivers most themselves? They can become quiet and pursue meaning within, not out there with relentless energy. When you know someone, you know their way, pace, rhythm, parameters and objectives.

10. There is always a battle between the desire to keep safe and to let go on their own.

lems. Insight is a problem in this population. Awareness of cognitive decline has become an important topic in the understanding of dementia. There are gradations of awareness. Very little has been done on the experience of a dementing person. Cohen, Kennedy and Eisdorfer (1984) hold that the dementing person goes through several stages: recognition and concern, denial, anger or sadness, maturation and departure from self. Recently, too, there is interest in people who are in the early stages of a dementia as they have awareness (Kennedy, 2000).

The technical term for loss of awareness is anosognosia. Several studies show an underestimation of the abilities by the dementing patient as compared to caregivers or actual performance (see Finkel,

1998). But there are problems here. Full anosognosia in a dementing patient accounts for about 15-25% of the cases (Reed, Jagust, & Coulter, 1993). Findings are also available showing no correlation between severity and anosognosia (Ott, Tate, Gordon, & Heindel, 1996). Few studies have evaluated factors that may affect the validity of self-reports of demented individuals. Cross informant consistency often depends on how the question is phrased. Clearly this has to do with stages of change, as well as elements specific to the dementing process (e.g., declarative versus procedural memory).

Awareness is not a global measure. Awareness is also an emergent function of brain changes. In one area, emotions, awareness is preserved relative to cognitive states. Feeling states do not require an awareness of loss, a memory of one's previous functioning, awareness of current functioning, or the ability to compare the two. Feeling states only demand that the person be aware of the moment. And, dementing persons appear to be aware of their emotions (Kennedy, 2000).

There is a question too as to whether this denial is "real" (an underlying brain disorder) or a defense. Prignatano (2001) believes that the failure of the person to appreciate the problems of cognition is the result of deficits in the heteromodal regions of the brain. The anterior regions of the brain influence thinking and feeling and have multiple connections to the limbic system. Improvement is marked by changes in both cognitive and affective areas. In this review, personality influences not only the symptom picture but also the degree of social integration. Personality influences the accommodation to the disease. Dependent people might become scared and feel totally abandoned; independent people deny and become more assertive and fear loss of control. According to Prignatano, focusing only on the cognitive side of things is a mistake. The focus needs to be on both what is learned and how learning takes place. The practice of neuropsychology and psychotherapy is important here.

We are, of course, addressing rehabilitation medicine. Over 75 years ago Shepherd Ivory Franz made a number of observations of relevance today regarding rehabilitation: each retraining effort must be individualized to the patient's cognitive impairments and personality (see Prignatano, 2001). Goldstein and colleagues (1997) especially noted that patients differ on the way they are affected by the struggle to adapt to the cognitive deficit (e.g., irritability), as well as by the tendency to avoid the struggle (isolation). It is also true that cognitive retraining improves the social integration of brain injured patients (Diller & Ben-Yishay, 1988).

Now it is evident that cognitive retraining improves neural reorganization.

In clinical application models, outcomes consistently demonstrate that the resident's cognitive and functional capabilities exist where not previously observed. The Clues Method (see Finkel, 1998) is one example. This is a system of clinical interventions applied to potentiate client capacities. Clients are seen as individuals: if you have visuo-spatial memory problems early, this becomes the area of problems later; if verbal, then verbal issues are at risk later. They are also seen as people where interventions can make a difference, despite frailty. Recently, Camp and colleagues had applied several techniques that address memory (spaced retrieval) (Brush & Camp, 1998), activity (Montessori methods) (Camp, 1999), and quality of life in severely demented patients to good effect.

It is argued then that rehabilitation can occur in an LTC facility, even with dementing residents. It is a whole person response. The rehabilitation of patients with higher cerebral dysfunctions caused by various brain regions requires that both cognitive and personality disturbances be addressed. Without studying the interaction of personality and cognitive disturbances as they emerge in patients at various stages after a brain problem, only a partial view of how the brain problem affects behavior is obtained.

Finally, we note one more thing. There is evidence that dementing patients do benefit from meaningful cognitive intervention (psychotherapy). Norberg (1996) showed that a dementing patient participating in meaningful cognitive intervention conversed at a higher level than those who were passive. Beck, Heacock, Mercer, Thatcher and Sparkman (1988) involved dementing patients in a cognitive training program based on the Thinking Skills Workbook. These subjects showed significantly more improvement in memory than a group of control subjects. Abraham, Neundorfer and Currie (1992) noted that cognitive nursing interventions, such as CBT group therapy and focused visual imagery group therapy, showed significant and lasting improvements in overall cognitive status in LTC facility residents with a slight to moderate cognitive impairment when compared with a comparison intervention of a discussion group. Hyer and Sohnle (2001) identified over 30 studies where the population was cognitively impaired.

Regarding the training, the following scale (Figure 1) was used. This is a model that addresses all the areas discussed relative to the resident. Caregivers can apply this measure. The level of cognitive status, degree of insight, capacity to inhibit problem behaviors (executive function), social skills, and type of personality constitute sufficient information for intervention. Residents are rated in each area. Caregivers can apply as needed. Over time, caregivers can develop their own cases to fit different types of residents, those high and low in the five categories and apply care accordingly.

Caregiver

> People with a high level of mastery live in a continual learning mode. They never arrive.
>
> –Senge

In addition to a psycho-philosophy, caregivers in an LTC facility require tending and information. An intervention that is multifactorial takes into account as many factors as possible that could impact on the QL. These include: emotional state, attitudes or beliefs (self-efficacy, control, etc.), social context, sensory-perceptual processing, and physiological state. Given these considerations, tasks like videotapes, computers, among others, become applicable. Most importantly is an approach that addresses the problem in a judicious and deliberative way. These are the technologies that involve "selective optimization with compensation" in a more programmed way. As noted above too, caregivers are confronted with the dual sword of excess overresponse (excess disability) or underresponse (Bortz & O'Brien, 1997). The central issue is what is necessary for the just right response.

We address two issues. One is a built-in template that applies to all caregiving equations, the placebo; the other involves necessary conditions for this to occur.

Power of the Caregiver

> It does help to believe in what you are doing.
>
> –Powell Lawton

FIGURE 1. Dementia Features

Cognitive Status	Mild	Moderate
Insight	Yes	No
Executive Function	Good	Poor
Social Skills	Good	Poor
Interpersonal Set	Independent	Dependent

For a drug to pass the FDA approval process it must be superior to placebo. This is 30%, or in psychiatry 40%, of the effect. The placebo response occurs when the patient receives messages from the environment that empower expectations and hope. These messages work in some fashion to alter the meaning of our state of health or illness. In effect, the body activates a pharmacy within. In fact, it can be argued that every time one person treats another with some substance/act, the person receives a message from the environment that triggers a placebo response. It is often in the early stages of an intervention that the caregiver (the placebo) communicates the message: the recipient knows that they are reacting better which reinforces later changes.

The key to the active placebo is that the caregiver believes in what they are doing, feels that they have an effective response array for care, and communicates this to the resident. What then potentiates the placebo? It involves the system support, personal confidence, a multifactorial armamentarium of care. The caregiver functions as an active treatment or placebo enhancer. The effect occurs in all caregiving and is most evident in a setting where a positive expectancy unfolds naturally. It works as a two-way street. The caregiver believes in themselves and in their work: the resident believes that the intervention is effective. In fact, if the caregiver believes in the effect, it is more likely to occur. We believe that the caregiver is a powerful force in the care of residents and can use their position for this purpose.

There is also the nocebo. This is the set of conditions that results from a sense of frustration and helplessness. How often have studies on this group of caregivers suggested this as a condition without using this term?

Information

An ideal for training is to provide the caregiver with just enough theory, information and training in a short period for a motivated application of care. As such, we teach only the basics of dementia, depression, and memory. From this we apply tasks that emphasize job satisfaction and simplicity.

In a general way, we believe that a kind of rehabilitation occurs, both restorative and compensatory (Hill, Backman, & Stigsdotter-Neely, 2000). Wilson et al. (1994) note that cognitive rehabilitation refers primarily to a process by which professionals work together with a client to optimize a client's level of functioning by alleviating, remediating, or circumventing deficits. Camp and colleagues (Camp, Koss, & Judge,

1999; Sterns & Camp, 1998) have argued for the use of cognitive rehabilitation for dementia patients.

Table 4 provides a summary of the research on what seems to be effective in the training of caregivers in an LTC facility. From here, we
proceed with the training. The core of our training modules is the ABC
model and the tenets of learning theory. This is the touchstone of all the
other learnings because it draws its power from simplicity, data, and
consistency.

We do not discuss here the "just sufficient" theory and content of dementia, depression, and memory (Table 1). In each, we apply a module
of a half-hour of didactics. For dementia we emphasize the behavioral
signs and symptoms ranging from forgetting to total care. The person
knows that this is a brain disorder. For residents who are agitated and
have problems due to dementia we teach a simple form of Montessori
(Camp, 1999). For depression we emphasize a brief assessment and
monitoring (MDS-driven), and two interventions, active listening and
positive activities. For memory, we use spaced retrieval (Brush &
Camp, 1998). The emphasis in each area is for simplicity, the use of 1-3
principles to be placed in a "toolbox" for care interventions.

Here, we address two issues on information.

Learning Model

The laws of learning allow for a further explication of the caregiver
dilemma. Use of standard learning models has also been applied and
found useful (Teri et al., 2000; Wertheimer et al., 1992). The work of
Teri and colleagues is noteworthy. The Seattle Protocol for Behavioral
Treatment of Depressed Patients is an example of how traditional therapies can be adapted for the dementia population (Teri, 1986; Teri &
Umoto, 1991). This is based on learning theory with the intent of identifying experiences which are enjoyable and increasing involvement. It is
educational and the focus is on maintenance of gains. The caregiver's
role is expanded as time passes.

Table 5 represents the core topics. We have expanded on the work of
Wertheimer et al. and Teri et al. to involve a broader view of rewards.
These are the basics of care that all caregivers should be familiar with
for good care.

Caregiver Supports

There are several relevant components of care. They involve the necessary information on the treatment of declining people. Caregivers

TABLE 4. Summary of Efficacy on Training

Does training work?
>   It works but only for a short time.
>   And, only in the area that was focused on.
>   There is a lack of generalization.

But,
>   Training is mandatory.
>   And, rehabilitation can occur.

Also,
>   Considered, sustained education seems to
>   positively affect morale and staff attitudes,
>   carer-resident communication, as well as
>   reduced psychotropic medication and restraint.

And finally,
>   No two caregivers are the same.
>   They require support especially under stress.
>   Teams work best especially with local control and
>   freedom to fail.

make a difference when certain conditions are present. These conditions are culled from several sources and suggest that the caregiver can act best when trained and comfortable in their role. They are in Table 6.

We provide a perspective on care in an LTC facility. Problems of course occur when the interaction calls for the resident to do something. Mostly this includes: toileting, dressing, transfer, turning, hygiene, or grooming. To this, Finkel (1998) identified resident factors associated with caregiver burden:

1. mild includes delusions and disruptive behaviors;
2. moderate includes severity of dementia, functional status, and cognitive status;
3. doubtful is type of dementia and duration of dementia.

Most pointedly, Reichman (2001a) added five factors that lead to resident problems: caregiver's behavior, behavior of other patients, overstimulation or understimulation of environment, and a lack of structure or cues.

With this as backdrop information we identify the caregiver behaviors that are often responsible for problems. These behaviors include: creating sudden or unexpected changes in the environment, instigating

TABLE 5. Summary of Reward Concerns

Laws of "Reward"
Reward good behavior
Do not reward bad behavior
Be tough on some bad behavior

Common Errors
Do not acknowledge good behavior
Punish good behavior
Reward negative behavior
Let real bad behavior go
Are not specific and clear

ABCs
Antecedents
Behaviors
Consequences

TABLE 6. Summary of Caregiver Supports

Feeling of support
No time pressure
Being trained
Ability to get help
Feeling confident
Feeling that one can fail
Rewards can be external or internal
    (value-based reward)

power struggles, placing excessive demands on the resident, being excessively critical, ignoring needs of the resident, being excessively controlling, repeated prompting or repeating resident, and being angry or irritable. This area is so important that Burgio and colleagues (Burgio & Stevens, 1999) apply a stress communication intervention that is used on-the-job with behavior forms and supervision.

Of course, care is in the hands of the most immediate caregiver. This is most often nursing personnel. They do the work of care in the LTC facility. This person is the central person in the care equation. They must be the principal actors and the ones motivated and trained. The tasks performed must have merit to the residents in and of themselves and attempt to lead somewhere, to better QL or behavior.

System

> . . . a culture becomes more caring and humane the more its citizens feel themselves to be a part of the problem that besets their lives. The only way to bring them close to such problems is to structure a culture where they deal with the problems at a person level.

–Gazzagana (1985, p. 198)

Care in an LTC facility is doable only if it is mandated, part of the routine, reimbursable, and effective (Camp, 2000). In effect, the system becomes the "body" under the direction of the "mind" of the caregiver. This program involves a commitment for care that has the support of the system. In the context of our model we advocate for conditions in Table 7.

In the service of the administration being on-board and committed to the task, there must be rewards for the staff. Training of behavioral principles must not only be taught but appreciated and seen as the method for change. Gains should be restricted to those tasks that are the focus of the program. The intervention must be targeted to the goal. Training must also "persevere" to be effective, especially with older people. This seems logical but is painfully underrepresented in programs.

Training then involves the interaction among the person, task, and technique. This is done judiciously over time with a human touch.

TABLE 7. Summary of Conditions for System Change

Care must be reimbursed.

Care must be supported.

Care must be effective and be subject to measurement.

Care must fit within the health care system.

There must be a multifactorial approach.

Training must be sustained.

Training is the interaction of person, technique and situation.

System must listen to staff and make changes.

Behavioral principles need to be used and monitored.

Camp (2000) notes that the key idea is to create linkages with staff and telescope the task for other purposes. This is restorative nursing. The learning methods are low tech, involving careful analysis, application and persistence. They may not always work, as time spent with the resident to have her brush her teeth may never reach completion. In time, effort may lead to self-initiated and better oral care but also other ADL involvement. It is the application of the behavioral principles to the task that matters. They are the "frontal lobes," if you will, of the declining patient. In the long run effective interventions involve science and human engineering, an infrastructure to handle this, and best practice standards.

CONCLUSION

We have argued that the caregiver is the key element of treatment in an LTC facility. We believe that for success this position needs to be made part of the system. For this to work, the caregiver requires much. In addition to feeling empowered, the caregiver needs training that is technologically apt, simple to use, rewarded, and ongoing. There must also be a sense of "team." Good training is the key to change. Whatever the exact model of training used, then, it should incorporate the elements identified here.

LTC facilities are hard places to be and to thrive. Camp calls this undertaking a "guerilla war." We have, however, specified reasons for optimism and change. We articulated a training process that emphasizes a psycho-philosophy that includes an understanding of our care ideas and training plan.

From the literature we know too that the care of a debilitating person who is dementing is part science and part art. There are, of course, differences in how care can apply to any LTC setting. There is agreement also. Addressing the American Association of Geriatric Psychiatrists, the president Reichman (2001b) noted that the primary goals of treatment for patients with AD are to improve quality of life and to maximize functional performance by enhancing cognition, mood, and behavior. The old way is through the one dimensional tool of medication; the new way is through the applied analysis of behavior as practiced by an informed and rewarded caregiver.

Chaos theory holds that life is essentially uncertain and without order. It is only when we step back from it that we can make sense of it. And so we devise guidelines or best practices. Currently, this (better) thinking about LTC facilities is evolving from a discussion on QL. We now know that the outcomes for a nursing home are different from those of a clinical trial.

That said, outcome studies need to be done. As an area we are distinctly overregulated and understudied. Bird (2000) noted :

> The overall conclusion is that the top-down approach that has driven the quest for a generalized drug or cognitive treatment needs to be supplemented by an equal or larger amount of effort that chips away at the clinical level. Much more research is required that focuses not on delaying or reversing the dementing process, but on methods for ameliorating the everyday behavioral and affective consequences of progressive cognitive loss. . . . Until this happens, psychosocial work on dementia at the clinical level will be based on unsupported assertion. (p. 264)

We end with the optimistic sense that we are converging to a point where key people in this area now believe that restorative change can occur for many, that the caregiver is the only game in town, and that quality indicators are in current discussion. We need this. After all, as Camp noted, "We have the resident for the rest of their life."

REFERENCES

Abraham, I. L., Neundorfer, M. M., & Currie, L. J. (1992). Effects of group interventions on cognition and depression in nursing home residents. *Nursing Research, 41*(4), 196-202.

Agich, G. (1993). *Autonomy and long-term care.* New York: Oxford University Press.

American Health Care Association (1990). The long-term care survey: Regulations, forms, procedures, guidelines. (Pub. no. 4697/UBP/2.5K/7/90.) Washington, DC: Author.

Austrom, M. G. (1996). Training staff to work in special care. In S. B. Hoffman & M. Kaplan (Eds.), *Special care programs for people with dementia* (pp. 17-35). Baltimore: Health Professions.

Austrom, M. G., Class, C. A., & Unverzagt, F. W. (1997, November). Life satisfaction, depression, and job satisfaction in long term care staff. Paper presented at the Annual Meeting of the Gerontological Society of America, Cincinnati, OH.

Baillon, S., Scothern, G., Neville, P. G., & Boyle, A. (1996). Factors that contribute to stress in care staff in residential homes for the elderly. *International Journal of Geriatric Psychiatry, 11*, 219-226.

Baldwin, N., Harris, J., Littlechild, R., & Pearson, M. (1993). *Residents' rights: A strategy in action for older people.* Aldershot, England: Avebury.

Baltes, M. M., Kindermann, T., Reisenzein, R., & Schmid, U. (1987). Further observational data on the behavioral and social work of institutions for the aged. *Psychology and Aging, 2,* 390-403.

Baltes, M. M., Neumann, E. M., & Zank, S. (1994). Maintenance and rehabilitation of independence in old age: An intervention program for staff. *Psychology and Aging, 9,* 179-188.

Baltes, M. M., & Wahl, H. W. (1991). The behavior system of dependency in the elderly: Interaction with the social environment. In M. Ory, R. P. Ables, & P. D. Lipman (Eds.), *Aging, health, and behavior* (pp. 83-106). Beverly Hills, CA: Sage.

Bates-Smith, K., & Tsukuda, R. A. (1984). Problems of an interdisciplinary training team. *Clinical Gerontologist, 2*(3), 66-68.

Beck, C. (1998). Psychosocial and behavioral interventions for Alzheimer's disease patients and their families. *American Journal of Geriatric Psychiatry, 6,* S41-S48.

Beck, C., Heacock, P., Mercer, S., Thatcher, R. N., & Sparkman, C. (1988). The impact of cognitive skills retraining on persons with Alzheimer's disease or mixed dementia. *Journal of Geriatric Psychiatry, 21,* 73-88.

Becker, G., & Kaufman, S. (1988). Old age, rehabilitation, and research: A review of the issues. *The Gerontologist, 28*(4), 459-468.

Bierman, A. S., Magari, E. S., Jette, A. M., Splaine, M., & Wasson, J. H. (1998). Assessing access as a first step toward improving the quality of care for very old adults. *Journal of Ambulatory Care Management, 21*(3), 17-26.

Bird, M. (2000). Psychosocial rehabilitation for problems arising from cognitive deficits in dementia. In R. D. Hill, L. Backman, A. & Stigsdotter Neely (Eds.), *Cognitive rehabilitation in old age* (pp. 249-269). New York: Oxford University Press.

Bonder, B. R. (1994). Psychotherapy for individuals with Alzheimer's disease. *Alzheimer's Disease and Related Disorders, 8*(3), 75-81.

Borson, S., Reichman, W. E., Coyne, A. C., Rovner, B., & Sakauye, K. (2000). Effectiveness of nursing home staff as managers of disruptive behavior: Perceptions of nursing directors. *American Journal of Geriatric Psychiatry, 8*(3), 251-253.

Bortz, J. J., & O'Brien, K. P. (1997). Psychotherapy with older adults: Theoretical issues, empirical findings, and clinical applications. In P. D. Nussbaum. *Handbook of neuropsychology and aging: Critical issues in neuropsychology* (pp. 431-451). New York: Plenum Press.

Bourgeois, M. S. (1991). Communication treatment for adults with dementia. *Journal of Speech and Hearing Research, 34,* 831-844.

Bourgeois, M., Beach, S., Schultz, R., & Burgio, L. (1996). When primary and secondary caregivers disagree: Predictors and psychosocial consequences. *Psychology and Aging, 11*(3), 527-537.

Bourgeois, M., Burgio, L., & Schultz, R. (1992, May). *Interventions to change caregiver and Alzheimer's patient outcomes.* Paper presented at the Association for Behavioral Analysis Conference. Alanta, GA.

Bourgeois, M., Burgio, L., Schultz, R., Beach, S., & Palmer, B. (1997). Modifying repetitive verbalizations of community-dwelling patients with AD. *The Gerontologist, 37*(1), 30-39.

Brod, M., Stewart, A. L., Sands, L., & Walton, P. (1999). Conceptualization and measurement of quality of life in dementia: The Dementia Quality of Life Instrument (DQoL). *The Gerontologist, 39*(1), 25-35.

Brodaty, H., & Gresham, M. (1992). Prescribing residential respite care for dementia: Effects, side-effects, indications and dosage. *International Journal of Geriatric Psychiatry, 7*(5), 357-362.

Brown, H. N., & Zinberg, N. E. (1982). Difficulties in the integration of psychological and medical practices. *American Journal of Psychiatry, 139*(12), 1576-1580.

Brush, J. A., & Camp, C. J. (1998). *A therapy technique for improving memory: Spaced retrieval.* Cleveland, OH: Menorah Park Center for Senior Living.

Burgio, L., Allen-Burge, R., Roth, D., Bourgeois, M., Dijkstra, K., Gerstle, E., & Bankester, L. (2001). Come talk with me: Improving communication between nursing assistants and nursing home residents during care routines. *The Gerontologist, 41*, 449-460.

Burgio, L. D., & Burgio, K. L. (1986). Behavioral gerontology: Application of behavioral methods to the problems of older adults. *Journal of Applied Behavior Analysis, 19*, 321-328.

Burgio, L. D., Engel, B. T., Hawkins, A., McCormick, L., & Scheve, A. (1990). Descriptive analysis of nursing staff behaviors in a teaching nursing home: Differences among NAs, LPNs, and RNs. *The Gerontologist, 30*, 107-112.

Burgio, L. D., & Stevens, A. B. (1999). Behavioral interventions in the nursing home: Motivating staff to apply a therapeutic model of care. In R. Schulz, G. Maddox, & M. P. Lawton (Eds.), *Annual review of gerontology and geriatrics*, Volume 18. New York: Springer Publishing.

Camp, C. (1999). *Montessori-based activities for persons with dementia.* Cleveland, OH: Menorah Park Center for Senior Living.

Camp, C. J. (2000). Clinical research in long term care: What the future holds. In V. Molinari (Ed.), *Professional psychology in long term care: A comprehensive guide* (pp. 401-423). New York: Hatherleigh Press.

Camp, C. J., Koss, E., & Judge, K. S. (1999). Cognitive assessment in late-stage dementia. In Peter A. Lichtenberg (Ed.), *Handbook of assessment in clinical gerontology. Wiley series on adulthood and aging* (pp. 442-467). New York: John Wiley & Sons, Inc.

Castleman, M., Gallagher-Thompson, D., & Naythons, M. (1999). *There's still a person in there: The complete guide to treating and coping with Alzheimer's.* New York: Putnam.

Chartock, P., Nevins, A., Rzetelny, H., & Gilberto, P. (1988). A mental health training program in nursing homes. *The Gerontologist, 28*(4), 503-507.

Cohen, D., Kennedy, G., & Eisdorfer, C. (1984). Phases of change in the patient with Alzheimer's dementia: A conceptual dimension for defining health care management. *Journal of the American Geriatrics Society, 32*(1), 11-15.

Cohen-Mansfield, J. (2000). Use of patient characteristics to determine nonpharmacologic interventions for behavioral and psychological symptoms of dementia. *International Psychogeriatrics, 12*(1), 373-380.

Cohn, M. D., Horgas, A. L., & Marsiske, M. (1990). Behavior management training for nurses aides: Is it effective? *Journal of Gerontological Nursing, 16*, 21-25.

Colenda, C. C., Streim, J., Greene, J. A., Meyers, N., Beckwith, E., & Rabins, P. (1999). The impact of OBRA '87 on psychiatric services in nursing homes: Joint testimony of The American Psychiatric Association and The American Association for Geriatric Psychiatry. *American Journal of Geriatric Psychiatry, 7*(1), 12-17.

Coons, D. H., Mace, N. L., Whyte, T., & Boling, K. (1996). *Quality of life in long-term care.* New York: Haworth.

Costa, P. T., & McCrae, R. R. (1988). Personality in adulthood: A six-year longitudinal study of self-reports and spouse ratings on the NEO personality inventory. *Journal of Personality and Social Psychology, 54,* 853-863.

Daniels, A. C. (1994). *Bringing out the best in people: How to apply the astonishing power of positive reinforcement.* New York: McGraw Hill.

del Bueno, D. J., Barker, F., & Christmyer, C. (1981). Implementing a competency-based orientation program. *Journal of Nursing Administration, 11,* 24-29.

de Santis Feltran, R. C. (1983). A study on the predictive validity of the DAT battery of specific aptitude tests. *Arquivos Brasileiros de Psicologia, 35*(1), 100-112.

Deming, W. E. (1986). *Out of crisis.* Cambridge, MA: MIT Press.

Diller, L., & Ben-Yishay, Y. (1987). Outcomes and evidence in neuropsychological rehabilitation in closed head injury. In H. S. Levin, & J. Grafman (Eds.), *Neurobehavioral recovery from head injury* (pp. 146-165). New York: Oxford University Press.

Dowd, J. (1975). Aging as exchange: A preface to theory. *Journal of Gerontology, 30,* 584-594.

Duffy, Michael (Ed.). (1999). *Handbook of counseling and psychotherapy with older adults.* New York: John Wiley & Sons, Inc.

Dupree, L. W., & Schonfield, L. (1998). Behavioral approaches with older adults. In M. Hersen, & V. Van Hasselt (Eds.) *Handbook of clinical geropsychology* (pp. 51-70). New York: Plenum.

Edberg, A. K., Hallberg, I. R., & Gustafson, L. (1996). Effects of clinical supervision on nurse-patient cooperation quality. *Clinical Nursing Research, 5,* 127-149.

Edberg, A. K., Nordmark Sandgreen, A., & Hallberg, I. R. (1995). Initiating and terminating verbal interaction between nurses and severely demented patients regarded as vocally disruptive. *Journal of Psychiatric and Mental Health Nursing, 2,* 159-167.

Faulk, L. (1988). Quality of life factors in board and care homes for the elderly: A hierarchical model. *Adult Foster Care Journal, 2*(2), 100-115.

Faulkner, A. O. (1985). Interdisciplinary health care teams: An educational approach to improvement of health care for the aged. *Gerontology & Geriatrics Education, 5,* 29-39.

Feil, N. (1999). Current concepts and techniques in validation therapy. [Chapter] In Duffy, Michael (Ed.) *Handbook of counseling and psychotherapy with older adults* (pp. 590-613). New York: John Wiley & Sons.

Feldt, K. S., & Ryden, M. D. (1992). Aggressive behavior: Educating nursing assistants. *Journal of Gerontological Nursing, 18,* 3-12.

Finkel, D. (1998). *Behavioral and psychological symptoms of dementia.* Macclesfield, England: Gardner-Caldwell Communications Unlimited.

Finkel, D., & McGue, M. (1998). Age differences in the nature and origin of individual differences in memory: A behavior genetic analysis. *International Journal of Aging & Human Development, 47*(3), 217-239.

Frazer, D. (1995). The medical issues in geropsychology training and practice. In B. Knight, L. Teri, P. Wohlford, & J. Santos (pp. 63-72). American Psychological Association: Washington, DC.

Fries, B. E., Hawes, C., Morris, J. N., & Phillips, C. D. (1997). Effect of the National Resident Assessment Instrument on selected health conditions and problems. *Journal of the American Geriatrics Society, 45*(8), 994-1001.

Goffman, E. (1959). The moral career of the mental patient. *Psychiatry, 22 May,* 123-142.

Goldstein, F. C., Strasser, D. C., Woodard, J. L., & Roberts, V. J. (1997). Functional outcome of cognitively impaired hip fracture patients on a geriatric rehabilitation unit. *Journal of the American Geriatrics Society, 45*(1), 35-42.

Hagen, B., & Sayers, D. (1995). When caring leaves bruises: The effects of staff education of resident aggression. *Journal of Gerontological Nursing, 21,* 7-16.

Hall, G. R., & Buckwalter, K. C. (1987). Progressively lowered stress threshold: A conceptual model for care of adults with Alzheimer's disease. *Archives of Psychiatric Nursing, 1*(6), 399-406.

Hallberg, I. R. (in press). Improving care quality through systematic reflective clinical supervision and planned individualized care: A controlled study in care given to demented patients. *Clinical Nursing Research.*

Hallberg, I. R., Holst, G., Nordmark, A., & Edberg, A. K. (1995). Cooperation during morning care between nurses and severely demented institutionalized patients. *Clinical Nursing Research, 4,* 78-104.

Hill, R. D., Backman, L., & Stigsdotter Neely, A. (Eds.) (2000). *Cognitive rehabilitation in old age.* New York: Oxford University Press.

Hinchliffe, A. C., Hyman, I., Blizard, B., & Livingston, G. (1992). The impact on carers of behavioural difficulties in dementia: A pilot study on management. *International Journal of Geriatric Psychiatry, 7*(8), 579-583.

Hinchliffe, A. C., Hyman, I. L., Blizard, B., & Livingston, G. (1995). Behavioral complications of dementia–Can they be treated? *International Journal of Geriatric Psychiatry, 10,* 839-847.

Hughes, C., Lapane, K., Mor, V., Ikegami, N., Jonsson, P., Ljunggren, G., & Sgadari, A. (2000, August). The impact of legislation on psychotropic drug use in nursing homes: A cross-national perspective. *Journal of the American Geriatrics Society, 48*(8), 931-937.

Hyer, L., & Sohnle, S. (2001). *Trauma among older people: Issue and treatment.* Philadelphia: Brunner/Routledge.

Hyer, L., & Sohnle, S. (2001). Training in a long-term care facility. Presentation at the 109th American Psychological Association, San Francisco, CA.

Kahana, E. F., & Kiyak, H. A. (1984). Attitudes and behavior of staff in facilities for the aged. *Research on Aging, 6,* 395-416.

Kane, R. L. (1998). Assuring quality in nursing home care. *Journal of the American Geriatric Society, 46,* 232-237.

Karuza, J., & Feather, J. (1989). Staff dynamics. In P. R. Katz, & E. Calkins (Eds.), *Principles and practice of nursing home care* (pp. 82-90). New York: Springer.

Kasteler, J. M., Ford, M. H., White, M. A., & Carruth, M. L. (1979). Personnel turnover: A major problem for nursing homes. *Nursing Homes, 28,* 20-27.

Kennedy, G. J. (2000). *Geriatric mental health care: A treatment guide for health professionals.* New York: The Guilford Press.

Kihlgren, M., Lindsten, I. G., Norberg, A., & Karlsson, I. (1992). The content of the oral daily reports at a long-term ward before and after staff training in integrity promoting care. *Scandinavian Journal of Caring Sciences, 6*(2), 105-112.

Lanctot, K. L., Bowles, S. K., Herrmann, N., Best, T. S., & Naranjo, C. A. (2000). Drugs mimicking dementia: Dementia symptoms associated with psychotropic drugs in institutionalized cognitively impaired patients. *Cns Drugs, 14*(5), 381-390.

Lawton, M. P. (1999). Measuring quality of life in nursing homes: The search continues. Invited address, divisions 34, 5, & 20, annual meeting of the American Psychological Association, Boston, MA: August 23rd.

Lichtenberg, P. A. (1994). *A guide to psychological practice in geriatric long-term care.* Binghamton, NY: Haworth Press.

Lichtenberg, P. A., & Duffy, M. (2000). Psychological assessment and psychotherapy in long-term care. *Clinical Psychology-Science & Practice, 7*(3), 317-328.

Lindsley, O. R. (1964). Geriatric behavioral prosthetics. In R. Kastenbaum (Ed.), *New thoughts on old age* (pp. 41-59). New York: Springer.

Logsdon, R. G. (2000). Enhancing quality of life in long term care. In V. Molinari (Ed.), *Professional psychology in long term care: A comprehensive guide* (pp. 133-159). New York: Hatherleigh Press.

Lombardo, N. B. E., Fogel, B. S., Robinson, G. K., & Weiss, H. P. (1995). Achieving mental health of nursing home residents: Overcoming barriers to mental health care. *Journal of Mental Health & Aging, 1*(3), 165-211.

Mathews, R. M., & Altman, H. (1997). Teaching nurse aides to promote independence in people with dementia. *Journal of Clinical Geropsychology, 3*, 149-156.

Mega, M. S., Cummings, J. L., Fiorello, T., & Gornbein, J. (1996). The spectrum of behavioral changes in Alzheimer's disease. *Neurology, 46*(1), 130-135.

Mintzer, J., Colenda, C., Waid, L. R., Lewis, L., Meeks, A., Stuckey, M., Bachman, D.L., Saladin, M., & Sampson, R. R. (1997). Effectiveness of a continuum of care using brief and partial hospitalization for agitated dementia patients. *Psychiatric Services, 48*(11), 1435-1439.

Mittelman, M. S. (2000). Effect of support and counseling on caregivers of patients with Alzheimer's disease. *International Psychogeriatrics, 12*(1), 341-346.

Mittelman, M.S., Ferris, S. H., & Shulman, E. (1996). A family intervention to delay nursing home placement of patients with Alzheimer's disease: A random controlled trial. *Journal of the American Medical Association, 276*(21), 1725-1731.

Mittelman, M. S., Ferris, S. H., Shulman, E., & Steinberg, G. (1995). A comprehensive support program: Effect on depression in spouse-caregivers of AD patients. *The Gerontologist, 35*(6), 792-802.

Molinari, V. (Ed). (2000). *Professional psychology in long term care: A comprehensive guide.* New York, NY: Hatherleigh Press.

Norberg, A. (1996). Caring for demented patients. *Acta Neurologica Scandinavica, 93*(165), 105-108.

Omnibus Budget Reconciliation Act (OBRA) of 1987, Public Law No. 100-203, Title IV, subtitle C, sections 4201-4206, 4211-4216, 101 Stat 1330-160 through 1330-220, 42 USC section 1395;-3(a)-(h) [Medicaid](1992).

Ott, B. R, Tate, C. A., Gordon, N. M., & Heindel, W. C. (1996). Gender differences in the behavioral manifestations of Alzheimer's disease. *Journal of the American Geriatrics Society, 44*(5), 583-587.

Pear, R. (2000). U.S. recommending strict new rules at nursing homes: Concern over staffing. *The New York Times,* July 23, Vol. CXLIX, 51, 458.

Penrod, J. D., Kane, R. A., & Kane, R. L. (2000). Effects of posthospital informal care on nursing home discharge. *Research on Aging, 22*(1), 66-82.

Perkins, M., Morton, M., & Ball, M. (1997). Quality care in personal care homes: Viewpoints of residents and providers in three Georgia counties. In C. A. Noble, &

R. J. F. Elsner (Eds.), *An odyssey in aging: Symposia from the 1997 student convention in gerontology and geriatrics.* Athens, GA: University of Georgia Press.

Phillips, C. D., Chu, C. W., Morris, J. N., & Hawes, C. (1993). Effects of cognitive impairment on the reliability of geriatric assessments in nursing homes. *Journal of the American Geriatrics Society, 41*(2), 136-142.

Phillips, C. D., & Hawes, C. (1992). Nursing home case-mix classification and residents suffering from cognitive impairment: RUG-II and cognition in the Texas case-mix data base. *Medical Care, 30*(2), 105-116.

Phillips, C. D., Morris, J. N., Hawes, C., & Fries, B. E. (1997). Association of the Resident Assessment Instrument (RAI) with changes in function, cognition, and psychosocial status. *Journal of the American Geriatrics Society, 45*(8), 986-993.

Phillips, C. D., Sloane, P. D., Hawes, C., Koch, G., Han, J., Spry, K., Dunteman, G., & Williams, R. L. (1997). Effects of residence in Alzheimer disease special care units on functional outcomes. *Journal of the American Medical Association, 278*(16), 1340-1344.

Pickney-Atkinson, V. J. (1980). Mastery learning model for an inservice nursing training program for the care of hypertensive patients. *Journal of Continuing Education in Nursing 11*, 24-29.

Pillemer, K., Hegeman, C. R., Albright, B., & Henderson, C. (1998). Building bridges between families and nursing home staff: The Partners in Caregiving program. *The Gerontologist, 38*(4), 499-503.

Post, S. G. (2000). Key issues in the ethics of dementia care. *Neurologic Clinics, 18*(4), 1011-1022.

Post, S.G., Ripich, D. N., & Whitehouse, P. J. (1994). Discourse ethics: Research, dementia, and communication. *Alzheimer Disease & Associated Disorders, 8*(Suppl 4), 58-65.

Prignatano, G. P. (2001). *Rehabilitation of higher cerebral functions and the patient's personality.* Phoenix, AZ: Barrow Neurological Institute Quarterly.

Pruchno, R. (1995). The role of family in clinical geropsychology. In B. Knight, L. Teri, P. Wohlford, & J. Santos (pp. 85-87). American Psychological Association: Washington, DC.

Qualls, S. H. (1988). Problems in families of older adults. In N. Epstein, & S. E. Schlesinger (Eds.), *Cognitive-behavioral therapy with families* (pp. 215-253). New York: Brunner/Mazel, Inc.

Reed, B. R., Jagust, W. J., & Coulter, L. (1993). Anosognosia in Alzheimer's disease: Relationships to depression, cognitive function, and cerebral perfusion. *Journal of Clinical & Experimental Neuropsychology, 15*(2), 231-244.

Reichman, W. E. (2001a). Meeting the needs of the patient with Alzheimer's diseases. *Clinical Geriatrics, 9*(2), 62-69.

Reichman, W. E. (2001b) Presentation to SDAT organization. American Association of Geriatric Psychiatrists. Bethesda, MD.

Rovner, B. W. (1994). What is special about special care units? The role of psychosocial rehabilitation. *Alzheimer Disease and Associated Disorders, 8*(1), S355-S358.

Rovner, B., Steele, C., & Folstein, M. (1996). A randomized trial of dementia care in nursing homes. *Journal of the American Geriatrics Society, 44*, 7-13.

Royall, D. R. (1994). Precis of executive dyscontrol as a cause of problem behavior in dementia. *Experimental Aging Research, 20*, 73-94.

Ryden, M. B. (1989). *Behavioral problems in dementia: A review of the literature.* Minneapolis, MN: University of Minnesota.

Saeman, H. (1992). What price prescription privileges? *Psychotherapy in Private Practice, 11*(1), 9-13.

Sbordone, R. J., & Sterman, L. T. (1983). The psychologist as a consultant in a nursing home: Effect on staff morale and turnover. *Professional Psychology, 14,* 240-250.

Schneider, L. S. (1996). Meta-analysis of controlled pharmacologic trials. *International Psychogeriatrics, 8*(3), 375-379.

Schnelle, J. F., McNees. P., Crooks, V., & Ouslander, J. G. (1995). The use of a computer-based model to disseminate an incontinence management program. *The Gerontologist, 35,* 656-665.

Schnelle, J. F., Newman, D. R., & Fogarty, T. (1990). Management of patient continence in long-term care nursing facilities. *The Gerontologist, 30,* 373-376.

Schnelle, J. F., Newman, D. R., Fogarty, T. E., Wallston, K., & Ory, M. (1991). Assessment and quality control of incontinence in long-term nursing facilities. *Journal of the American Geriatrics Society, 39,* 165-171.

Schnelle, J. F., Ouslander, J. G., & Cruise, P. A. (1997). Policy without technology: A barrier to improving nursing home care. *Gerontologist, 37,* 527-532.

Schwartz, A. (1984). Staff development and morale building in nursing homes. *The Gerontologist, 14,* 50-54.

Segal, Z., Williams, J., & Teasdale, J. (2002). *Mindfulness-based cognitive therapy for depression: A new approach to preventing relapse.* New York: Guilford.

Smith, H. L., Discenza, R., & Saxberg, B. O. (1978). Administering long-term care services. *The Gerontologist, 18,* 159-166.

Smith, M., Buckwalter, K. C., Garand, L., Mitchell, S., Albanese, M., & Kreiter, C. (1994). Evaluation of a geriatric mental health training program for nursing personnel in rural long-term care facilities. *Issues in Mental Health Nursing, 15,* 149-169.

Smyer, M. A., Cohn, M., & Brannon, D. (1988). *Mental health consultation in nursing homes.* New York: New York University Press.

Smyer, M.A., Shea, D. G., & Streit, A. (1994). The provision and use of mental health services in nursing homes: Results from the National Medical Expenditure Survey. *American Journal of Public Health, 84*(2), 284-287.

Snyder-Halpern, R., & Buczkowski, E. (1990). Performance-based staff development: A baseline for clinical competence. *Journal of Nursing Staff Development,* 7-11.

Stein, S., Linn, M. W., & Elliot, E. M. (1986). The relationship between nursing home residents' perceptions of nursing staff and quality of nursing home care. *Journal of Physical and Occupational Therapy, 4,* 143-156.

Sterns, H. L., & Camp, C. J. Applied gerontology. *Applied Psychology: An International Review, 47*(2), 175-198.

Stevens, A., Burgio, L. D., Burgio, K. L., Paul, P., Tanner. D., & Driver, D. (1996, November). Effects of a behavioral supervision model on CNS behavioral skill use. Paper presented at the annual meeting of the Gerontological Society of America, Washington, DC.

Stewart, A., & King, A. (1994). Conceptualizing and measuring quality of life in older populations. In R. Ables, H. Gift, & M. Ory (Eds.), *Aging and quality of life: Charting new territories in behavioral science research* (pp. 27-56). New York: Springer.

Sunderland, T. (2000). *Identification and diagnosis of behavioral disturbances in dementia.* Worcester, MA: Athina Diagnostics.

Sunderland, T., & Silver, M. A. (1988). Neuroleptics in the treatment of dementia. *International Journal of Geriatric Psychiatry, 3*(2), 79-88.

Teri, L. (1986). Severe cognitive impairments in older adults. *Behavior Therapist, 9*(3), 51-54.

Teri, L., Logsdon, R. G., Peskind, E., Raskind, M., Weiner, M. F., Tractenberg, R. E., Foster, N. L., Schneider, L. S., Sano, M., Whitehouse, P., Tariot, P., Mellow, A. M., Auchus, A. P., Grundman, M., Thomas, R. G., Schafer, K., & Thal, L. J. (2000). Treatment of agitation in AD: A randomized, placebo-controlled clinical trial. *Neurology, 55*(9), 1271-1278.

Teri, L., & Logsdon, R. (1991). Cognitive-behavioral interventions for treatment of depression in Alzheimer's patients. *The Gerontologist, 31,* 413-416.

Teri, L., & Umoto, J. (1991). Reducing excess disability in dementia patients: Training caregivers to manage patient depression. *Clinical Gerontologist, 31,* 49-63.

Vaccaro, F. J. (1988). Application of operant procedures in a group of institutionalized aggressive geriatric patients. *Psychology and Aging, 3,* 22-28.

Verhaegen P., Marcoen, A., & Goossens, L. (1992). Improving memory performance in the aged through mnemonic training: A meta-analytic study. *Psychology and Aging, 7*(2), 242-251.

Vygotsky, L. S., & Rieber, R. W. (1997). *The collected works of L. S. Vygotsky, Vol. 4: The history of the development of higher mental functions.* New York: Plenum.

Waxman, H. M., Carner, E. A., & Berkenstock, G. (1984). Job turnover and job satisfaction among nursing home aides. *The Gerontologist, 24,* 503-509.

Wertheimer, J., Boula, J. G., Brull, J., & Gut, A. M. (1992). Learning processes in dementia. *International Journal of Geriatric Psychiatry, 7*(3), 161-172.

West, R. L., Welch, D. C., & Yassuda, M. S. (2000). Innovative approaches to memory training for older adults. In R. D. Hill, L. Backman, & A. Stigsdotter Neely (Eds.) *Cognitive rehabilitation in old age* (pp. 81-105). New York: Oxford University Press.

Williams, D. P., Wood, E. C., Moorleghen, F., & Chittuluru, V. C. (1995). A decision model for guiding the management of disruptive behaviors in demented residents of institutionalized settings. *The American Journal of Alzheimer's Disease, May/June,* 22-29.

Wilson, B. A., Baddeley, A., Evans, J., & Shiel, A. (1994). Errorless learning in the rehabilitation of memory impaired people. *Neuropsychological Rehabilitation, 4,* 307-326.

Zarit, S. H., Dolan, M. M., & Leitsch, S. A. (1998). Interventions in nursing homes and other alternative living settings. In I. H. Nordhus, I. Hilde, & G. R. VandenBos (Eds.), *Clinical geropsychology* (pp. 329-343). Washington, DC: American Psychological Association.

Zeiss, A. M., & Steffen, A. M. (1996). Interdisciplinary health care teams: The basic unit of geriatric care. In L. L. Carstensen, & B. A. Edelstein (Eds.), *The practical handbook of clinical gerontology* (pp. 423-450). Thousand Oaks, CA: Sage.

Zgola, J. M. (1999). *Care that works: A relationship approach to persons with dementia.* Johns Hopkins University Press.

Zinn, J. S., Brannon, D., & Weech, R. (1997). Quality improvement in nursing care facilities. Extent, impetus, and impact. *American Journal of Medical Quality, 12,* 51-61.

SECTION THREE: ETHICAL AND CONFIDENTIALITY QUANDARIES

Informed Consent in the Long Term Care Setting

Martin D. Zehr, PhD, JD

SUMMARY. Informed consent, considered as either an ethical construct or legal requirement, is a concept with which any healthcare professional should have a thorough familiarity prior to working with patients in any type of care setting. The evolution of informed consent during the twentieth century has resulted in the adoption of a patient-oriented approach which mandates the provision of full disclosure of relevant treatment information, under circumstances in which the patient's voluntary participation in the treatment protocol is made explicit. It is also assumed that the healthcare professional will make an inquiry,

Martin D. Zehr is affiliated with Research Medical Center, Kansas City, MO, and Central Missouri State University (E-mail: MDZehr@HealthMidwest.org).

Portions of this article were presented as part of the symposium "Confidentiality in Long-Term Care" at the annual convention of the Gerontological Society of America, Washington, DC, November 2000.

[Haworth co-indexing entry note]: "Informed Consent in the Long Term Care Setting." Zehr, Martin D. Co-published simultaneously in *Clinical Gerontologist* (The Haworth Press, Inc.) Vol. 25, No. 3/4, 2002, pp. 239-260; and: *Emerging Trends in Psychological Practice in Long-Term Care* (ed: Margaret P. Norris, Victor Molinari, and Suzann Ogland-Hand) The Haworth Press, Inc., 2002, pp. 239-260. Single or multiple copies of this article are available for a fee from The Haworth Document Delivery Service [1-800-HAWORTH, 9:00 a.m. - 5:00 p.m. (EST). E-mail address: getinfo@haworthpressinc.com].

whether informal or otherwise, to ensure that the informed consent to treatment is being obtained from a competent individual. Healthcare professionals in long term care settings, whether in the role of employees or consultants, should be cognizant of special circumstances with such patients, including specific statutory requirements, which result in ethical and legal obligations for practice which may not be applicable to patient populations generally. *[Article copies available for a fee from The Haworth Document Delivery Service: 1-800-HAWORTH. E-mail address: <getinfo@haworthpressinc.com> Website: <http://www.HaworthPress.com> © 2002 by The Haworth Press, Inc. All rights reserved.]*

KEYWORDS. Ethics, informed consent, long term care, legal capacity

The clinician whose work entails a substantial amount of practice in long term care settings with geriatric patients must adapt to a complicated structure of clients, services, payers and disciplines, in addition to the operational constraints of the particular facility, which are not routinely encountered in a typical outpatient setting or even in a general medical setting. Long term care, increasingly defined in terms of a continuum of services and interventions ranging from minimal ADL assistance to 24-hour skilled nursing and complete guardianship, requires a sensitivity to a myriad of ethical concerns which may, at times, lead to conflicts with routine institutional behavior in long term care settings (Moye & Zehr, 2000). Primary among the ethical issues which are likely to be encountered in a disproportionate frequency in long term care settings are those related to informed consent with regard to diagnostic and treatment interactions between clinicians and residents. It is nevertheless notable that, even among clinicians who indicate a special interest in geriatric patient care, education with respect to informed consent issues is not a topic which attracts special interest, as evidenced by a recent survey of psychologists attending continuing education workshops on geropsychology issues (Norman et al., 2000). Respondents in this survey indicated their particular interests in a number of specific topics relevant to working with older adults and, while some ethical concerns were listed, e.g., end-of-life decision-making, the subject of informed consent while working with geriatric patients was conspicuous by its absence. Informed consent, however, presents special challenges for clinicians working with a geriatric population in long term care settings which warrant inclusion in any educational protocol purporting to provide even minimal preparation in clinical gerontology.

All healthcare professionals in this era are undoubtedly aware of their obligation to provide informed consent as a prerequisite to initiating any measure or procedure which could reasonably be construed as "treatment." However, the meanings and implications of informed consent are as varied as the situations which invoke its consideration. It is therefore imperative that each clinician have as explicit a notion of the ethical and legal underpinnings of informed consent as possible, at least to the extent that, when a potential treatment protocol requires more than a cursory explanation to the patient, an internalized checklist or algorithm can be summoned to provide adequate guidance in the particular situation. From an ethical standpoint, informed consent is based, in our society, on values including beneficence and patient autonomy, which can nevertheless represent seemingly competing bases for clinician-patient interactions in the specific case. It is usually assumed, however, that patient autonomy, or self-determination, requires access, to the extent possible, to all available information relevant to the treatment alternatives being considered. Implicit in this requirement is the assumption that the clinician, in turn, is thoroughly familiar with the treatment alternatives, including non-treatment, and their respective implications for the patient's physical and psychological well-being, and that the clinician is capable of communicating the details of each treatment alternative in a manner which maximizes the probability that the patient can indeed make a choice based on an "informed understanding" of the alternatives.

In a long term care setting, in addition to the usual ethical imperative that the clinician understand and implement treatment based on the tenets of the doctrine of informed consent, there must be a heightened sensitivity to considerations of cognitive capacity, if not legal capacity, because informed consent cannot, by definition, be conveyed by any individual who cannot understand the consequences of any potential choice of treatment. With the older patients who typically reside in long term care facilities, there is also the increased probability that the healthcare professional will be required to address treatment questions to proxy caregivers who may or may not be present, e.g., legal guardians or designated healthcare powers of attorneys, and that the clinician will have to acquire a familiarity with institutional policies which have a direct impact on informed consent for all covered residents, e.g., contractual admission policies which require the patient's consent to review of medical records by outside consultants contacted by agency medical staff at their discretion. In a long term care setting, the relationship between the agency and the professional, whether in the role of employee or outside consultant, may also dictate an additional obligation regarding familiarity with applicable statutory measures designed explicitly to enhance informed consent for residents. A primary example of the latter is the Patient Self-Determination Act (PSDA), enacted by Congress in 1990, which requires federally-funded healthcare providers to, among other things, inform the patient of his or her right to execute an advance directive for healthcare decisions and to offer written information pertaining to statutory or institutional policies regarding their ability to accept or deny treatment. Clinicians, with their assumption of responsibility for acting in such a manner as to maximize patient autonomy, could conceivably find themselves in the position of advocates for patients who have not been accorded their rights under the PSDA and therefore have not been provided with the opportunity to provide informed consent for certain end-of-life treatment decisions. Indeed, at least two formal studies of the implementation of the PSDA, a statewide survey of nursing homes in Connecticut (Bradley et al., 1997) and an examination of compliance with the provisions of the PSDA in New York City (Mezey et al., 1997), have indicated that residents of long term care facilities are often denied legally required information which would presumably enhance their opportunity to provide informed consent in certain treatment situations. The denial of rights in this situation is particularly disturbing when considered in conjunction with evidence indicating that many long term care facility residents with a formal diagnosis of dementia continue to demonstrate sufficient decisional capacity to make a reasonable choice of a healthcare proxy. In one applicable study it was in fact shown that thirty-nine percent of residents of a long term care facility with a dementia diagnosis made healthcare proxy decisions that were "consistent with and comparable to those of their non-demented peers" (Sansone et al., 1998).

Finally, the healthcare professional working in the long term care setting must develop a sensitivity to more basic considerations which have an obvious impact on the individual's capacity to provide informed consent, i.e., ordinary changes in the ability to process treatment information which are the byproduct of the aging process and require accommodation but which do not affect legal capacity or cognitive capacity generally (Park, Morrell & Shifren, 1999). The professional working with residents in a long term care facility should, then, develop an enhanced understanding of the doctrine of informed consent which has greater relevance and practical value insofar as work with the typically older adults living in these facilities is concerned.

EVOLUTION OF THE INFORMED CONSENT DOCTRINE

Informed consent, from a legal perspective, has been a part of the legacy of the English common law upon which our own judicial system is based for at least three centuries. In a case decided in 1767 titled *Slater v. Baker and Stapleton*, an English court specifically observed that it was "improper" to initiate a medical treatment, in this case, surgery, "without consent." This breach of duty to the patient was based on the theory that the patient had been subjected to an unconsented touching, which, from a formalistic legal analysis, is the equivalent of an assault and battery. If, however, the patient had registered no complaint under these circumstances, consent would be implied and, therefore, from a strictly legal standpoint, not actionable. This "simple" consent for treatment did not impose any obligation upon the treating party to actually "inform" the recipient of anything other than the option of choosing the intended treatment or refusing it.

Only much later, in the United States, did courts develop, through a series of state cases, the modern legal doctrine of informed consent, which requires three basic components as a predicate to decisions regarding treatment:

1. disclosure of information regarding the proposed treatment by the healthcare professional;
2. voluntary choice of treatment alternatives by the patient; and
3. sufficient competence of the patient to comprehend both the nature and consequences of the proposed treatment alternatives.

Simple consent was supplanted in the legal context by the requirement of an informed consent which was based on the idea that patients had the right to receive sufficient information upon which a meaningful choice could be made regarding treatment options (Appelbaum, Lidz & Meisel, 1987). Simultaneously, these court decisions replaced the notion of potential caregiver liability based on an unwanted battery with a reliance on claims based in negligence (Morton, 1987), that is, courts recognized a fiduciary, or trust obligation, by virtue of the healthcare professional's status vis-à-vis the patient, which mandated the professional's acting in good faith and in the best interests of the patient. In this context, the best interests of the patient include a deference to the patient's right to act independently and a tacit rejection of the paternalistic notion that the clinician's judgement itself is the final arbiter of this standard. Instead, any questions regarding the actuality of informed consent in a clinical situation must be evaluated from the patient's standpoint. A closer look at the three required components, cited above, from the patient's perspective, is therefore warranted to elaborate the current status of the construct in professional practice.

DISCLOSURE

In one of the first modern-era cases addressing the subject of informed consent, the Kansas Supreme Court, in a 1960 decision in *Natanson v. Kline*, stated that patients must be informed regarding the nature and purposes of a proposed course of treatment, its potential benefits and risks, any available alternative treatments, and their associated risks (Grisso & Appelbaum, 1998a). In general terms, these requirements constitute the basis for adequate disclosure as a component of informed consent today, although, in one important respect, the basis for judging disclosure has changed. In *Natanson*, the court indicated that the amount of information that professionals were required to disclose to the patient would be assessed by comparison with that which a "reasonable" member of the profession would discuss with patients in a similar situation. This standard has gradually been discarded in a number of jurisdictions, however, and replaced by a patient-oriented standard of disclosure, i.e., a requirement that the clinician provide the patient with as much information as the "reasonable" patient would want to know in order to make an informed treatment decision (Darr, 1997). This latter criterion is obviously more in accord with the underlying assumption that patients should have the right to act with an optimal degree of independence that is effectively precluded when the clinician decides what the patient needs to know. From an operational standpoint, the patient-oriented standard also recognizes the inherent relevance of the patient's questions, as these are presumably generated in pursuance of his or her attempt to attain the "reasonable" patient standard prior to making a treatment choice. Courts have not yet, in any widespread manner, taken the next logical step, i.e., adopting a standard which would always require the clinician to furnish as much treatment-related information as a *particular* patient would want to know, but, from a strictly ethical standpoint, it is reasonable to assume that any healthcare worker who professes an interest in the dignity and autonomy of the patient would routinely make an effort to ascertain and address the specific concerns of the patient contemplating treatment choices or the refusal of treatment. The reasonable patient standard is sometimes referred to as the "materiality standard," that is, a requirement that the clinician disclose any and all information regarding treatment alternatives which would "materially affect" a patient's decision (Smith, 1996). Because, however, it is virtually impossible to determine either the amount or type of information which will "materially affect" a particular patient's choice of treatment, the prudent clinician should make every attempt to create an atmosphere in which the patient feels that his questions are welcome, making sure to solicit questions when none are forthcoming.

The law in most jurisdictions recognizes an exception to the requirement of disclosure embodied in a concept called *therapeutic privilege*, under which physicians are permitted to withhold information from patients when disclosure itself may be harmful. Invoking this privilege on a regular basis, however, begs the obvious question, what is the basis for deciding what is potentially harmful? Widespread reliance on this concept as a basis for less than full disclosure of relevant information would appear to subvert the whole notion, from the patient's perspective, of a right to be apprised of the information required to make an informed treatment choice. As an illustration, consider the situation, commonly encountered in a long term care facility, in which a clinician, following a formal evaluation, reaches the conclusion that a particular resident's behavior and symptoms are consistent with an early-stage dementia, likely on the basis of Alzheimer's disease. Under the concept of therapeutic privilege, the clinician could arguably justify withholding this diagnostic conclusion from the patient, reasoning that the patient in the early stage of a progressive dementia process would likely be able to comprehend the implications of the diagnosis and therefore would, from a psychological standpoint, become devastated when apprised of this determination. On the other hand, the patient in these circumstances, whose judgement may be intact and who may be well aware of their mild cognitive deficits, may be precluded, as a direct result of the exercise of therapeutic privilege, from participation in any present or future treatment protocol which could have a medically significant impact on his condition. In this day and age particularly, in which Internet Web sites abound with useful information relevant to any imaginable topic, invocation of therapeutic privilege as an exception to the informed consent doctrine may have the unintended and potentially deleterious consequence of depriving the patient (and caregivers) of information regarding both present and forthcoming treatments which are at the time unfamiliar even to the primary clinician. Under such circumstances one of the primary tenets of the informed consent doctrine, the requirement that the patient be informed of potential alternative treatment approaches, will have been indisputably violated. In addition, failure to disclose diagnostic information on the basis of therapeutic privilege in this situation might have a detrimental impact on the patient's ability to initiate advance planning measures, e.g., conveying a durable power of attorney and arranging for a possible future change in living circumstances. Thus, invocation of therapeutic privilege can have significant negative and unintended consequences for the ultimate well-being of the patient and should be relied upon only in rare instances (Zehr, 1998). The anticipated harm to be avoided through reliance on therapeutic privilege in situations like this must be weighed against the long range implications for the patient's well-being. In any event, most commentators consider therapeutic privilege to be the most controversial exception to the informed consent doctrine (Kapp, 1992), one which should be relied on only in rare cases, and even then presumably after consulting a colleague to obtain an independent opinion regarding the decision to withhold information in the treatment setting.

Full disclosure in an institutional setting also requires that patients be apprised of the possible uses of information elicited from the patient in the course of treatment. Especially when treatment consists of some form of counseling or psychological intervention, patients should be made aware, at the outset of the proposed therapeutic relationship, of the limits of confidentiality, the types of records kept in the course of treatment, and the rights of others, including institutional personnel or healthcare reimbursement agents, to obtain access to recorded information (Ebert, 1993). Because such disclosure can have an inhibiting effect insofar as the individual's decision to enter into counseling is concerned, it is obviously material to the patient's treatment choice and, therefore, is required. It should be noted in this regard, however, that, contrary to commonly-held belief, empirical research tends to support the conclusion that likelihood of patient consent to enter a proposed course of treatment actually tends to increase as a function of the amount and type of information disclosed relevant to treatment increases (Sprung & Winick, 1989).

Full disclosure of the relevant information associated with particular treatment alternatives should not be interpreted to mean a mere recitation of the known facts and probabilities associated with each choice. There is no ethical prohibition against the clinician's expression of a preference for a treatment option, or even active encouragement to choose a treatment, provided that the advice to do so is not presented in a manner which could be reasonably viewed by the patient as a form of coercion. Indeed, where a longstanding relationship based on trust and mutual respect exists between the patient and healthcare professional, there may exist a justified expectation that the treatment preference of the clinician be expressed and explained to the patient, as exercise of the patient's choice certainly includes the option to rely on the opinion of the trusted professional. Nevertheless, the clinician should also be sensitive to the possibility that the implication may be communicated, whether intended or not, that treatment is contingent on acquiescence to the healthcare professional's delineation of alternatives.

VOLUNTARINESS

In the context of informed consent, it is vital that the patient's independent decision-making be free from any undue coercive influences. No patient, of course, should be subject to overt threats to initiate a course of treatment in direct opposition to his or her expressed wishes, but most constraints on the voluntary nature of treatment choices in a healthcare setting are likely to either be subtle, to the extent that even the patient is largely unaware of their impact, or to exist with the tacit acceptance of the patient, in which case acceptance of the coercive influence may be interpreted, in the larger context, as voluntary acceptance of the influenced treatment choice. The clinician who works regularly with older adults in a long term care setting should therefore develop an awareness of the factors which might constrain a resident's tendency to make particular treatment choices, especially because some of these influences can be minimized, thereby enhancing the resident's ability to make voluntary choices which most closely conform with his or her considered preferences. Factors enumerated by Kapp (1992) which likely limit the voluntary nature of patient choices in these settings include

1. involuntary commitment status;
2. an eagerness to please staff and other residents;
3. susceptibility to threats or inducements resulting from physical or mental disability;
4. inability to obtain access to independent advice or consultation.

A lack of available treatment choices, a situation common in the case of behavioral healthcare in long term care facilities, can also be considered in a sense to be a coercive condition, but this is a type of constraint which is not usually considered as representing anything other than one of the ordinary, often unavoidable, constraints of living.

Outside influences, of course, can have a dramatic influence on a patient's choice of treatment regimen or level of cooperation with the rules of the long term care setting. A spouse or relative, for example, may insist on, and the patient may assent to, a course of treatment which the patient might not otherwise choose, but choices made under such conditions are not usually viewed as undue influences on treatment choices, because the source of the major outside influence is part of the fabric of the patient's life, i.e., the life circumstances which are the direct result of the individual's cumulative life choices. Some of these so-called "outside influences" can, moreover, appear to represent values and methods related to decision making which directly contradict the assumptions of respect for individual autonomy that are the basis for the requirement of informed consent. Clinicians working with patients from some cultural and ethnic backgrounds, for example, may find that important decisions which are usually assumed to be the prerogative of the individual are made through such means as deference to a patriarchal leader in the extended family or through a communal decision process in which the individual patient's role is, in effect, minor. Decisions made from such ethnic-cultural perspectives are not to be dismissed out of hand simply because the mechanisms which generate them appear to undermine the values of individual autonomy which are the basis for the legal requirements of informed consent. As illustrated in the work of Ramon Valle, much of which is based on experience with Hispanic families dealing with the dementing illness of a member, these ethnic and cultural considerations, if accepted by the patient, may in some instances require explicit incorporation of wider family involvement from the beginning of the process of choosing a treatment regimen than would otherwise be the case (Valle, 1998). The clinician who ignores or attempts to minimize the wider family involvement in these instances is, in effect, attempting to impose his or her own values on the family structure and the patient, risking the possible result that both the patient and other family members reject both the clinician and his recommendations.

As noted above, voluntary consent may be inferred in specific situations when the patient does not register any objection to initiation of a treatment, particularly in a long term care setting in which acceptance of certain discretionary staff actions is made a precondition of admission. Even in such instances, however, the healthcare professional should be wary of assuming a wider latitude of authority in clinician-patient interactions than that which would be applicable in an outpatient setting. For one thing, explicit institutional policies, or habitually accepted staff behavior affecting patient rights, may in fact constitute direct violation of statutory provisions applicable to patient rights. The lack of compliance with the provisions of the PSDA in an institutional setting, as discussed earlier, is an example of the latter. Aside from formalized requirements which recognize specific patient rights, however, there is an additional consideration which should serve as the impetus for the healthcare worker to act consistently in a manner that evinces an intention to keep the patient as well-informed as is practicable regarding every aspect of treatment or institutional policy which has implications for the patient's well-being. Specifically, the desire to foster conditions which support the creation and maintenance of a therapeutic relationship, especially where treatment may consist of an extended series of consecutive contacts, such as those which comprise a counseling relationship or other form of psychological intervention, necessitates the occasional rejection of the doctrine of implied consent, even in circumstances where it is legally defensible. Sharing of patient-related information in such circumstances, in which disclosure is not mandated, can facilitate the reciprocal and open exchange of the type of patient information which can serve as the basis for a productive therapy relationship. Finally, although implied consent may be applicable with respect to the actions of the clinician employed directly by the facility, thus obviating the requirement of obtaining a separate informed consent prior to initiating treatment, the professional who works in the facility on a consultative basis must usually obtain a separate informed consent before any services are provided (Lichtenberg et al., 1998).

COMPETENCE

The requirement that patients have sufficient cognitive (and legal) capacity to understand the treatment alternatives presented to them as a basis for making a meaningful decision is a commonsense notion, which nevertheless is problematic when attempts are made to apply statutory guidelines in specific instances. Clinicians, particularly those who work with older adults in long term care settings, will invariably encounter situations in which they will be called upon to provide information upon which these ultimately legal determinations will be based; therefore, it is incumbent on the healthcare professional to have at least a rudimentary understanding of the concept. Capacity in a legal context is typically defined or described in reference to its absence, such as in the following statutory definition of an incapacitated person, in a civil, as opposed to a criminal, frame of reference as:

> one who is unable by reason of physical or mental condition to receive and evaluate information or to communicate decisions to such an extent that he lacks capacity to meet essential requirements for food, clothing, shelter, safety, or other care such that serious physical injury, illness, or disease is likely to occur. (Section 475.010 Revised Statutes of Missouri, 1985)

Such legal definitions incorporate the notion of capacity as a unitary, indivisible concept although, in practice, the legal system commonly recognizes separate competencies or degrees of competency, as, for example, in provisions for conservatorship, in which authority for making financial decisions is legally conferred to another, versus all-encompassing guardianships. Statutes in most states have been adopted in the last two decades which incorporate references to specific types of disabilities and degrees of cognitive incapacity, and the legal system has now become more amenable to the use of data from the behavioral sciences which describe, for example, various types of memory deficits and their implications for actual functioning in everyday situations (Anderer, 1990). The clinician who works with those elder patients in a long term setting who are most likely to be subject to inquiries regarding their capacity to perform certain functions, including the analysis of information related to a treatment choice and the subsequent communication of a choice, should always keep in mind that there is never an isomorphic relationship between a particular set of data, even that obtained through the use of formal, objective testing instruments and a determination of legal capacity. In the study cited earlier by Sansone and his colleagues (Sansone et al., 1998), for example, it was found that thirty-six percent of demented residents of a long term care center with a Folstein Mini-Mental State Exam score below 15 demonstrated the capacity to either consistently designate a healthcare proxy or state a decision not to name one. Likewise, the diagnosis of a neurodegenerative condition known to have a significant effect on cognitive functioning, e.g., Alzheimer's disease, is not, by itself, the equivalent of a determination regarding the individual's capacity to function independently, including the capacity to make treatment decisions (Grisso, 1986). Capacity, from the legal perspective, is always a situationally-based concept, such that, it is perfectly conceivable that an individual with a specific pattern of cognitive deficits could be determined to be capable of independent functioning in one setting and judged to be legally incapacitated in other settings. Such determinations are further complicated by the extent of the individual's awareness of the nature and extent of his or her cognitive deficits. Thus, while an individual may exhibit pronounced memory deficits in conjunction with a diagnosis of Alzheimer's disease, if he simultaneously demonstrates an acute awareness of these deficits, it is quite possible that he can initiate or consent to compensatory measures, e.g., reliance on the help of a trusted friend, in order "to meet essential requirements." A lack of the requisite awareness, however, may preclude the institution of compensatory measures and thus render the individual practically and legally incapacitated. The number and complexity of the demands inherent in the patient's living circumstances can also constitute an important, if not decisive, factor in any determination of capacity to function autonomously. Thus, for example, an individual with significant cognitive deficits may nevertheless be capable of independent functioning if the routine demands of his or her living situation are few in number and relatively simple of accomplishment, whereas an individual with a similar degree and pattern of deficits may be rendered completely incapacitated insofar as his or her ability to fulfill even the routine demands associated with a position as CEO of a corporate entity. For all of these reasons, it should be apparent that the development of a reliable algorithm as a basis for a universally applicable standard of capacity, particularly in the legal sense, is an impossibility. This conclusion is no less valid in the context of a discussion of capacity as one of the three components of decision-making for the conveyance of informed consent in a treatment setting.

Despite the difficulties inherent in any attempt to apply research-based findings to legal issues involving questions of competency, or capacity, circumscribed efforts have yielded potentially useful information relevant to specific situations. Daniel Marson and his colleagues have, for example, shown that deficits in semantic memory and word fluency measures are associated with competency status for different legal standards, with specific reference to the capacity to consent to treatment (Marson et al., 1995a, b, 1996). These researchers assessed the ability of normal older control subjects and patients with probable Alzheimer's disease, when presented with two clinical vignettes requiring decisions regarding medical treatment, to respond in a manner indicating the following progressively complex legal standards:

1. The capacity to *evidence* a treatment choice, regardless of the appropriateness of the decision.

2. The capacity to make the *reasonable* treatment choice.
3. The capacity to *appreciate* the emotional and cognitive consequences of a treatment choice.
4. The capacity to provide *rational reasons* for a treatment choice.
5. The capacity to *understand* the treatment situation and choices (Marson et al., 1995a, p. 951).

Although this series of studies clearly indicated the predictive value of neuropsychological test measures for the assessment of the various levels of capacity, the results of these studies showed that, for the most stringent legal standard, which required an "understanding" of the treatment situation, measures of conceptualization ability and of visual confrontational naming (or semantic memory) were better predictors of level five competence than was short term memory per se. Thus, even with significant short term memory impairment, patients may provide relatively consistent choices indicating adequate comprehension of the treatment situation and alternatives. Such patients could conceivably be deemed competent insofar as their ability to provide informed consent in a treatment situation is concerned while simultaneously, as a result of significant short term memory impairment, be unable to meet some of the routine demands of daily life without assistance or reliance on compensatory mechanisms. The work of Marson and his colleagues underscores the problem of attempting to use formal testing to address what are, ultimately, legal determinations. It nevertheless indicates that objective assessment of cognitive functions which provides normative-based evidence of a particular individual's pattern of deficits can assist the trier of fact, i.e., the court, or, in the long term care setting, the facility administrator, when attempting to ascertain whether the patient-resident is capable of informed consent. Clearly, while no objective assessment instrument can reasonably be expected to incorporate all of the individual, situational and treatment information variables in a manner which adequately represents the complexity of their interaction in the specific clinical situation from which a question of informed consent arises, attempts at devising formal tests of competency to consent to treatment have shown their usefulness as an adjunct to clinical observation of patient behavior. Pruchno et al. (1995), for example, devised a brief, reliable assessment tool which was validated with residents in a nursing home facility and shown to have predictive value with reference to the criterion measure of a psychologist's evaluation of competence to participate in decisions about medical care. A more comprehensive instrument designed for the same purpose was published by Thomas

Grisso and Paul Appelbaum (1998a), pioneers in the study of psy-cho-legal concerns with both patients in healthcare settings and individuals who are the subject of proceedings in the criminal justice system. The MacArthur Competence Assessment Tool for Treatment (MacCat-T; 1998b) is the product of a decade of work by Grisso and Appelbaum in the MacArthur Civil Competence Project, a program of research whose primary focus was the study of informed consent and patients' decision-making capacities. The MacCat-T itself consists of a structured interview schedule which is designed to elicit information that directly addresses the following elements of informed consent to treatment:

1. *understanding* of treatment-related information, focusing on categories of information that must be disclosed as required by the law of informed consent.
2. *appreciation* of the significance of the information for the patient's situation, focusing on the nature of the disorder and the possibility that treatment could be beneficial.
3. *reasoning* in the process of deciding upon treatment, focusing on the ability to draw inferences about the impact of the alternatives on the patient's *everyday* life.
4. *expressing a choice* about treatment (Grisso & Appelbaum, 1998b, p. 1).

The authors themselves emphasize that the MacCat-T should be utilized in conjunction with a broad range of clinical information and that the derived scores from administration of the instrument do ". . . not translate directly into determinations of legal competence or incompetence." Nevertheless, such attempts cannot help but provide the clinician with a method of consistently investigating and addressing those elements of a resident's cognitive capacity which are most directly relevant to both clinical and legal aspects of the informed consent construct. The ability to supplement clinical observations with objective data in a situation in which decisions have a dramatic impact on an important individual right, to accept or reject a proposed treatment, should be welcomed by healthcare professionals who find themselves in the position of having to provide, what is hopefully, an informed opinion regarding the resident's capacity to provide informed consent. The difficulty of ascertaining the capacity of the individual to provide informed consent exclusively on the basis of clinical observations is underscored by work which indicates that, when questions of choice of treatment are posed to surrogate decision-makers, who in most cases have known the patient for extended periods of time, those surrogates could correctly guess the patient's choice at only a chance level (Suhl et al., 1994). In the latter situation the surrogates presumably do not possess the level of training of the clinician who is addressing the question at hand with at least an internalized training-based framework, but such finding nevertheless supports the notion that inclusion of an objective instrument designed to address the specific question of informed consent in the armamentarium of the clinician should be strongly considered.

Surrogate or proxy decision-makers for residents in long term care facilities are, of course, entitled to be apprised of the same information that would otherwise be presented to the resident prior to initiation of a treatment protocol, despite the fact that practical considerations will often render communication of the required information problematic. The doctrine of implied consent or the explicit contractual terms that are endorsed as a precondition of admission to the long term care facility may have a mitigating effect on the need to keep the surrogate apprised of minor day-to-day adjustments in the resident's treatment regimen, but it is nevertheless advisable, even when wide legally-based latitude exists in such cases, to make a special effort to contact the surrogate, who may be a legal guardian or power of attorney, and inform that individual of contemplated treatments as they are being considered. Exceeding the strictly legal requirements of informed consent is likely to have some of the same benefits when working with the surrogate as with the patient, i.e., creation and maintenance of an involved, cooperative relationship between the parties. Finally, in this regard, it should be noted that the subject of informed consent can arise vis-à-vis the proxy decision-maker when the resident of the long term care facility is a member of a population which is the focus of research efforts. With respect to research with patients suffering from varying degrees of Alzheimer's disease, for example, it has long been realized that there are special ethical problems regarding obtaining informed consent from both patients and proxy decision-makers (High, 1993). In such cases it is imperative that the legal surrogate have as much understanding of the risks, benefits and nature and extent of patient involvement as the competent patient would be entitled to know, including advisement of the right to terminate participation at any time. It is also advisable in such situations to make an attempt to discuss the same information directly with the patient, as it is likely that many patients will understand some or all of the requirements of study participation and the attempt, at a minimum, will likely increase the probability that the patient will participate in conformance with the requirements of the particular study.

REQUIRED INFORMATION FOR INFORMED CONSENT

Once the determination has been reached that the resident/patient meets the threshold of competency sufficient for the potential conveyance of informed consent, the disclosure and voluntariness requirements must be met before the informed consent is complete. Incomplete disclosure of the critical elements of a proposed treatment, or the failure to disclose what may, from the patient's perspective, be a more palatable alternative, can result in a consent which is neither informed and, therefore, not truly voluntary. While most healthcare professionals will undoubtedly be familiar with the critical elements that constitute informed consent, it is nevertheless worthwhile to review a cursory listing of these, following the suggestions on this subject provided by Kapp (1992):

1. Diagnosis. The patient for whom a treatment is proposed should presumably be aware of the malady or problem which is the impetus for the proposed treatment or intervention, not only by name, if a diagnostic label has been designated, but in terms of the symptom complex associated with the diagnosis. In particular, when a psychiatric disorder is the focus of therapeutic efforts, the patient or proxy should be apprised of the set of behaviors which the intervention is designed to address.

2. Nature and purpose of the proposed intervention. The clinician should discuss with the patient, in language which is clear and intended to be as comprehensible to the patient as is practicable, the mechanisms and desired goals or effects of the treatment.

3. Risks, consequences, and participation demands of the treatment or procedure. The patient should be apprised of any and all known potential adverse side effects of the proposed treatment regimen, their known frequency, and risks associated with death, disability or discomfort if applicable. As a general rule, it is advisable to err on the side of more disclosure. Expectations regarding patient behavior and any associated constraints during the course of the treatment should also be disclosed.

4. Probability of treatment or intervention success. The patient should be informed regarding the known chances of a successful outcome for similarly situated patients who have undergone the same treatment under similar circumstances, as well as the reasonably anticipated benefits of treatment.

5. Alternatives. The patient should be apprised of known alternative treatments of the same problem or condition and their associated costs, benefits, risks and probabilities of success, even when access to such

treatments may render them, from a practical standpoint, as only dubious alternatives.

6. Result anticipated if nothing is done. The status quo is a form of treatment alternative which entails its own specific risks and consequences.

7. Limitations on the professional or the facility. Any relevant legal, clinical, ethical or other limitations which may have an impact on the ability to provide the proposed treatment should be disclosed prior to initiation of the procedure.

8. Opinion of the practitioner. As noted above, there is nothing inherently unethical about the professional's communication of his or her own opinion regarding the efficacy or desirability of the proposed treatment and, in practice, the patient may actually desire the frankly expressed evaluation of the clinician's opinion in this regard. Caution should be exercised, however, to ensure that any opinion discussed with the patient is given in a manner which is devoid of any suggestion of coercion or undue influence. When possible, it is recommended that the patient be given a specified amount of time to consider the proposed treatment, thus underscoring the fact that participation is voluntary, providing the patient with an opportunity to consider questions that he may wish to raise with the clinician, and allowing the patient to consult with anyone whose opinion he or she might regard as critical prior to reaching a decision.

Ideally, each of the above considerations can be addressed by the professional who seeks to obtain informed consent from a patient, and, in any but emergency situations, it is unlikely that the clinician cannot be availed of an adequate opportunity to address these issues in satisfactory detail, which should be assessed from the patient's standpoint, except where the patient is not predisposed to ask any questions. In any case, from a strictly legal standpoint, the professional who addresses each of these elements on a routine basis when discussing proposed treatment interventions with a patient, and takes the additional precaution of documenting the discussion and informed consent in the patient's records, has taken a major step in reducing the probability of any future liability attaching to the question of informed consent. Also, as most clinicians are aware, for many treatment interventions there already exist specific or boilerplate consent forms designed both for the protection of the institution as well as to ensure that the particular patient has actually been provided with an opportunity to convey informed consent. Even under such circumstances, however, it is advisable to supplement an endorsed written consent with a discussion of its implications, since these may not be readily apparent to the patient. Ultimately, in any situation which calls for a consideration of informed consent, ethical and therapeutic considerations should motivate the clinician to go beyond the strictly legal requirements of informed consent applicable in the long term care setting.

CONCLUSIONS

Informed consent to treatment requires full disclosure of relevant treatment information to a competent individual under circumstances which, explicitly and otherwise, inform the patient that his or her participation in the proposed treatment is voluntary. Each of the components of informed consent, full disclosure, voluntariness, and the competence of the patient whose consent is being solicited, requires a careful analysis of the patient, the circumstances in which the consent is being sought, and the professional's ability to adequately communicate the types of information which the patient must receive and understand as a prerequisite to informed consent. While no universally applicable objective measures exist upon which the clinician can rely as a guarantee that minimal requirements have been met for informed consent, there are nevertheless legal and ethical guidelines which, if routinely addressed by the practitioner, can maximize the probability that the requirements of informed consent, especially from the patient's perspective, can be adequately addressed. It should be kept in mind, however, that, for the clinician, the ability to assess the patient's perspective necessitates an awareness of, and sometimes deference to, the cultural and ethnic context from which the patient acts or expresses preferences, whether for a specific treatment alternative or a healthcare proxy decision-maker. Finally, it is imperative that the practitioner not only be familiar with the elements of informed consent, but also attempt, in order to maximize the probability of achievement of therapeutic objectives, to ensure that more than the minimal legal requirements of informed consent are met, i.e., that every possible attempt is made to act in a manner consistent with the ethical basis for informed consent, the desire to protect, to the extent possible, the ability of the patient to function independently by making his or her treatment choices.

CASE STUDY

Mr. L, a widower, was recently relocated to a long term care facility, at the urging of his daughter, to facilitate recovery from a hip injury which continues to preclude normal ambulation and execution of routine ADLs in his home. He participates in physical therapy on a daily basis and is reported to be making regular progress toward the goal of ambulation with a walker, at which time he will be discharged from the care center to return home. During the course of Mr. L's treatment, Dr. W, a psychologist who sees residents in the facility for counseling and diagnostic work on an as-needed, contractual basis, encounters him on occasion in the lobby area and they engage in general conversation.

Dr. W, during a number of such casual contacts, observes that Mr. L appears to be clinically depressed and often has little or no recollection of prior recent contacts, that he often repeats himself in conversation with no apparent awareness of his repetition, and that, despite having lived in the facility for two months, he still requires assistance with directions or help from his roommate in order to find his room. Dr. W decides, subsequent to one such encounter, to accompany Mr. L to his room, at which time he conducts an informal mental status exam in the course of a general conversation. Immediately thereafter, Dr. W initiates a conversation with Mr. L's roommate, also present in the room, in order to obtain more specific information regarding any behavioral anomalies or evidence of cognitive deficits which he may have observed. Convinced that Mr. L may be demonstrating behavior consistent with an early-stage dementia, Dr. W then proceeds to enter a notation in Mr. L's medical chart stating that, in his opinion, Mr. L, as a direct result of cognitive impairment, lacks sufficient mental capacity to care for himself independently, and therefore should not be released from the facility until such time as a guardian has been appointed for him in order to insure that his basic care needs are met in a reliable manner. He also makes a record of his closing remarks to Mr. L, during which Dr. W advises him that he is going to make a formal request for initiation of treatment of Mr. L's depression. He states in his note that Mr. L made no response to the latter remarks.

Consider the following questions in reference to the above scenario and the preceding discussion of ethical issues relevant to informed consent in the long term care setting.

1. During their initial contacts in the care facility, would it be reasonable to assume that Mr. L's participation in conversation was voluntary, and that the observations made by Dr. W in the course of these conversations were obtained with the informed consent of Mr. L?

2. Was informed consent, in any form, obtained from Mr. L prior to the meeting and discussion with Dr. W conducted in his room at the facility?

3. What problems, with respect to informed consent issues, arise in the course of the discussion held in the patient's room between Dr. W, Mr. L, and his roommate?

4. What ethical dilemmas and questions are inherent in Dr. W's recording of the note, and its content, in Mr. L's medical record?

5. What suggestions do you have for approaching a similar situation in a long term care facility which would minimize the possibility of inadequate informed consent and simultaneously insure that adequate attention is paid to the resident's healthcare needs?

REFERENCES

Anderer, S.J. (1990). A model for determining competency in guardianship proceedings. *Medical and Psychological Disability Law Reporter, 14*, 107-114.

Appelbaum, P.S., Lidz, C.W., & Meisel, A. (1987). *Informed consent: Legal theory and clinical practice.* New York: Oxford University Press.

Bradley, E., Walker, L., Blechner, B., & Wetle, T. (1997). Assessing capacity to participate in discussions of advance directives in nursing homes: Findings from a study of the Patient Self Determination Act. *Journal of the American Geriatrics Society, 45*, 79-83.

Darr, K. (1997). *Ethics in health services management.* (3rd Edition). Baltimore: Health Professions Press.

Ebert, B.W. (1993). Informed consent. Board of psychology update. *California Department of Consumer Affairs,* No. 3, January, 1997.

Grisso, T. (1986). *Evaluating competencies.* New York: Plenum Press.

Grisso, T. & Appelbaum, P.S. (1998a). *Assessing competence to consent to treatment: A guide for physicians and other health professionals.* New York: Oxford University Press.

Grisso, T. & Appelbaum, P.S. (1998b). *MacArthur Competence Assessment Tool for Treatment (MacCat-T).* Sarasota, FL: Professional Resource Press.

High, W.M. (1993). Advancing research with Alzheimer disease subjects: Investigators' perceptions and ethical issues. *Alzheimer Disease and Associated Disorders, 8,* Informed Consent 33 Supp. 4, 66-74.

Kapp, M.B. (1992). *Geriatrics and the law: Patient rights and professional responsibilities.* (2nd Edition). New York: Springer.

Lichtenberg, P., Crose, R., Fraser, D., Smith, M., Kramer, N., Rosowsky, E., Molinari, V., Qualls, S., Stilwell, N., Salamon, M., Hartman-Stein, P., Duffy, M., Parr, J., & Gallagher-Thompson, D. (1998). Standards for psychological services in long term care facilities. *The Gerontologist, 38,* 122-127.

Marson, D., Chatterjee, A., Ingram, K., & Harrell, L. (1996). Toward a neurologic model of competency: Cognitive predictors of capacity to consent in Alzheimer's disease using three different legal standards. *Neurology, 46,* 666-672.

Marson, D., Cody, H., Ingram, K. & Harrell, L. (1995). Neuropsychologic predictors of Alzheimer's disease using a rational reasons legal standard. *Archives of Neurology, 52,* 955-959.

Marson, D., Ingram, K., Cody, H., & Harrell, L. (1995). Assessing the competency of patients with Alzheimer's disease under different legal standards. *Archives of Neurology, 52,* 949-954.

Mezey, M., Mitty, E., Rappaport, M., & Ramsey, G. (1997). Implementation of the Patient Self-Determination Act (PSDA) in nursing homes in New York City. *Journal of the American Geriatric Society, 45,* 43-49.

Morton, W.J. (1987). The doctrine of informed consent. *Medicine and Law, 6,* 117-125.

Moye, J. & Zehr, M. (2000). Resolving ethical challenges for psychological practice in long-term care. *Clinical Psychology: Science and Practice, 7,* 337-344.

Norman, S., Ishler, K., Ashcraft, L., & Patterson, M. (2000). Continuing education needs in clinical geropsychology: The practitioner's perspective. *Clinical Gerontologist, 22,* 37-50.

Park, D.C., Morrell, R.W., & Shifren, K. (Eds.) (1999). *Processing of medical information in aging patients: Cognitive and human factors perspectives.* Mahwah, NJ: Lawrence Erlbaum Associates, Inc.

Pruchno, R., Smyer, M., Rose, M., Hartman-Stein, P., & Henderson-Laribee, D. (1995). Competence of long-term care residents to participate in decisions about their medical care: A brief, objective assessment. *The Gerontologist, 35,* 5, 622-629.

Sansone, P., Schmitt, L., Nichols, J., Phillips, M., & Belisle, S. (1998). Determining the capacity of demented nursing home residents to name a health care proxy. *Clinical Gerontologist, 19,* 35-50.

Smith, G.P. II (1996). *Legal and healthcare ethics for the elderly.* Washington, DC: Taylor & Francis.

Sprung, C.L. & Winick, B.J. (1989). Informed consent in theory and practice: Legal and medical perspectives on the informed consent doctrine and a proposed reconceptualization. *Critical Care Medicine, 17, 12,* 1346-1354.

Suhl, J., Simons, P., Reedy, T., & Garrick, T. (1994). Myth of substituted judgement: Surrogate decision making regarding life support is unreliable. *Archives of Internal Medicine, 154,* 90-96.

Valle, R. (1998). *Caregiving across cultures: Working with dementing illness and ethnically diverse populations.* Washington, DC: Taylor & Francis.

Zehr, M. (1998). Memory dysfunction in neurodegenerative disease: Ethical and legal issues. In A. Troster (Ed.), *Memory in neurodegenerative processes: Biological, cognitive and clinical perspectives,* 377-389. New York: Cambridge University Press.

Psychologists' Multiple Roles in Long-Term Care: Untangling Confidentiality Quandaries

Margaret P. Norris, PhD

SUMMARY. Psychologists consulting in long-term care settings face unique challenges in protecting the confidentiality of their clients. In multidisciplinary health service facilities, the psychologist typically provides direct therapy services to clients, while at the same time they coordinate their treatment efforts with numerous other health service providers. The psychologist must balance the confidentiality of their clients with their collaborative role as a member of a treatment team. This article will summarize confidentiality standards of various professional organizations, discuss the issues involved in these multiple roles, suggest guidelines that psychologists may use to resolve conflicts, and present brief scenarios that illustrate confidentiality dilemmas. Recommended practices include (1) informing clients at the initiation of services about communication procedures of the facility (e.g., progress notes, treatment team meetings); (2) obtaining agreements about what types of information will and will not be communicated in these forums, as well as what information patients want shared or protected from family members; (3) establishing a practice of providing general rather than specific information to staff; (4) adopting the "need to know" principle, i.e., restricting

Margaret P. Norris is Associate Professor, Texas A&M University.

Portions of this paper were presented as part of a symposium on "Confidentiality in Long-Term Care" at the annual convention of the Gerontological Society of America, Washington, DC, November 2000.

[Haworth co-indexing entry note]: "Psychologists' Multiple Roles in Long-Term Care: Untangling Confidentiality Quandaries." Norris, Margaret P. Co-published simultaneously in *Clinical Gerontologist* (The Haworth Press, Inc.) Vol. 25, No. 3/4, 2002, pp. 261-275; and: *Emerging Trends in Psychological Practice in Long-Term Care* (ed: Margaret P. Norris, Victor Molinari, and Suzann Ogland-Hand) The Haworth Press, Inc., 2002, pp. 261-275. Single or multiple copies of this article are available for a fee from The Haworth Document Delivery Service [1-800-HAWORTH, 9:00 a.m. - 5:00 p.m. (EST). E-mail address: getinfo@haworthpressinc.com].

all communication to information that is essential to the facility's care and treatment of the patient. *[Article copies available for a fee from The Haworth Document Delivery Service: 1-800-HAWORTH. E-mail address: <getinfo@haworthpressinc.com> Website: <http://www.HaworthPress.com> © 2002 by The Haworth Press, Inc. All rights reserved.]*

KEYWORDS. Confidentiality, long-term care, ethics, geropsychology practice

Psychologists working in long-term care settings face unique challenges in protecting the confidentiality of their clients. In multidisciplinary health service facilities such as skilled nursing homes, the psychologist typically provides direct therapy services to patients, while at the same time coordinates treatment efforts with numerous other health service providers. Psychologists must balance client confidentiality with their collaborative role as a member of a treatment team. This article will summarize confidentiality standards of various professional organizations, discuss the issues involved in these multiple roles, suggest guidelines that psychologists may use to resolve conflicts, and present brief scenarios that illustrate confidentiality dilemmas.

CONFIDENTIALITY REGULATIONS AND STANDARDS

A number of professional organizations regulate confidentiality standards including the American Psychological Association, various state and federal agencies, the Center for Medicare and Medicaid Services (CMS) (formerly Health Care Finance Administration, HCFA), and the Health Insurance Portability and Accountability Act (HIPAA). In addition, Psychologists in Long-Term Care has recommended and published ethical standards. The policies and regulations of these organizations are reviewed below.

The American Psychological Association (1992) publishes the *Ethical Principles of Psychologists and Code of Conduct* to reflect the values of the profession. The following codes pertain to confidentiality with italics added to highlight germane issues in long-term care settings:

Article 5.05 Disclosures. (a) Psychologists disclose confidential information without the consent of the individual only as mandated by law, or where permitted by law for a valid purpose, such as (1) *to provide needed professional services to the patient or the individual* or organizational client, (2) *to obtain appropriate professional consultations,* (3) to protect the patient or client or others from harm, or (4) to obtain payment for services. . . .

Article 5.06 Consultations. When consulting with colleagues, (1) psychologists *do not share confidential information that reasonably could lead to the identification of a patient,* client, research participant, or other person or organization with whom they have a confidential relationship unless they have obtained the prior consent of the person or organization *or the disclosure cannot be avoided,* and (2) they share information *only to the extent necessary to achieve the purposes of the consultation.*

An implicit assumption of these guidelines is that the practice setting is a traditional outpatient office in which the psychologist is providing services that are independent of any ancillary health care services that the client may also be receiving. For example, consulting with professionals without revealing the identification of the client is reasonable in the context of obtaining professional supervision for difficulties in one's caseload. However, consultation in inpatient settings without disclosing the patient's identity is not feasible. As indicated by the italics, several aspects of these codes can be interpreted as offering greater flexibility in the unique circumstances of long-term care settings. The codes state that consultation may take place for obtaining other professional services for the patient, that consultation may reveal the identity of the patient when the disclosure cannot be avoided, and that the only information disclosed is that which is necessary for the purposes of consultation. Interestingly, the revision of APA's *Ethical Principles of Psychologists and Code of Conduct,* which is currently underway, still does not explicitly address confidentiality standards in institutional settings, whether these are hospitals, long-term care facilities, or other sites (*APA Monitor,* February 2001).

In addition to the national standards of APA, psychologists are also regulated by their state licensing boards as well as state and federal laws. Of course, it is beyond the scope of this article to review standards and laws of all 50 states. Those regulations for the state of Texas are reviewed below in order to illustrate to the reader the differences that may exist between state and APA guidelines, in the hope and expectation that all psychologists will seek out and become familiar with their individual state standards and laws.

The Rules and Regulations of the Texas State Board of Examiners of Psychologists (Texas State Board of Examiners of Psychologists, 2000) states:

> Article 465.12 Privacy and Confidentiality. (g) Licensees may share information for consultation purposes without a consent only to the extent necessary to achieve the purposes of the consultation and *excluding information that could lead to the identification of the patient or client.*

Again, this regulation does not realistically apply in inpatient settings where consultation with other staff is inherent to patient care and can not take place anonymously. However, knowledgeable psychologists practicing in Texas also know Texas law pertaining to confidentiality (Shuman, 1997):

> Article 5561-h (4) (b) Exceptions to the privilege of confidentiality, in other than court proceedings, allowing disclosure of confidential information by a professional, exist only to the following . . . (6) to other professionals and personnel under the direction of the *professional who are participating in the diagnosis, evaluation, or treatment of the patient/client.*

Thus, Texas state law allows for the very type of consultation that may be pertinent in the context of inpatient settings where multiple health care professionals are treating the patients.

Two organizations, CMS and Psychologists in Long-Term Care (PLTC), address issues of confidentiality that specifically apply to geropsychology services. In contrast to the limitations on consultation posed by other organizations, CMS *requires* psychologists to consult with the patient's physician (Health Care Finance Administration, 2000):

> . . . *contingent upon the patient's consent,* [the clinical psychologist] will attempt to consult with the patient's attending or primary care physician *in accordance with accepted professional ethical norms, taking into consideration patient confidentiality. . . .* The clinical psychologist must notify the physician within a reasonable time that he/she is furnishing services to the patient. Additionally, the clinical psychologist must document, in the patient's medical record, the date the patient consented or declined consent to con-

sultations, and the date of the consultation. . . . The only exception to the consultation requirement for clinical psychologists is in cases where the patient's primary care or attending physician refers the patient to the clinical psychologist.

This CMS policy applies to all Medicare beneficiaries, regardless of place of services. Fortunately, CMS gives consideration to professional ethical norms and to the patient's right to refuse the consultation. Unfortunately, however, the psychologist is required to document when a patient declines the consultation with their physician. Such documentation in the patient's medical chart effectively notifies the physician that the patient is receiving psychological services. Even more perilously, this documentation notifies the physician of the patient's discomfort with revealing information to their physician. Both inherently contradict the patient's right to privacy. Consequently, psychologists may consider placing this documentation in patient records that are not accessible to the patient's physician.

The professional organization Psychologists in Long-Term Care (PLTC) published *Standards for Psychological Services in Long-Term Care Settings* (Lichtenberg et al., 1998). Recognizing the gap in the application of APA and state ethical codes to long-term care settings, PLTC established standards for psychological service delivery in this distinct setting. These are recommended professional standards rather than mandatory regulations and rules, which geropsychologists may adopt in their practice principles. The standards affirm that patients in long-term care facilities have the same rights to confidentiality regarding psychological services as all other patients. The standards also address issues germane to the unique context of providing psychology services in a multidisciplinary inpatient setting:

a. Confidentiality standards must be consistent with the reporting/charting regulations within which the facility must operate. If a conflict arises, the psychologist strives to work with the facility to achieve maximum consistency.

b. Confidentiality standards should allow for the demands of the psychologist's role as an active member of an institutional treatment team that shares pertinent information with other health professionals.

c. Finally, a new federal law, HIPAA, will affect psychologists' treatment of confidentiality issues in profound ways. HIPAA was put into law to govern how patient records are handled, shared, and protected in the health care system. On April 13, 2003, all health care entities (including psychologists) must comply with three rules: the transaction rule, the security rule, and most importantly, the privacy rule.

The privacy rule protects the confidentiality of Protected Health Information (PHI), which is any health information that identifies the individual, including both physical and mental health information. Psychologists must obtain patients' consent prior to using PHI for the purposes of treatment, payment, or health care operations. Most importantly, the HIPPA privacy rule gives special consideration to psychotherapy notes, defined as "Notes recorded in any medium by a health care provider who is a mental health professional documenting or analyzing the contents of conversation during a private counseling session or a group, joint, or family counseling session and that are separated from the rest of the individual's medical record" (American Psychological Practice Organization, 2002a). Authorization to release psychotherapy notes is more explicitly defined than consent to release PHI. Authorization will require: a specific definition of the information/notes to be disclosed, to whom the information is going, the purpose of the disclosure, an expiration date, the right to revoke the authorization, and the right to not authorize the disclosure.

The privacy rule also identifies information that is not protected under the psychotherapy notes definition. This information is likely to define the documentation that psychologists will use in inpatient settings such as nursing homes and other LTC facilities. The exempted information includes the counseling start and stop times, modality of treatment, frequency of treatment, results of clinical tests, diagnosis, functional status, treatment plans, symptoms, prognosis, and progress. It is important to keep in mind, however, that such information will still be considered PHI; thus, documentation of such information in patient medical charts will require the patient's consent.

The details of the HIPAA rules are far more complicated than can be covered in this article. Readers are advised to stay abreast of HIPAA rules. APA is providing members with essential HIPAA information (American Psychological Practice Organization, 2002b) and will continue to do so, especially through the APA Practice Organization's practitioner portal, which will be available on the Internet.

In conclusion, psychologists working in long-term care settings must take into account confidentiality regulations and standards by various organizations. Aspects of these policies are consistent, whereas others are contradictory; some do not apply well to inpatient settings, yet others specifically address the need for geropsychologists to coordinate their treatment efforts with other disciplines and colleagues involved in patient care. All the guidelines clarify that long-term care residents receiving psychological services have the same rights to confidentiality as all other mental health clients. However, the limitations to confidentiality are not explicit in many situations. Psychologists must decide what information should be communicated when charting progress notes and reporting in treatment team meetings. The PLTC ethical standards acknowledge that psychologists maintain an active role in the treatment team by "sharing pertinent information with other health professionals," yet balancing this role with the ethical principles of patient confidentiality may inevitably be ambiguous.

CONFIDENTIALITY DILEMMAS IN LONG-TERM CARE

Four issues characterize the confidentiality issues that psychologists face in long-term care settings: balancing the multiple roles of the psychologist, deciding on the method for obtaining consent, establishing the capacity of a patient to give consent, and obtaining patient information without the patient's consent.

Multiple Roles of Psychologists

The psychologist typically has at least three roles in inpatient settings such as skilled nursing homes. First, the psychologist is providing direct services to the older residents. Secondly, the psychologist is typically hired by the facility as either a consultant or employee; therefore, there are obligations to the system and the other health care providers in the organization. Third, services to older adults are often more embedded in the broader context of the family than is the case for young and middle-aged patients (Qualls, 2000).

To illustrate, conflicts may arise between the psychologist's commitment to the both patient and to the LTC facility when patients tell the psychologist about concerns with the quality of care they are receiving. For example, the psychologist must decide what appropriate actions should be taken if their patient reports that the medication nurse has not been dispensing their pain medication to them. This situation is further complicated if the patient asks the psychologist to not take this matter further because the patient fears retaliation. Given such a serious report of patient neglect, the psychologist must first reach a conclusion about the possible veracity of the patient's report. Is the patient capable of remembering from day to day if they have been given their medicine? Is the patient's relationship with the staff influencing their report in any way? If there is reason to believe the patient's report is bona fide, the psychologist is obligated to pursue the matter further, and to do so hopefully after securing the patient's release or assuring them that their identity can be protected. Similar dilemmas arise when patients complain to the psychologist that they are waiting for lengthy periods for the staff to respond to their call button, that an aide has been disrespectful to them, or they are planning a transfer to another facility but do not want the staff to know. The cases of Lynn and Harry, illustrating conflicts between the psychologist's role to the patient and the staff, are also detailed below.

Conflicts arising from the psychologist's services to both the patient and their families can be equally convoluted. On many occasions, plans and decisions made by the older patient have a direct impact on family members. Placement in the facility, for example, is commonly a decision made with family or sometimes exclusively by the family. Psychologists in long-term care facilities are often asked to see patients who are angry with their family for placing them in the facility. The patient's ability to live independently is often viewed quite differently by the patient and their family. In contexts other than placement, obtaining patient information from family members is often necessary. Particularly in cases of dementia, critical personal history about the patient may be more accurately obtained from family members than from the patient.

Because of these multiple roles, psychologists are often faced with the question of "Who is the client?" Is it the patient, the staff, the family, or all three? Certainly there is no one answer that applies in all cases. In some circumstances, individual psychotherapy may take place with little need for communication with other parties. In other circumstances, the staff, family, and even other residents' (e.g., via improving appropriate socialization) are integral pieces of the psychology services.

Methods for Obtaining Informed Consent

A second dilemma facing psychologists working with long-term care patients concerns the method of receiving consent for services and for releasing information to others. In almost all cases, explanations must be more simply and clearly stated to long-term care patients than typical patients seen in outpatient settings. Written consent is the customary standard in the discipline. However, some long-term care residents may respond more favorably to verbal consent. Older patients, particularly those who are medically frail, may find consent forms difficult to read and understand. Providing a signature may not even be possible for some nursing home residents. Some older adults may be distrustful or concerned about signing documents. For example, it is not uncommon for long-term care residents to state that their son or daughter signs all forms for them, which obviously defeats the purpose of a confidentiality agreement. Psychologists must recognize situations in which written consent will hinder rather facilitate the consent process. These situations should be documented in the patient's record along with alternate courses of action that may be taken (e.g., verbal consent, contacting family, consulting with their physician), as described below.

Patient Capacity to Give Consent

A third dilemma inherently common in long-term care settings concerns the question of whether a patient has the capacity to consent to the release of information to others. Research is sparse in instructing psychologists at what point of cognitive impairment a patient loses the capacity to give consent to release information about their treatment. This issue has been addressed more from a legal perspective than a scientific one. As long-term care residents become more impaired, services often become less individually oriented and more systemic, involving nurses, nurses aides, activity and physical therapists, and others. These systemic services are inherently delivered in coordination with other health professionals who must be informed of the patient's mental status and emotional needs. Readers are referred to Zehr's chapter, "Informed Consent in the Long-Term Care Setting," in this volume for detailed coverage of patient capacity.

Obtaining Information Without Patient Consent

A final confidentiality predicament in long-term care settings is one that appears to be largely ignored in the professional literature. That is, do confidentiality issues extend beyond the domain of *releasing* patient information and perhaps also include *obtaining* patient information? The ethical standards for releasing patient information have been widely addressed; however, it is also common for psychologists to obtain patient information from others without the patient's consent–a possible conflict that typically remains unexamined. The premise of confidential therapy is that it is a private process between the therapist and the client. In most outpatient settings, the psychologist rarely has access to information about the patient other than the information the patient chooses to disclose. In long-term care settings (and other inpatient or multidisciplinary outpatient facilities), the psychologist typically learns quite a lot about the patient without their knowledge or consent. For example, a psychologist is often asked to see a patient after being informed of some problematic incident such as noncompliance in physical therapy, arguments with another resident or staff, throwing lunch trays, being sexually inappropriate with staff, and so on. The referral information may also be merely the tip of the iceberg. The psychologist may be given a litany of past behavior problems, private medical information, descriptions of relationships with staff and family, and other staff's views of the patient and their problems. If the psychologist addresses these issues with the patient, as they are often asked to do, the patient is made aware that the psychologist has been talking to staff. This discussion may raise the patient's concern about the extent of these conversations and whether the psychologist can be trusted to keep information private. It can be difficult to convince a patient that even though the psychologist knows what others are saying about the patient, the psychologist is not, in turn, sharing the patient's personal disclosures with others.

RECOMMENDED PRACTICES AND ILLUSTRATIVE CASES

The first basic and rather uncomplicated recommendation for psychologists treating long-term care residents is that all patients should be informed at the initiation of services about communication procedures of the facility such as progress notes and treatment team meetings. This practice should be universally practiced, while accommodating the cognitive functioning level of the patient. Additional recommended practices are more complex because they serve to protect the confidentiality of the long-term care patient, while at the same time, they allow the psychologist to function as a member of a health team. Examples are given to illustrate application of these guidelines.

Psychologists should obtain agreements about the type of information that will and will not be communicated to staff. This agreement is not simply established at the initiation of services, but is considered an ongoing process throughout treatment to address new issues and whether they will or will not be shared with staff.

Case of Lynn

Lynn was a 73-year-old divorced woman referred for treatment of depression by her physician in a multidisciplinary outpatient medical center. Lynn lived independently in an apartment complex for seniors. She was involved in numerous social activities although her level of participation fluctuated according to her mood variations. She enjoyed good health other than diabetes. Lynn's son, who lived in the same community, was her only immediate family.

As stated above, the issues of confidentiality in this type of setting are not unlike those encountered in long-term care settings. The center holds bimonthly treatment team meetings attended by physicians, nurses, a social worker, nutritionist, physical therapist, psychologist, neuropsychologist, and director of an activity program. The problems discussed in the team meetings, in accordance with the agreement between the patient and the psychologist, included the patient's level and symptoms of depression, her response to antidepressant medication, the waxing and waning of her social activities, and her struggles with diet and exercise after her diabetes worsened, requiring insulin injections. Examples of issues not discussed in team meetings included an incident of a conflict between the patient and a nurse in the center, and her frustration at one point with her medical care influencing in her decision to see another physician for a second opinion. Both of these issues appeared to be driven, in part, by irritable mood and somatic concerns since her insulin treatment was begun. Although she initially wanted some of this information "resolved" in the treatment team, a discussion with the patient helped her understand the risk of worsening her relationship with the medical staff (who were frustrated with her behavior and irritable mood).

Psychologists should obtain agreements about what types of information will and will not be communicated with family members.

Case of Sara

Sara was a 39-year-old African American woman with multiple sclerosis who was referred for problems adjusting to her recent nursing home placement. This case illustrates these confidentiality issues in long-term care settings are not restricted to older patients.

Sara's placement in a skilled care nursing facility stemmed from her declining health status and loss of independent functioning. The placement resulted in her separation from her husband and two sons who lived approximately 50 miles away from the nursing home. Sara and her family were from a small rural town and a conservative southern culture that emphasized conformity to traditional morals. Staff became concerned about Sara's emotional state because she was expressing guilt and despair about not being able to care for children at home, as well as anger at her husband. She had accused her husband of having an extramarital affair and openly spoke with staff about this issue. Her husband adamantly denied it, asserting to staff that she was delusional, and staff tended to respond to Sara with the assumption that the affair was a delusion.

Early in therapy, Sara requested that her psychologist assist her in making her husband understand that she no longer wanted a relationship with him. In speaking with the psychologist, the husband expressed feeling torn between his devotion to his wife and his desire for a sexual relationship. He openly discussed his distress that she "had not been in my bed" for years and his anguish that he very much wanted a marital relationship. The conversation raised doubts about whether Sara's accusations were delusional, as insisted by her husband. Nevertheless, it was also clear that the truthfulness of either the patient's and the husband's contentions could not be definitively known. Without reference to the conversation, the psychologist cautioned staff to refrain from passing judgment on the veracity of either Sara's or her husband's allegation.

Over the course of the next several months, the husband's regular visits dropped off substantially, which raised questions about his degree of commitment to her. Sara communicated that she no longer considered him family and he should not be informed of her care and health status. Several important issues were not discussed with her husband. For example, as Sara adjusted to the nursing home, she quickly lost interest in her children, again suggesting that the family unity was in a fragile state. Her husband was not told of Sara's emotional disengagement from her children because it was feared that he would tell the children in a retaliative manner. Also with the intent of protecting the client's confidentiality, he was not informed of the patient's noncompliance with staff's suggestion for more socialization and participation in activities. The husband had expressed annoyance about her withdrawal prior to placement. This problem was respected as Sara's private emotional issue. In contrast, her husband was informed, as required by state law, when she was transferred to the hospital following a rapid decline in her health.

Establish the practice of providing general rather than specific information in medical records. Psychology service progress notes in medical records should serve the important purpose of helping the patient's caregivers understand the patient's needs and hopefully foster greater empathetic care from others (Moye, 2000).

Case of Harry

Harry was a 75-year-old divorced male referred for depression one month after admission to the nursing home. Since his divorce 3 years ago, he had resided in the independent apartment division of a multi-level care facility for older adults. He reported close ties to his only daughter and 3 granddaughters. Contact with his ex-wife was rare. Harry had congestive heart failure and diabetes, which had worsened due to his obesity and past alcohol use. He was a retired bank executive with large financial resources that he had dispensed to his daughter.

In therapy, Harry discussed issues of marital discord including multiple extramarital affairs. He expressed no regret over the affairs but terrible sorrowfulness that his wife decided to leave him–not because of the affairs, Harry believed, but because he had given large monetary gifts to a mistress. Currently, the patient had only intermittent contact with his daughter who was the family contact person for the nursing home. The patient requested that the psychologist contact his daughter to express his wishes that she visit him more frequently. Staff members were also seriously concerned about his depressed state and were hopeful that increased family contact would help alleviate his depression. When the psychologist contacted his daughter, she informed the psychologist that on one occasion many years ago her father sexually molested his granddaughter when he was intoxicated. As pointed out in the above case of Lynn, it was not possible for the psychologist to discern the veracity of the allegation. Regardless of whether the abuse occurred, it was clear the daughter believed it had and she felt much bitterness toward her father. The staff needed to know that she should not be urged to visit; however, they did not need to know the details of this family conflict and the reason for the daughter's disengagement. To inform staff of the need to not push for more family visits, the chart note read, "It was clear from my discussion with the patient's daughter that she needs to maintain some restrictions in their relationship and her visits are not likely to increase."

Adopt the "need to know" principle, i.e., restrict all communication to information that is essential to the care and treatment of the patient.

Often there are occasions in which the psychologist should make a distinction between what information is recorded in the medical chart, what information is verbally communicated, and whether actions should be taken to minimize conflicts.

To illustrate, as Harry's depression resolved, he spoke in therapy of his desire for a sexual relationship and had identified a staff member and a volunteer about whom he was having explicit sexual fantasies. The chart note made vague reference to distress over interpersonal and relationship issues in order to help all nursing staff understand that he was distraught. The staff did not need to know, however, that Harry was dwelling on sexual feelings or to whom his feelings were directed. In contrast, the two individuals needed to be informed at an appropriate level to modify their behavior with Harry. The female staff member was cautioned that Harry did not always interpret affection the way it was intended and she understood to maintain a professional demeanor with him. The volunteer was a woman whose motivation to visit with residents appeared to be, in part, driven by her own emotional needs for social intimacy and she tended to be overtly but appropriately affectionate with residents. She was simply asked to see other residents in need of companionship without explaining Harry's personal concerns.

CONCLUSIONS

Psychologists consulting in long-term care settings need to understand the unique challenges in protecting the confidentiality of their clients. Whether the setting is inpatient or outpatient, and in virtually all multidisciplinary health service facilities, the psychologist has multiple roles in serving their patients, numerous other health service providers and the facility, as well as family members. The psychologist treating medically frail patients must also recognize that the process for obtaining a release of confidential information may need modifications such as simple explanations and verbal consent. The capacity of patients to decide whether they want information released to others must be assessed. And, the psychologist must be cognizant of the inpatient circumstances that impart far more patient information without the patient's explicit consent than is typical of outpatient settings. A number of recommendations are offered to assist the psychologist facing these confidentiality quandaries, including informing the patient of communication standards in the facility and deciding with the patient what specific information will be disclosed to staff and family members. When information is divulged to others, the psychologist must be cautious about particularly sensitive topics such as sexuality, finances, and relationships with staff and family, in order to avoid breaching privacy. Finally, communication should take into account the principles of conveying general information, which the caregivers need to know in order to enhance the collaborative efforts of multiple professionals treating and caring for the patient. A vitally important closing remark is that the imminent HIPAA privacy rule will soon regulate much of the confidentiality issues faced by psychologists working in LTC settings.

REFERENCES

American Psychological Association (2001, February). Ethical principles of psychologists and code of conduct: Draft for comment. *Monitor on Psychology, 32 (2)*, 77-89.

American Psychological Association (1992). Ethical principles of psychologists and code of conduct. *American Psychologist, 47*, 1597-1611.

American Psychological Practice Organization (2002a). Special HIPAA Compliance Issue. *Practitioner Focus, 14*(1), p. 5.

American Psychological Practice Organization (2002b). Getting Ready for HIPAA: A Primer for Psychologists. Washington DC: Author

Health Care Finance Administration (2000, June 1). Requirements for consultation. *Medicare Part B Newsletter, 00-006*, p. 12.

Lichtenberg, P.A., Smith, M., Frazer, D., Molinari, V., Rosowsky, E., Crose, R., Stillwell, N., Kramer, N., Hartman-Stein, P., Qualls, S., Salamon, M., Duffy, M., Parr, J., & Gallagher-Thompson, D. (1998). Standards for psychological services in long-term care facilities. *The Gerontologist, 38*, 122-127.

Moye, J. (2000). Ethical issues. In V. Molinari (Ed.), *Professional psychology in long-term care* (pp. 329-348). New York: Hatherleigh.

Qualls, S. (2000). Working with families in nursing homes. In V. Molinari (Ed.), *Professional psychology in long-term care* (pp. 91-112). New York: Hatherleigh.

Shuman, D. W. (1997). *Law and mental health professionals: Texas* (2nd ed.). Washington DC: American Psychological Association.

Texas State Board of Examiners of Psychologists (2000). *Psychologists Licensing Act and Rules and Regulations of the Texas State Board of Examiners of Psychologists*. Austin: Author.

Confidentiality and Informed Consent versus Collaboration: Challenges of Psychotherapy Ethics in Nursing Homes

Michael Duffy, PhD, ABPP

SUMMARY. Conventional prescriptions for ethical psychotherapy practice are largely based on outpatient, office-based procedures. Maintaining confidentiality and insuring informed consent in nursing homes, however, becomes considerably more complex. These are situations in which following ethical norms inflexibly will detract from quality of care. This article discusses the conflict of values and ethics that can sometimes exist. Case examples are used to illustrate the tension between confidentiality and optimal therapeutic strategy; between informed consent and urgent needs of the patient. *[Article copies available for a fee from The Haworth Document Delivery Service: 1-800-HAWORTH. E-mail address: <getinfo@haworthpressinc.com> Website: <http://www.HaworthPress.com> © 2002 by The Haworth Press, Inc. All rights reserved.]*

KEYWORDS. Psychotherapy, ethics, confidentiality, informed consent, conflict of values

Michael Duffy is affiliated with the Counseling Psychology Program at Texas A&M University.

Address correspondence to: Michael Duffy, Counseling Psychology Program, Texas A&M University, Department of Educational Psychology, College Station, TX 77843.

Portions of this paper were presented as part of the symposium "Confidentiality in Long-Term Care" at the annual convention of the Gerontological Society of America, Washington, DC, November 2000.

[Haworth co-indexing entry note]: "Confidentiality and Informed Consent versus Collaboration: Challenges of Psychotherapy Ethics in Nursing Homes." Duffy, Michael. Co-published simultaneously in *Clinical Gerontologist* (The Haworth Press, Inc.) Vol. 25, No. 3/4, 2002, pp. 277-292; and: *Emerging Trends in Psychological Practice in Long-Term Care* (ed: Margaret P. Norris, Victor Molinari, Suzann Ogland-Hand) The Haworth Press, Inc., 2002, pp. 277-292. Single or multiple copies of this article are available for a fee from The Haworth Document Delivery Service [1-800-HAWORTH, 9:00 a.m. - 5:00 p.m. (EST). E-mail address: getinfo@haworthpressinc.com].

Over the past two decades, confidentiality regulations in psychotherapy have become increasingly restrictive and stringent. For example, waiver of confidentiality is increasingly specific: release of information is restricted to *named individuals*, the *type of information* is specified (written documents, unilateral verbal communication, shared verbal communication), the *purpose of the communication* is spelled out, and a period of time for the waiver is identified. There are also tighter guidelines for information sharing between clinical colleagues working in the same agency. Whereas, many years ago, colleagues felt free to consult and share information about clients, now there is a stricter emphasis on "need to know," and any discussion is preferably accompanied by a written release.

Most psychologists welcome this increased emphasis on the confidentiality of clients and have felt at odds with the violation of this confidentiality in the legal world (by subpoena) and the very loose maintenance of confidentiality often encountered in the general world of health care. However, such high standards are considerably more easily maintained in the quiet and orderly world of the outpatient psychotherapy office than in the hurly burly world of a typical nursing home where good mental health care depends on effective and strategic working relationships with the various members of the health care staff (Halter, 1999).

The ethical question becomes, can, in fact, ethical psychotherapists not communicate and collaborate with members of staff who can effectively (not intentionally) undo the therapeutic work achieved by the therapist? This predicament is especially dangerous when the optimal therapeutic strategy with a given patient is not obvious to the general staff person–when the preferred approach is *counterintuitive* and will need an explanation to caregivers, if they are to support healthy change. Caregivers, for example, are often reactive or overly sympathetic and have difficulty assuming an empathic understanding of the resident's problem. For example, hypochondriacal patients may be helped better by counterintuitive soothing support rather than by the intent to convince them that they are not sick. We need to bear in mind that the caregivers most directly involved in patient care, and therefore most impact the quality and the effectiveness of care, are the least trained among the staff.

The parallel ethical challenge is insuring informed consent within the nursing home context. Again, informed consent can be more clearly and easily obtained in the world of a private consulting office where clients are relatively clear as to the purpose of psychotherapy and are motivated to seek change. This situation is much less the case in nursing homes: residents often do not see themselves as needing psychotherapy or mental health services, and among cognitively impaired patients their ability to render an informed consent may be questionable. It may be the case that the older adult in the nursing home is not the best judge of actual mental health needs and may therefore make decisions or obstruct services that may be necessary for their well-being and even survival.

In a recent discussion with the chair of the committee charged with revising the APA code of ethics, I raised these questions, asking whether the committee is giving attention to special contexts, such as nursing homes, in which the maintenance of confidentiality and informed consent becomes more complex than in conventional service delivery settings (Duffy, 2000). Indeed, the committee had discussed these special contexts and felt that there may be a need in the revised code to include a clause indicating that in these special contexts such as nursing homes, hospitals, and several institutional children's settings, the norms for confidentiality and informed consent may need to be understood and interpreted in a more flexible, context-related manner. A recent draft (APA Ethics Committee, 2001) of the APA ethics code revision process appeared to include such flexibility. We also discussed the highly relevant contemporary trend for psychologists to work in primary care settings, which are quite likely to be multidiscipline and integrated in nature. Psychologists providing mental health services in comprehensive family clinics, for example, are interfacing continually with other specialties such as pediatrics, geriatrics, and family practice. To provide integrated mental health services in this context, requiring a flexible and effective method of both providing services to patients and also protecting confidentiality and insuring informed consent for services, becomes a complex but critical task.

A series of case examples will illustrate the tension that frequently exists between formal ethical regulations and the exigencies of nursing home practice. A psychotherapist treating a nursing home resident may have personal information about the patient's personality and developmental experiences that is clearly confidential. The therapist may also know that not sharing this information with nurse aides, for example, will enable well-intentioned but *countertherapeutic* treatment of the older adult. Ethical norms require silence; moral concern for the well-being of the patient requires communication! Ethical norms require a clearly articulated and written version of informed consent; moral concern for the well-being of the patient requires rapid intervention in a case where clearly articulated consent may be an ideal rather than a possible reality.

A CASE THAT TESTS THE LIMITS

A recent case will illustrate these complex issues of informed consent and confidentiality in a long-term care context. The resident was a man in his early eighties who had suffered two major strokes and who, by a previous assessment (not available), appeared to have definable cognitive impairment, probably of the vascular type. The staff were concerned that the resident was being noncooperative both with physical therapy directed at his rehabilitation and also with the various social activities provided for his well-being. There was concern by the administration staff that he may be significantly depressed and it was also felt, given his disinterest in female-oriented activities, that he would work best with a male therapist. In line with my practice of gathering as much collateral information as possible about a patient, I arranged a meeting with the social services coordinator and the resident's sister who held a limited guardianship of his health care and financial matters. It transpired that my patient was an ex-military man who had well-articulated and intolerant views about mental health and all things psychological. His sister was quite unsure that he would be willing to work with me, as indeed were other members of the staff who had found him to be relatively intransigent in accepting professional help. His sister suggested to me that I meet my patient "incognito" so that I would be able to help without raising the specter of psychological services or psychotherapy, which would likely generate his opposition. I empathetically replied to the sister that I certainly understood why she would suggest this method and that basically that she had a good understanding of her brother's reaction. I told her, however, which she completely understood, that my need to develop an informed consent from the patient was an important part of my professional responsibility. I let her know, however, with some amount of humor, that I agreed with her that meeting her brother with a "white coat, scalpel, and MMPI or a long legal written consent form would not do the trick"! We agreed that I would have an informal, naturalistic visit with her brother in which our conversation would both inform him as to my identity and purpose without, hopefully, raising unnecessary and undue opposition. This plan transpired quite well. I met with the patient alone and after some greeting, let him know that I was a doctor who worked with older adults who were at times distressed. I had come by to check up on his well-being and at the request of his family and staff who were concerned about his mood. I indicated that we would try to find out whether this concern was justified. I left the door of the room ajar after noticing his distinct aversive reaction when I closed it upon entering. I initially remained standing and eventually (with his permission) perched on the edge of the bed while carrying on our conversation–which quickly became an exploration of some key aspects of his background including his married life. One hypothesis of the social service coordinator was that he was suffering from unresolved grief over the death of his wife several years earlier. At the end of about twenty minutes of conversation in which he responded quite well and seemed to forget his apprehension, I asked if it would be alright for me to come back again to visit in a few days to check on how he was doing. He seemed quite willing to have me do so which became the entrée to a series of bi-weekly, initially, and eventually weekly meetings.

It transpired over the course of our interviews and through the use of the Geriatric Depression Scale (Yesavage, Brink et al., 1983) that my client was without any evident signs of depression and also seemed to have adjusted quite well to the loss of his spouse after a lifelong and very close marital relationship. They had had no children and had a shared life with a considerable amount of travel and social engagement in a number of countries associated with his work and career in the military. It was also evident in clinical interviews that there were some cognitive impairments–mostly memory and misidentification of even close relatives. It became clear to me in our conversations that my client was by temperament and personality type inclined to be more introverted than extroverted. Indeed, he was a good example of the less well-known "social introvert" pattern where introversion co-exists with good social skills. Even though he had led an active and skilled social life along with his outgoing wife, he had probably always been more introverted by temperament, internally-oriented and quiet, happy with his own company. He might well be described as one of those persons identified in the classic Cummings and Henry (1960) on disengagement in which they found that older persons who were socially disengaged were also able to maintain a high morale. This personality finding seemed pertinent to the referral questions and the need to confer with staff. It seemed likely that my client was disinclined to be involved in largely female-oriented social activities in the nursing home and was usually more interested in quiet contacts with other residents limited to lunch time and dinner. He was disinterested in most of the activities and was quite vocal and at times aggressive in refusing to be a part of these activities. He even experienced physical therapy as intrusive and while the physical therapist was quite skilled and related to him very well, his lack of cooperation made the work difficult. My hypothesis at this point was confirmed through collateral information from several persons including the patient's sister, the physical therapist, the activity director and the social service coordinator. Since it also seemed likely that the continuing pressure to be socially engaged was probably exacerbating his behavioral difficulties and even mood, then communicating with the various caregivers would be imperative in providing for my client's well-being. In a series of brief conversations with the staff, I gave my impressions that he was not depressed but disinterested in activities and encouraged them to entertain a different viewpoint about the need to engage him routinely in the social activities program. I indicated that he likely had never been inclined to engage with other persons in this manner and would be unlikely to do so at this point in his life. It was particularly interesting that the activities director certainly shared and agreed with these positions, but, however, mentioned his likely conflict with administrators and state inspectors who looked for evidence of social activities. State inspectors are frequently not close enough to the subtle aspects of cases to recognize that general regulations about well-being and the need for activities may not apply in a rigid fashion to all residents. It has been my experience over a long period of time that activity directors are the first to recognize, in line with the Cummings and Henry classic study (1960), that not all residents can be pushed into social activities and that such behavior is counterindicated in many cases.

This case, I believe, illustrates well the complexities of maintaining confidentiality and adequate informed consent in the complex world of a nursing home. To insist on a formal and perhaps rigid manner of insuring informed consent in a manner similar to outpatient psychotherapy would almost definitely have precluded the provision of services at all. It is also seems clear that the therapeutic well-being of this resident could only be protected by: (a) receiving collateral affirmation of my clinical impressions from staff, particularly nurse aides, who were intimately familiar with the resident, and (b) that a more subtle and accurate understanding of the dynamics of this situation would need to be communicated to the caregivers. It is, I believe, a clear example of my earlier suggestion that not to communicate with other persons would have been therapeutically and ethically hazardous. Also, as is typical in nursing homes, there were difficulties with this resident both in the areas of eyesight and reading which would have made it difficult to examine a formal consent form and also there were issues of cognitive impairment that would raise questions about his ability to consent. Since his sister had a limited guardianship for healthcare, it can be argued that there was no imperative to gain consent from the resident. However, as with conducting psychotherapy with children who have no legal entitlement to consent, we usually seek *assent,* as an ethical way of ensuring that our client is as informed as is possible.

A final comment on this case: sometimes our typical vigilance in protecting confidentiality and informed consent can lead to an overcorrection, which essentially interferes with the effective provision of services. I am reminded of the situation of novice psychotherapists who can make such a big issue of the constraints and limits of confidentiality and of informed consent that they actually raise concerns in a client's mind rather than reassure. Or this same overcorrection can occur in informing the client of audio- or videotaping that is required for psychotherapy supervision. The novice therapist may so emphasize the informed consent aspect of the recording that it precisely raises anxieties on the part of the client that would not otherwise have been present.

ETHICAL PRINCIPLES VERSUS ETHICAL REGULATIONS

In a recent oral examination of a doctoral student, I was struck by the contrast between understanding of principles versus regulations. The student was clearly well-versed and articulate in the current ethical regulations contained in both the state licensure board requirements and the national APA code of ethics. She was well able to answer questions that tested her knowledge of regulation. However, I noticed that when asked to comment on the ethical *principles* that formed the basis for particular regulations, she was virtually unable to respond. This struck me as a clear example of the disconnection that often exists between an ethical principle and a particular ethical regulation that grows out of this principle. On this basis, this means that a psychotherapist would tend to follow regulations in a relatively rigid manner and be unable to adjust to varied contextual circumstances. Understanding the underlying principle gives a greater capacity to *generalize* from case to case–and therefore a caregiver is able to think through the *intrinsic meaning* of the principle in circumstances that differ, especially in the complex world of long-term care (Karasu, 1991).

THE SITUATION OF COMPETING VALUES

Another ethical quandary that faces the psychotherapist is that even when we attend to fundamental principles we may be confronted with a situation in which *more than one* ethical principle or value is at stake.

This is clearly the case in the complex world of institutional, multidisciplinary health care services. Clearly, in the situations mentioned earlier, the rights of the client for confidentiality and to be ensured of informed consent are beyond question. However, equally pressing are ethical obligations to provide a high quality service to the client. Working in complex environments like nursing homes throws up situations in which there is a potential conflict of values, and, therefore, ethical situations. In the case we discussed earlier, holding to a rigid regulation on confidentiality and informed consent might preclude providing much needed and relevant service to the patient. However, understanding the ethical principles underlying these can help the therapist determine which value is predominant in these circumstances.

Fundamentally, the trajectory of appropriate behavior begins with basic morality, which involves avoiding evil and doing good. This basic moral stance is applied to the situation of professional work and generates a more focused set of ethical principles that avoid evil and maximize good for our clients such as their need for privacy and confidentiality, their need to be informed of the meaning and scope of our services, and the high quality of those services. Over time, these principles find shape and form in a series of specific regulations that guide the management of the principles; so, for example, as mentioned in the introduction, the principle of confidentiality has been regulated in some fairly specific and increasingly precise, if constraining, ways. Finally, these ethical regulations, often codified in our licensure board materials, also become the subject of legal constraints that involve possible legal proceedings when violated such as the prohibition of sexual contact between therapist and client, and the obligation to report child and older adult abuse. This trajectory from morality to legal constraint is certainly meaningful and necessary; however, it is also the sphere in which most rigid and legalistic thinking begins to emerge within human experience, and even within professional practice. The reliance on regulation and legal constraint can, in fact, obviate the presence of truly moral principles. An example will illustrate this point. During the course of a therapeutic relationship the therapist may discover issues which suggest that the client might best be referred to another therapist. These issues might include conflict of interest, dual relationship, or personality incompatibilities, which interfere with the progress of therapy. The therapist is then required by regulation to carefully prepare the client for the referral and to make an appropriate referral including following up on the positive outcome. It is the case, however, that a therapist may be in perfect compliance with these behavioral ethical regulations and procedures but in fact internally be guilty of emotionally abandoning this client–being motivated more by disinterest and dislike than the well-being of the client. The difference is in the *intentionality* of the therapist. Even though this is a nonvisible and subtle dimension of therapy, in my experience such "shifting off" of a client can have subtle but distinct effects upon the client's well-being. The therapist's documentation may have been "squeaky clean" in conforming behaviorally to ethical regulations, but the therapist has in fact violated an internal ethical principle in failing to attend always to the well-being of the client.

THE FUNDAMENTAL ETHICAL PRINCIPLE: CLIENT WELL-BEING

Given the complexity, psychotherapy, behaving in a way that consistently preserves ethical principles, is complicated in many ways. At times it is difficult to clarify the ethical principle of importance in a given situation. At other times it seems that the ethical regulation will protect the legal status of the therapist but may not contribute to the well-being of the client. In yet other situations, competing ethical principles and values as described above confront the therapist. In these circumstances it may be helpful to focus on what might be described as the fundamental ethical principle, namely, client well-being. We can perhaps state this principle as follows: in any ethical situation, the safest and clearest decision will be that which protects the well-being of our client even at the cost of risking our own well-being. This is in accord with the classical position taken by Freud in defining treatment boundaries. He suggested the "principle of abstinence" which implied that no therapeutic alliance can develop with the patient if the therapist does not abstain from using the patient for his or her own personal gratification (Simon, 1991). Being helpful to another human being is inherently gratifying and will always remain so; however, over time, the therapist learns to be driven by a more altruistic motivation–namely, the well-being of the client. All decisions about treatment approaches and techniques can be made by an answer to the clear question: is this approach or technique chosen for the well-being of the client (versus the interest or gratification of the therapist)? This principle also becomes helpful in many other related treatment decisions such as when and when not to use self-disclosure, when to talk versus when to listen, when to use a technique, etc. Given this fundamental ethical principle, these questions also are more easily answered. We self-disclose when it is to the benefit and in tune with the needs of the client. We talk when the client benefits from our talking and listen when the client benefits from our listening. We use a particular technique (e.g., hypnosis) not because it is gratifying or trendy, but because it benefits the client. Consistent empathic attention to the experience of our client will help clue us to the appropriateness of ethical and treatment decisions.

This fundamental ethical principle of client well-being is certainly no new discovery. This fundamental altruism is the basic guide for moral behavior present in many rational and religious systems as well as professional standards. It is certainly a hallmark of Judaism and Christianity and most world religions where specific commandments/prescriptions are subsumed under the first, highest and ultimately only commandment, "to love one another." Therapeutic relationships are perhaps ideally a perfect example of empathic intimacy in which the well-being of clients predominates and guides all treatment decisions. With this concept in mind, we can approach several of the complex ethical problems that occur as we attempt to ensure confidentiality and informed consent in nursing homes. What follows is a series of situations in which formal and written informed consent or waivers of confidentiality are either impossible or would probably eliminate the possibility of providing mental health services to our clients.

Extended Family Therapy

When providing psychotherapy in the nursing home, it is frequently important and indeed unavoidable to work systemically with members of the extended family (Hohmann-Marriott, 2001). When providing clinical supervision in the nursing home, I soon ask trainees who are working with individual residents to remember to "look up from the bedside," in order to notice members of the resident's family system and other influences. Work that focuses entirely on the defined problem of a resident may miss a complete understanding of the forces that shape the problematic behavior. For example, it may sometimes be more effective for the resident to receive a well-placed strategic phone call from an absent adult child than to undergo a long-term course of psychotherapy for depression (Duffy, 1986). To work in this way, however, is not always straightforward. Sometimes the resident, while critically needing contact with family members, expresses unwillingness to make that contact or have the therapist make the contact. Also, we may know that the traditional informed consent and confidentiality statements do not explicitly encompass the wider world of the extended family (Beahrs and Guthrie, 2001). However, in each of these circumstances we may be aware that, in our best professional judgement, the road to recovery must involve some therapeutic interaction with extended family members. It is not unusual for us to find an older resident of the nursing home with an ever-present daughter whom she seems not to even notice or appreciate while being continually absorbed by a loved but emotionally non-present daughter who seldom visits. Resolution of such dynamic quandaries becomes an important ingredient of therapeutic strategy and cannot be avoided.

Agitated Behavior

Sometimes when we work routinely in nursing homes, we may become involved in emergency or urgent treatment which certainly falls outside the continuum of informed consent and confidentiality that exists in our regular office outpatients. An example of this situation is when we encounter on a nursing home corridor a patient in agitated condition and very clearly distressed. Not infrequently, we are aware the staff's reaction to such situations may not always be therapeutic. Nursing home aides, for example, will at times exacerbate agitated behavior in demented patients by ill-judged attempts to physically restrain. Based on the fundamental ethical principle described earlier, we would certainly be willing to intervene and offer our services. In such situations both our understanding of the dynamics of demented behavior and our anxiety and agitation management skills will be of great service. However, the intervention is needed immediately. If we choose to intervene we would certainly be doing so without the benefits of informed consent (even verbal consent) and would be operating in a public space without any protection of conventional confidentiality. Clearly, our decision must be immediate and the use of the fundamental principle described above may help resolve this conundrum. I suspect that most therapists would choose to intervene in such circumstances and concern themselves with the niceties of ethical regulations later. While such choices generally will receive the support of both staff and later of residents, they are not without some risk of liability. It is certainly possible, should the outcome not be perfect, that either family or resident might choose to bring a claim against the therapist. This is the minimal risk that accompanies the choice for altruistic empathy in such cases.

Grieving

Grieving is another situation in which psychotherapy may need to extend the usual confidentiality norms to help family, staff, or volunteers understand a resident's situation and needs. Untrained caregivers often either emotionally avoid the grieving resident or simplistically give large dosages of reassurance–both of which can prolong grieving and risk comorbid depression. The situation is further complicated in that grieving is often hidden and may go unnoticed.

Grieving for predictable losses is an ever present but often avoided issue in the life of a nursing home. Grieving may not only be for the conventional issue of loss of a loved one but also for the loss of a thousand freedoms that has occurred when an older adult moves from the autonomous life of a private residence into the inevitable constraints of institutional life. Overnight, they have lost innumerable moments of personal discretion such as: when to rise and go to bed, what to eat and when to eat, the disposition of personal finances, the loss of control over one's personal environment, such as personal furniture, belongings, clothing, etc. In these circumstances there is an inevitable process of grieving that may result in symptomatic behavior such as anxiety and depression, but which is poorly understood by both nursing home staff and the resident themselves. With regard to the loss of loved ones, or even roommates, the pervasive tradition in long-term care is to follow one of two predictable response patterns: either to ignore the loss of a loved one or roommate (which is easier when the roommate has died in hospital as the result of an acute care episode) or to follow a pattern of easy reassurance in which staff, fellow residents and family seek to reassure the resident that "everything will be all right, just wait and see." In the dynamics and personality problems of some residents, such approaches can be especially deleterious. Those of us who have personally experienced such avoidant or simplistic reassuring behaviors will be aware that they rarely have therapeutic effect in moving through the grieving process, and it is important to help family members and staff to better understand the resident's needs. In training paraprofessionals (Crose, Duffy, Warren, and Franklin, 1987), I have become aware that a first major stage in therapeutic skill is to *move beyond the intuitive tendency* to reassure in the face of difficulty. In fact, the *therapeutic direction is counterintuitive*, namely, to allow the person to experience and work through the painful experience is more likely to bring closure to the grieving than well-intentioned but empty reassurances.

Faced with such well-intentioned, but countertherapeutic, patterns among nursing home staff, family members, and other residents, the psychotherapist must choose to either ignore this unhelpful behavior or make an attempt to redirect the helpers into a more productive approach. This may involve engaging staff, family members and even residents in conversations that would push beyond our conventional sense of limits of confidentiality. This willingness to provide consultative help to the helpers is outside the bounds of practice in a traditional outpatient private practice setting. However, in the complex world of the nursing home, where multiple influences work for and against the well-being of residents, it may become imperative to attempt to influence the behavior of collateral helpers. Again, the primary ethical principle comes to our help. Given that we provide those surrounding us with only general and essential information about the grieving person, we can often direct their helping into a more therapeutic mold. Thus, we may be able to help the avoidant roommate to allow their grieving partner to keep talking and venting. Alternatively, it may help the "reassuring" roommate to recognize that a person will best transition through grief when being allowed to express the pain as it exists without the interference of inappropriate reassurance.

Cognitive Impairment

Gaining meaningful informed consent from residents who have some degree of cognitive impairment is a challenge (Ratzan, 1986; Dymek, Achison, Harrell and Marson, 2001). The presence of formal legal guardianships is surprisingly rare and, when available, is often of only minimal help. In many cases, we attempt to communicate to our residents the nature and purpose of our interventions, but we are only too aware that such an attempt may be quite limited. And, with regard to limits of confidentiality, as mentioned earlier, it may be unethical for us not to inform staff members of a more appropriate way to manage the behavior of a demented resident. It is desirable that staff understand some critical information: the sources of agitation; the emotional memory trigger-points that disturb residents; a critical developmental experience that explains a resident's strong reaction to caregiving; circumstances of abuse or neglect in earlier life that may have led to distrustful or hoarding behavior. The capacity of staff to deal with residents empathetically may depend precisely on the more accurate and complete information that only the therapist can provide. To fail to do so may put the resident at risk of being compromised by countertherapeutic behavior on the part of the staff. The work of the therapist on one or two occasions a week is being systematically *undone* by the nonempathic (but well-intentioned) behavior of staff during the remainder of the week.

Hypochondriacal Behavior

A similar circumstance prevails with dealing with hypochondriacal behavior. Teaching staff therapeutic responses to hypochondriacal patients requires some degree of disclosure to the staff. It is common for staff to treat patients with hypochondriacal behavior in an intuitively obvious manner. Namely, this involves a two-phase process in which the initial reactions of caregivers to the patient are *sympathetic* (note, not empathic) and after several frustrated attempts to be sympathetic, caregivers, including family physicians, frequently become frustrated and back off while assuring the patient that they do not need any further assistance because they are clearly not sick. This *psychologically distancing* behavior has a reverse therapeutic effect. It precisely increases the degree of anxiety and felt need on the part of the patients to clamor for reassuring closeness through their symptomatic behavior. A counterintuitive approach, on the other hand, is much more likely to be successful in reducing symptomatic behavior. In this case, the fundamental therapeutic principle is to *move psychologically "toward" the person,* based on an understanding of the underlying dynamics of this symptomatic behavior as a need for closeness and reassurance. In this revised scenario the physician or psychotherapist will *encourage* the person to make frequent and routine (brief) contact with them–even beyond the patient's expectation–and will often find that this results in a reduction in anxiety with a comparable reduction in psychosomatic symptoms. In this case it again becomes imperative for the psychotherapist to confer informally and tactfully with the variety of care providers including nurse aides, family members, and even physicians. Such collaborative and comprehensive behavior clearly falls outside the usual bounds of confidentiality limits and tests the therapist's willingness to put the client's well-being ahead of liability consciousness.

Refusal of Services

It is not unusual in nursing homes for patients to refuse psychological services, as well as medical and nursing services (Moye, 2000). It is certainly ethically legitimate and defensible for the psychotherapist to accept this behavior without demur and consequently provide no services–persons have a perfect right to refuse help, without explanation. But, as we might suspect, persons who refuse psychological services are sometimes those who need them most, even to a degree that threatens life itself. In the case of seriously depressed residents who may be making unhealthy attempts to end their life through refusing to eat or through noncompliance with medication, there may be an altruistic imperative at least to make an attempt to deliver services. And it is often the case that the experienced psychotherapist may often be successful where others may fail. Therefore, we know that if we are willing to operate outside the safe bounds of conventional informed consent then we are quite likely to benefit the patient–even to the extent of saving a life (Speilman, 1986). In such circumstances, the therapist once again needs to decide whether to accept the safety of conventional informed consent or take the risk of acting in the best interests of the client even if it stretches the concept of consent. Clearly, in cases of imminent danger of death, therapists in all contexts are willing to intervene and are usually protected by law. However, in many cases in the nursing home, the suicidal intent is masked and it cannot be identified clearly as the basis for action that is outside the bounds of informed consent. Also, in such cases, of course, the need to inform other health care providers also will extend beyond the conventional range of confidentiality. With both issues, the fundamental ethical principle comes to bear once again that the well-being of the resident or client is more fundamental as a moral imperative than the avoidance of liability by the therapist.

CONCLUSION

We have conceptualized ethical behavior in the nursing home through a series of case examples which suggest that the context of long-term care may "stretch" an overly rigid interpretation of ethical principles of informed consent and confidentiality. To operate in such an environment in a therapeutic manner requires some flexibility and risk-taking on the part of a psychotherapist. It seems clear that what matters in such behavior is an understanding of the fundamental principles, or indeed fundamental principle of moral behavior. Unless such principles form the basis for clinical judgement, a psychotherapist will be unarmed in dealing with the complexities of a large, sometimes chaotic, multidiscipline setting in which residents are frequently impaired in their ability to give consent and understand the limits of confidentiality.

REFERENCES

Beahrs, J.O. and Guthrie, T.G. (2001). Informed consent in psychotherapy. *American Journal of Psychiatry*, 158(1), 4-10.

Crose, R., Duffy, M., and Warren, J. (1987). Project OASIS: Volunteer mental health professionals serving nursing home residents. *The Gerontologist*, 27, 359-362.

Cummings, E. and Henry, W.E. (1960). *Growing old: The process of disengagement.* New York: Basic Books.

Duffy, M. (1986). The techniques and contexts of multigenerational therapy. *Clinical Gerontologist*, 5, 347-362.

Duffy, M. (2000). Personal Communication, October, Washington, DC. APA Ethics Committee (2001) Ethics Code, Draft 5. Washington, DC: APA.

Dymek, M.P., Achison, P., Harrell, L. and Marson, D.C. (2001). Competency to consent to medical treatment in cognitively impaired patients with Parkinson's disease. *Neurology*, 56(1), 17-24.

Halter, J.B. (1999). The challenge of communicating health information to elderly clients. In D.C. Park and R.W. Morrell (Eds.), *Processing of medical information in aging patients: Cognitive and human factors perspectives*, 23-28. Mahwah, NJ: Lawrence Erlbaum Associates, Inc.

Hohmann-Marriott, B.E. (2001). Marriage and family research: Ethical issues and guidelines. *American Journal of Family Therapy*, 29(1), 1-11.

Karasu, T.B. (1991). Ethical aspects of psychotherapy. In S. Bloch and P. Chodoff (Eds.), *Psychiatric ethics* (2nd Ed.), 135-166. Oxford, UK: Oxford University Press.

Moye, J. (2000). Mr. Frank refuses surgery: Cognition and values in competency determination in complex cases. *Journal of Aging Studies*, 14(4), 385-401.

Ratzan, R.M. (1986). Communication and informed consent in clinical geriatrics. *International Journal of Aging and Human Development*, 23(1), 17-26.

Simon, R.I. (1991). The practice of psychotherapy: Legal liabilities of an "impossible" profession. *American Psychiatric Press Review of Clinical Psychiatry and the Law.* Washington, DC: American Psychiatric Press.

Speilman, B.J. (1986). Rethinking paradigms in geriatric ethics. *Journal of Religion and Health*, 25(2), 142-148.

Yesavage, Brink et al. (1983). Development and validation of a geriatric depression scale: A preliminary report. *Journal of Psychiatric Research*, 17, 37-49.

Index